HEALTHCARE MANAGEMENT

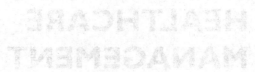

HEALTHCARE MANAGEMENT

Kieran Walshe and Judith Smith (eds)

Open University Press

Open University Press
McGraw-Hill Education
McGraw-Hill House
Shoppenhangers Road
Maidenhead
Berkshire
SL6 2QL
England

email: enquiries@openup.co.uk
world wide web: www.openup.co.uk

and Two Penn Plaza, New York, NY 10121–2289, USA

First published 2006

A catalogue record of this book is available from the British Library

ISBN10: 0 335 22119 X (pb)   0 335 22120 3 (hb)
ISBN13: 978 0 335 22119 6 (pb)   978 0 335 22120 2 (hb)

Library of Congress Cataloging-in-Publication Data
CIP data applied for

Typeset by RefineCatch Limited, Bungay, Suffolk
Printed in Poland EU by OZGraf S.A. www.polskabook.pl

This book is dedicated to the many writers and thinkers on health policy and management whose ideas have influenced us, both as managers and as academics: to people like Henry Mintzberg for his writings on the nature of management and how managers learn; Rosemary Stewart for her pioneering work on healthcare management; Rudolf Klein for his insights into the politics of healthcare; Chris Ham for his skilful policy analyses – and many others.

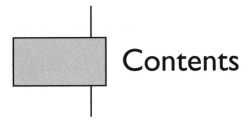

Contents

Figures

Tables

Boxes

Contributors

Dr Lawrence Benson works at Manchester Business School's (MBS), Centre for Public Policy and Management as a Lecturer in Healthcare and Public Sector Management. His main research interests to date are workforce redesign, healthcare regulation, clinical and managerial networks and partnership working in primary care.

Dr Ruth Boaden is Senior Lecturer in Operations Management at Manchester Business School. Her research interests cover a wide range of areas within health services management including electronic health records, re-engineering, operating theatre management and scheduling, patient safety, the management of emergency admissions, bed management and chronic disease management. Her main areas of interest are in quality and improvement and the use of industrial methods within the NHS and she emphasises the application of research in practice in all she does.

Carol Brooks is co-owner and director of a change management consultancy working across the public sector. She holds a Visiting Fellow position at Manchester Business School, where she is Course Director for the suite of Doctors in Management programmes. Carol has a background in healthcare management, education, training and workforce planning. She is also a non-executive director in a large acute hospital trust. She has an academic background in organisational psychology.

Dr Naomi Chambers is a Senior Fellow in the Centre for Public Policy and Management at Manchester Business School, and is currently Director of Executive Education for the school. Her research and teaching interests include primary care, comparative health management and board development. She was a non-executive director on a health authority and subsequently a primary care trust for ten years from 1996.

Deborah Davidson is a Senior Fellow at the Health Services Management Centre, University of Birmingham where she leads the department's work in organisational development and leadership. Prior to this she worked at King's College London as Director of Educational

Programmes at the Institute for Applied Health and Social Policy and from 1989 to 1998, as Executive Director of a leading edge mental health charity in north London that focused on work with black and ethnic minority communities.

Dr Jennifer Dixon is the Director of Policy at the King's Fund. She has researched and written widely on healthcare reform in the UK and internationally. Her background is in clinical medicine and policy analysis and she has a PhD in health services research. She was a Harkness Fellow in New York in 1990, the policy advisor to the Chief Executive of the National Health Service between 1998 and 2000, and is currently a board member of the Audit Commission and the Healthcare Commission.

Dave Evans is a nurse by profession and worked in the NHS for over 18 years in a number of senior management posts within the acute sector. He was Project Director for the Kidderminster Treatment Centre following which he was appointed as Hospital Director. In 2005 he joined Durrow, a management consultancy specialising in strategic health planning and project management. In addition he established his own consultancy, PSPC – people, space, process, change (info@pspc.org.uk). Dave regularly speaks at conferences both in the UK and overseas.

Dr Tim Freeman is Lecturer in Health Policy in the Health Services Management Centre at the University of Birmingham, where he is responsible for the department's doctoral programme. Previously, he worked as a researcher for Save the Children Fund and the Sainsbury Centre for Mental Health, and has worked as a manager in the NHS. He teaches and publishes widely on topics related to governance, performance management and quality improvement.

Dr Jon Glasby is Head of Health and Social Care Partnerships and a Senior Lecturer at the Health Services Management Centre, University of Birmingham. A qualified social worker by background, he is also a board member of the national Social Care Institute for Excellence and programme director of what is believed to be the UK's first MSc in Managing Partnerships in Health and Social Care.

Dr Neil Goodwin is a UK NHS manager and leadership academic. He has operated at chief executive level for over 20 years and is currently chief executive of the Greater Manchester strategic health authority, the largest strategic body in the English NHS. Neil is also visiting professor of leadership studies at Manchester Business School and a fellow of Durham University. He is a board member of the European Health Management Association and the author of *Leadership in Healthcare: A European Perspective*.

Andrew Hine joined KPMG at the end of 2004. During a 13-year NHS career Andrew worked at all levels of the NHS and managed services from specialist acute to community hospitals and including primary care, mental health and learning disability services. He has also worked on secondment to the civil service within the Welsh Office Health Department.

Dr Paula Hyde is a Senior Lecturer in Leadership and Experiential Learning, Manchester Business School, The University of Manchester. Paula's main research interests are workforce modernisation in the NHS, HR and performance and the effects of organisational structures and systems on individual behaviours at work. Current projects study HRM and performance in healthcare and skills mix changes in health systems.

Kim Jelphs currently works as a Senior Fellow at the Health Services Management Centre, University of Birmingham. She has worked in the NHS for 25 years and has held senior clinical posts in both the acute and primary care sectors. Her role as a clinical director in an NHS trust saw her leading clinical governance in an innovative way, with some processes and tools receiving national recognition. She has a wide and varied experience of working with individuals, teams and organisations across many sectors.

Professor Justin Keen is Professor of Health Politics and Information Management at the University of Leeds. He has also worked at Brunel University, the National Audit Office and the King's Fund, London. His principal research interests are in the governance of health and social care services and the effects of information technologies on clinical practice.

Dr Helen Lester is a Reader in Primary Care in the Department of Primary Care and General Practice at the University of Birmingham. She has a particular interest in primary care mental health, health inequalities and mental health policy. Helen is the expert lead for the national review of the GP contract Quality and Outcomes Framework in England.

Dr Anne McBride is a Senior Lecturer in Employment Studies, Manchester Business School, The University of Manchester. Anne's main research interests are workforce modernisation in the NHS, gender relations at work and public sector industrial relations. Current projects study local healthcare workforce developments in the context of national government policies and initiatives, for example, skills mix changes in health systems.

Dr Ruth McDonald is a Research Fellow at the National Primary Care Research and Development Centre, University of Manchester. She is a health economist by background and has published widely on matters pertaining to the management and organisation of health services and is the author of *Using Health Economics in Health Services. Rationing Rationally?*

Dr Shirley McIver joined the Health Services Management Centre at Birmingham University in 1993. She coordinates the Public and Patients as Partners Programme which carries out research, consultancy and education in the area of public and user involvement. She is also programme director for the MSc Managing Quality and Service Improvement in Healthcare.

Ann Mahon is Senior Fellow and Director of Postgraduate Programmes at the Centre for Public Policy and Management, Manchester Business School (MBS). She directs and contributes to a range of postgraduate and executive education programmes and directs the public health and healthcare management course unit on the MSc Healthcare Management at MBS.

Professor Steve Onyett is Senior Development Consultant for the National Institute for Mental Health in England development centre for the south west (NIMHE-SW) and Visiting Professor at the Faculty of Health and Social Care at the University of the West of England. Steve is a strong advocate of the application of clinical know-how to organisational change and partnership working, and has worked as practitioner, service development consultant, manager, trainer and researcher. In his current role he leads on issues concerning leadership and teamworking, particularly with respect to the promotion of social inclusion.

Helen Parker is a Senior Fellow at the Health Services Management Centre at the University of Birmingham. Prior to this she spent over 20 years working in the NHS in both clinical and senior management posts, and for most of that period working in primary care. Helen is also a director of a city centre hostel for the homeless.

Professor Edward Peck is Director of the Health Services Management Centre at the University of Birmingham. He is interested in organisational development and his edited volume entitled *Organisational Development in Healthcare* was published by Radcliffe (2005). He also researches policy implementation and his book *Beyond Delivery: Policy Implementation as Organisational Settlement and Sense-Making* – co-authored book with Perri 6 – was published by Palgrave Macmillan in 2006.

Suzanne Robinson is a Lecturer in Health Economics and Healthcare Management at the Health Services Management Centre, University of Birmingham. Her main research interests span the range of health economics and healthcare policy, with special interests around funding healthcare systems and methodological issues around approaches to valuing health states for use in economic evaluation.

Dr Ann Shacklady-Smith is Director of the Masters in Public Administration and Senior Fellow in Public Management within the Centre for Public Policy and Management at Manchester Business School. Ann has an extensive background in teaching, research and consultancy in management development and change within education and local government. Her research interests include critical reflection in learning, and the use of action research and appreciative inquiry methods for implementing whole-of-organisation change. She has worked in business schools within the UK and New Zealand, with state sector organisations in Malaysia, and as a consultant with government ministries, local authorities and the voluntary sector.

Judith Smith is Senior Lecturer and Director of Research at the Health Services Management Centre at the University of Birmingham. She has been involved in health services research since the mid-1990s, before which she worked as a senior manager in the NHS. Judith's research interests are concerned with the organisation and management of primary care, health commissioning, and international health policy. She is a board member of the European Health Management Association and holds visiting research fellowships at the Australian National University and the Victoria University of Wellington.

Anne Tofts co-founded Healthskills in 1996 following 20 years as an NHS operational manager, regional organisation development manager and advisor at the Department of Health. Anne facilitates strategy and leadership development with health and care organisations, working with front-line clinicians and policymakers.

Professor Tom Walley is Professor of Clinical Pharmacology at the University of Liverpool, a consultant physician in the NHS and director of the NHS Health Technology Assessment Programme

Professor Kieran Walshe is Professor of Health Policy and Management at Manchester Business School where he also co-directs the Centre for Public Policy and Management. He is also research director of the NHS service delivery and organisation research programme and deputy editor of the *International Journal for Quality in Health Care*. His research interests concern quality and performance in public services, regulation and inspection, organisational failure and turnaround, and policy evaluation and learning.

Dr Juliet Woodin is a Senior Fellow at the Health Services Management Centre, University of Birmingham. Prior to joining HSMC she worked as a senior manager in the NHS and was Chief Executive of Nottingham Health Authority from 1995 to 2002. Her early career was as a researcher and lecturer in public policy.

Preface

A good rule of thumb for authors is that you should write books that you yourself really want or need to read. So it was for this book. Having run a wide range of postgraduate programmes for healthcare managers in the UK ourselves, and having worked with colleagues involved in this area in other European countries, the USA, Canada, Australia and New Zealand, we knew there simply wasn't a comprehensive, research-based book which provided a foundation for postgraduate study of health policy and management. There were policy books, and management books, but none that brought the two together – and certainly not in a way that was appropriate for an international readership. Moreover, we also worked on development programmes with many senior and middle managers who had enormous experiential learning, but struggled to set that in a wider, more theoretical context. We thought they needed a book like this too.

As with all good ideas, when we pointed out the need for a book like this to other people, they suggested that we should get on and write it. This seemed to make sense at first, but we quickly realised that we simply didn't have the breadth of knowledge and expertise that was demanded by such an ambitious project. However, we were aware that between us we knew people who could contribute the appropriately expert material for the book we envisaged.

To our delight, when we approached those colleagues rather tentatively to ask them to contribute to this book, they shared our enthusiasm for the idea, and were prepared to invest their time and effort in writing chapters to a demanding timescale. It is remarkable that it took just eight months from us designing the book and approaching chapter authors to delivering the final text to our publishers. This has allowed us to make the content about as up to date as it could be in what is (as we emphasise in the book) a complex and fast-changing world.

We owe a great deal to the contributors to this book and hope that they are as pleased as we are with the overall result of our collective effort (and that they will forgive us for rather assertive project management). But we owe as much to Amy Bevell and Lyndsey Jackson who were really in charge of making sure both that chapter authors and editors stuck to the deadlines and delivered on time. Editing this book has truly been a pleasure, and that is due in no small measure to Amy and Lyndsey's work in coordinating, advising, administering and sometimes harassing (in the nicest possible way) all the contributors, including ourselves.

Kieran Walshe
Judith Smith

May 2006

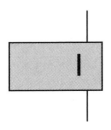

1 Introduction: the current and future challenges of healthcare management

Kieran Walshe and Judith Smith

Introduction

The purpose of this book is to support the learning and development of practising managers in healthcare organisations and health systems, and those undertaking postgraduate study on programmes concerned with health policy, health management and related areas. Increasingly those two groups overlap – more and more managers undertake a masters degree as part of their intellectual and career development, and we strongly believe in the power of the interaction between academic and experiential learning that this brings. No one learns to be a manager in a classroom, or from a book. Management is learnt by doing, by experiencing the challenges and opportunities of leadership (Mintzberg 2004). But the best and most successful managers are reflective practitioners – profoundly aware of their own behaviours, attitudes and actions and their impact on others and on the organisation, and able to analyse and critically review their own practice and set it in a wider context, framed by appropriate theories, models and concepts (Peck 2004). The future leaders of our healthcare systems need to be able to integrate theory and practice, and to have the adaptability and flexibility that comes from really understanding the nature of management and leadership.

This chapter sets the context for the book, by first describing the challenges of the political and social environment in which healthcare systems and organisations exist, and how that environment is changing. It then describes some of the particular challenges of those organisations – some of the characteristics and dynamics which make healthcare organisations both so interesting and so difficult to lead. Then the chapter sets out the structure of the rest of the book and explains how we anticipate that it might be used, both in support of formal programmes of study and by managers who simply want to develop and expand their own understanding and awareness.

Healthcare systems, politics and society

In most developed countries, the healthcare sector is anything from 8% to 15% of the economy, making it one of the largest industries in any state – bigger generally than education, agriculture, IT, tourism or telecommunications, and a crucial component of wider economic performance. In most countries, around one worker in ten is employed in the healthcare sector – as doctors, nurses, scientists, therapists, cleaners, cooks, engineers, administrators, clerks, finance controllers – and, of course, as managers. This means that almost everyone has a relative or knows someone who works in healthcare, and the healthcare workforce can be a politically powerful group with considerable influence over public opinion. Almost everyone uses health services, or has members of their family or friends who are significant healthcare users, and everyone has a view to express about their local healthcare system.

In many countries, the history of the healthcare system is intertwined with the development of communities and social structures. Religious groups, charities, voluntary organisations, trade unions and local municipalities have all played important roles in building the healthcare organisations and systems we have today, and people in those communities often feel viscerally connected to 'their' hospitals, community clinics, ambulance service, and other parts of the healthcare system. They fundraise to support new facilities or equipment, and volunteer to work in a wide range of roles which augment or support the employed healthcare workforce. That connection with the community also comes to the fore when anyone – especially government – suggests changing or reconfiguring healthcare provision. Proposals to close much loved community hospitals, or to reorganise district hospital services, or to change maternity services are often professionally driven, by a laudable policy imperative to make health services more effective, safe and efficient. But when evidence of clinical effectiveness and technocratic appraisals of service options collide with popular sentiment and public opinion, what matters is usually not 'what works' but what people want.

For many local and national politicians, health policy and the healthcare system offer not only opportunities to shine in the eyes of the electorate when things are going well, but also threats to future electoral success when there are problems with healthcare funding or service provision and people look for someone to hold to account. Many of the problems that constituents bring to politicians in their local offices concern healthcare services, and politicians are closely in touch with and aware of the attitudes and beliefs of the public about their local health service. While they will happily gain political benefit from the opening of a new facility, or the expansion of clinical services, they will equally happily secure benefit by criticising the plans of 'faceless bureaucrats' in the local healthcare organisation for changes in healthcare services, argue that there are too many managers and pen-pushers, and wax nostalgically about times past when hospitals were run by doctors and nurses and matron was in charge.

Finally, for the press, TV and radio media, both locally and nationally, the healthcare system is an endless source of news stories, debates and current affairs topics. From patient safety to MRSA and bird flu, from dangerous doctors to hospital closures, from waiting lists to celebrity illnesses, the healthcare system is news. Big healthcare stories can command pages of news coverage in national dailies and repeated presentation on TV news bulletins, while at a local level it would be rare to find a local newspaper which did not have some content about local hospitals, clinics or other healthcare services in every issue. Healthcare organisations can use the level of media interest to their advantage, to raise public awareness of health issues and to communicate with the community, but they can also find themselves on the receiving end of intense and hostile media scrutiny when things go wrong.

In other words, healthcare organisations exist in a turbulent political and social environment, in which their actions and behaviours are highly visible and much scrutinised. Leadership and management take place in this 'goldfish bowl', where their performance and process can be just as important as their outcomes. But if that were not enough, in every developed country the healthcare system is subject to four inexorable and challenging social trends:

- the demographic shift;
- the pace of technological innovation;
- changing user and consumer expectations; and
- rising costs.

The only certainty is that if it is difficult to make the sums add up for the healthcare system today, these pressures mean it will be even harder to do so tomorrow.

The demographic challenge is that because people are living longer the numbers of elderly and very elderly people are rising fast – and those people make much heavier use of the healthcare system. People may live longer, but they cost more to keep alive, they are more likely to have complex, chronic health conditions, and their last few months of life tend to be more expensive. A further dimension to this demographic challenge is the rising incidence of chronic disease in the wider population of developed countries. The World Health Organisation suggests that this is a direct result of risk factors such as tobacco use, physical inactivity and unhealthy diets (WHO 2005).

The second challenge is related to the first in that it reflects an increasing ability to control chronic disease and thus extend life – the pace of technological innovation. Most obviously in pharmaceuticals, but also in surgery, diagnostics and other areas, we keep finding new ways to cure or manage disease. Sometimes that means new treatments which are more effective than (and usually more expensive than) the existing ones. But it also means new treatments for diseases or problems which we simply could not treat before. Previously fatal conditions become treatable, and interventions to slow the progress of disease or manage its impact become more available.

This in turn connects with and feeds the third challenge – changing user and consumer expectations. People want more from the health service than their parents did. They are not content to be passive recipients of healthcare, prescribed and dispensed by healthcare providers at their convenience. Accustomed to ever-widening choice and sovereignty in decisions in other areas of life – banking, shopping, housing, education – they expect to be consulted, informed and involved by healthcare providers in any decisions that affect their health. They are better informed, more articulate and more likely to know about and demand new and expensive treatments.

The first three challenges are in large measure responsible for the fourth – rising costs. Each of them contributes to the constant pressure for more healthcare funding. However much governments or others increase their spending, it never seems to be enough. In almost every other area of the economy, productivity is rising and costs are falling through competition and innovation. We have better, faster, cheaper computers, cars, consumer goods, food, banking and so on, yet in healthcare costs are stubbornly high and continue to rise.

In short, the social, political and economic context in which healthcare organisations have to exist is often a hostile, fast-changing and pressured environment. Managers and leaders strive to balance competing, shifting and irreconcilable demands from a wide range of stakeholders – and do so while under close public scrutiny. The task of leadership in healthcare organisations – defining the mission of the organisation, setting out a clear and consistent vision, guiding and incentivising the organisation towards its objectives, and ensuring safe and high quality care – is made much more challenging by the social, economic and political context in which they work.

Healthcare organisations and healthcare management

Organisations are the product of their environment and context, and many of the distinctive characteristics and behaviours of healthcare organisations result from some of the social, political and economic factors outlined above. However, some also result from the nature of the enterprise – healthcare itself. The uniquely personal and personalised nature of health services, the special vulnerability and need for support and advocacy of patients, the complexity of the care process, and the advanced nature of the technologies used, all contribute to the special challenges of management in healthcare organisations.

Of course, we should be cautious that this does not lead us to be parochial or narrow-minded in our understanding of what we do, or of what we can learn from other sectors and settings. We are all prone to exceptionalism, believing that our job, organisation, profession or community is in some ways uniquely different. It gives us an excuse for why we perform less well. Our patients are sicker, our facilities less modern, our community is disadvantaged, our clinicians are more difficult or disengaged. It also provides the perfect reason for not adopting new ideas from elsewhere – it would not work here, because here is different. Healthcare systems and organisations have a strong tendency to exceptionalism, which needs to be challenged on a regular basis. Healthcare organisations are large, complex, professionally dominated entities providing a very wide range of highly tailored and personalised services to large numbers of often vulnerable users. But those characteristics are shared in various degrees by local authorities, police and emergency services, universities, schools, advertising agencies, management consultancies, travel agencies, law firms and other organisations. Healthcare is nevertheless different, and three important areas of difference deserve some further consideration: the place of professions, the role of patients, and the nature of the healthcare process.

For managers entering healthcare organisations from other sectors – whether from other public services, commercial for-profit companies or the voluntary sector – one of the first striking differences they notice is the absence of clear, hierarchical structures for command and control, and the powerful nature of professional status, knowledge and control. Sir Roy Griffiths, who in the 1980s led a management review of the NHS in the UK, famously wrote in his report about walking through a hospital looking vainly for 'the person in charge' (Griffiths 1983). But to do so would be to miss the point, which is that healthcare organisations are professional bureaucracies in which more or less all the intellectual, creative and social capital exists in the frontline workers – clinicians of all professions, but particularly doctors. Like law firms and advertising agencies, it makes no sense to try to manage these talented, highly intelligent individuals in ways that are reductionist, or which run counter to their highly professionalised self-image and culture. This does not mean that they should be unmanaged – just that the processes and content of management and leadership need to take account of and indeed embrace the professional culture. Things get done not through instruction or direction, but by negotiation, persuasion, peer influence and agreement. Leaders make skilful use of the values, language and apparatus of the profession to achieve their objectives, and learn to lead without needing to be 'in charge'.

The people who use healthcare services, whether you call them patients, users, consumers or whatever, are ordinary people, but they are not like the consumers of many other public or commercial services. First, there is a huge asymmetry of power and information in the relationship between a patient and a healthcare provider. Even the most middle-class, well-informed, internet-surfing patient cannot acquire the detailed knowledge and expertise which comes with clinical practice. Very few patients are prepared to go against the explicit advice of senior clinicians, and many patients actively seek to transfer responsibility for decision making to those professionals. 'Tell me what you think I should do, doctor.' At some level, patients have to be able to trust that healthcare providers are competent, and to take their advice on important decisions about their health. No amount of performance measurement, league tables, audit or regulation can substitute for this trust.

Secondly, when people become patients and use healthcare services they are often at their most vulnerable and are much less able to act independently and assertively than they would normally be. They may be emotionally fragile following an unwelcome diagnosis of disease, and physically weakened by the experience of illness or the effects of treatment. When lying flat on a wheeled trolley, feeling nauseous and in pain, surrounded by the unfamiliar noise and clatter of an emergency department and frightened by sudden intimations of mortality, we are at our most dependent. We are not well placed to exercise choice, or to assert our right to self-determination. We want and need to be cared for – a somewhat unfashionable and paternalistic notion which does not sit comfortably with concepts of the patient as a sovereign consumer of health services. This all means that healthcare organisations, and those who lead them, have a special responsibility to compensate for the unavoidable asymmetry of power and information in their relationships with patients, by providing mechanisms and systems to protect and advocate for patients, seek their views, understand their concerns, and make services patient centred.

Despite all the high technology medicine, complicated equipment and advanced pharmaceuticals available today, the healthcare process itself is still organised very much as it was a hundred years ago. It is a craft model of production in which individual health professionals ply their trade, providing their distinctive contribution to any patient's treatment when called upon. This is not mass production. Healthcare organisations such as hospitals are much more like marketplaces than they are like factories, with the patients moving from stall to stall to get what they want, not being whisked smoothly along on a conveyor belt from start to finish. Fundamentally, it is an unmanaged and undocumented process. Usually there is no written timetable or plan showing how the patient should move through the system, and no one person acts as 'process manager', steering and coordinating the care that the patient receives and assuring quality and efficiency. This model has endured because of its flexibility. The patient care process can be endlessly adapted or tailored to the needs of individual patients, the circumstances of their disease, and their response to treatment. But the complexity of modern healthcare processes, with multiple handovers from one healthcare professional to another, the ever-accelerating pace of care as lengths of stay get shorter and shorter, and the risks and toxicity of many new healthcare interventions (the flip side of their much greater effectiveness) all mean that the traditional model is increasingly seen as unreliable, unsafe, and prone to error and unexplained variation (Walshe and Boaden 2005). Increasingly, healthcare organisations use care pathways, treatment plans and clinical guidelines to bring some structure and explicitness to the healthcare process. Techniques for process mapping and design, commonplace in other sectors, are increasingly used not just to describe the healthcare process but in so doing to identify ways in which it can be improved (McNulty and Ferlie 2004). Like any area where custom, practice and precedent have long reigned supreme, healthcare processes are often ripe for challenge. Why does a patient need to come to hospital three times to see different people and have tests before they get a diagnosis? Can't we organise the process so that all the interactions take place in a single visit? Why are certain tasks only undertaken by doctors or nurses? Could they be done just as well by other healthcare practitioners? Gradually, the healthcare process is being made more explicit, exposed for discussion debate and challenge, and standardised or routinised in ways that make the delivery of healthcare more consistent, more efficient and safer.

In conclusion, there is one other important feature of healthcare organisations. Whether they are government owned, independent not-for-profits, or commercial healthcare providers, they all share to some degree a sense of social mission or purpose concerned with the public good (Drucker 2006). The professional values and culture of healthcare are deeply embedded, and most people working in healthcare organisations have both an altruistic belief in the social value of the work they do and a set of more self-interested motivations to do with reward, recognition and advancement. Similarly, healthcare organisations – even commercial, for-profit entities – do some things which do not make sense in business terms, but which reflect their social mission, while at the same time they respond to financial incentives and behave entrepreneurially. When exposed to strong competitive pressures, not-for-profit and commercial for-profit healthcare providers behave fairly similarly, and their social mission may take second place to organisational survival and growth. The challenge, at both the individual and organisational level, is to make proper use of both sets of motivations, but not to lose sight of the powerful and pervasive beneficial effects that can result from understanding and playing to the social mission.

About this book and how to use it

No book can contain everything on a particular subject, but in this case we have made a valiant attempt to provide a general textbook on healthcare management which covers most of the territory needed both for postgraduate study and for those interested in reading for their own development. The 27 chapters of the book which follow this introduction and overview are split into three main parts as follows.

Part 1: Setting the context

Chapters 2 to 6 aim to set out the wider political, social and economic context in which healthcare organisations exist. These chapters provide the 'big picture' which helps to explain the way that those organisations behave and what they do, remembering that, as observed earlier, organisations are very much a product of their environment and context. This section covers the politics of health and the health policy process (Chapter 2); healthcare financing and funding (Chapter 3); healthcare systems, provision and service delivery (Chapter 4); healthcare technologies and innovation (Chapter 5); health and well-being and the wider public health context (Chapter 6).

Part 2: Managing healthcare organisations

The middle section of the book aims to cover some of the specifics of healthcare management – issues and topics which are particular to the business of healthcare itself. It starts with three chapters about managing in different healthcare sectors – primary care (Chapter 7), acute care (Chapter 8) and mental health (Chapter 9). It then goes on to tackle a range of other subjects including service and capital development (Chapter 10); planning and strategic direction (Chapter 11); commissioning and contracting (Chapter 12); healthcare information systems and technology (Chapter 13); the healthcare workforce (Chapter 14); working with clinicians (Chapter 15); the governance of healthcare organisations (Chapter 16); partnership working with other agencies (Chapter 17); performance management and improvement (Chapter 18).

Part 3: Management theories, models and techniques

The third section of the book moves on to tackle a range of subjects where we feel theories, ideas, models, frameworks or techniques developed in the field of business and management can and should be brought to bear on the area of healthcare management. It starts with chapters on leadership (Chapter 19); organisational development (Chapter 20); and personal effectiveness (Chapter 21). It then continues with a series of practically focused chapters on managing change (Chapter 22); managing resources (Chapter 23); working in teams and managing people (Chapter 24); understanding user perspectives (Chapter 25); quality improvement (Chapter 26); research, evaluation and evidence-based management (Chapter 27).

Making sense of this substantial volume of materials and ideas is itself a challenge, and so we conclude in Chapter 28 by mapping out what we feel are some of the lessons about complexity, change and creativity in healthcare leadership and management which we would draw from the book as a whole.

While the content of each chapter has led its design, we have asked our authors to follow a broadly consistent format in order to make the materials in the book as useful and readable as possible. You will therefore find each chapter is structured into around five or six sections, and we make liberal use of figures, tables, charts and diagrams to illustrate the content. Each chapter finishes with the following:

- **Summary box** containing key points drawing together the main messages from the chapter.
- **Self-test exercises** designed to help you to apply the content of the chapter and your learning to your own organisations. The exercises generally consist of a number of questions which we suggest you use as the basis either for personal reflection or for discussion with colleagues.
- **References and further reading** with details of books, reports, journal articles and other materials referenced in the chapter or intended to provide background reading for you on the topic.
- **Websites and resources** where you might seek further information. We have done our best to ensure these are as up to date as possible, but bear in mind that content on the internet does change rapidly and so some links could no longer be current.

Finally, we would welcome comments about and ideas for improvement of this book. Whether you use it casually for your own development or more intensively as part of a postgraduate programme of study, we would like your feedback. Please email either one of us at kieran.walshe@man.ac.uk or j.a.smith.20@bham.ac.uk.

References and further reading

Drucker, P. (2006) *Managing the Nonprofit Organisation*. London: HarperCollins.

Griffiths, R. (1983) *Report of the NHS Management Inquiry*. London: Department of Health and Social Security.

McNulty, T. and Ferlie, E. (2004) *Reengineering Healthcare: The Complexities of Organisational Transformation*. Oxford: Oxford University Press.

Mintzberg, H. (2004) *Managers not MBAs*. London: Prentice Hall.

Peck, E. (2004) *Organisational Development in Healthcare: Approaches, Innovations, Achievements*. Oxford: Radcliffe Medical Press.

Walshe, K. and Boaden, R. (eds) (2005) *Patient Safety: Research into Practice*. Maidenhead: Open University Press/McGraw Hill.

World Health Organisation (WHO, 2005) *Preventing Chronic Diseases: A Vital Investment*. Geneva: WHO

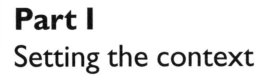

Part I
Setting the context

2 The politics of healthcare and the health policy process: implications for healthcare management

Jennifer Dixon

Introduction and overview

All governments in the developed world have a firm interest in shaping the healthcare industry. There are several reasons for this. Healthcare expenditures of a variety of payers, not least government, are significantly large and pressures on these expenditures are high. Since governments are major payers, they are accountable in a highly visible way for expenditure, not least at the ballot box. Every voter is a potential user of healthcare. Care and supplies are purchased from powerful corporate bodies or professional groups. There is a large difference in knowledge between providers (and their suppliers) and users (and often payers) of care, which may result in excessive care and avoidable costs. The healthcare sector employs a large number of people: for example, in the National Health Service (NHS) in England 1.3 million people out of a population of 49.1 million. The nature of healthcare is such that it is highly emotive and features frequently in the media, for there are distinct ideological and moral issues on which political parties are likely to disagree, for example, who pays for care (such as the individual, the employer, the government) and the factors which improve performance in health systems (for example, direct or indirect government intervention or market incentives). For these reasons, healthcare is rarely out of the sights of politicians.

It is no surprise then that governments and other payers regularly try to reform the healthcare sector. Managers working in provider or commissioning bodies are often at the receiving end of what might seem to be arbitrary and burdensome change. In doing their job it is important for them to understand, and therefore possibly predict, the pattern of reform that impinges on their work, partly to be able to plan better for change and where appropriate to attempt to modify the type and level of specific interventions.

This chapter focuses on reform which is the direct result of government action. It starts by examining how healthcare reforms come about and the main factors which shape them. It goes on to examine briefly the broad pattern of reforms in the healthcare sector across Europe. Then, using the example of the NHS in England, it outlines the menu of policies now being developed and implemented, and tries to weave a narrative around these changes in order to predict future change, thus attempting to assess the power of managers to shape reforms in future.

The dynamics of reform in the health sector

Why change occurs

In a lucid and sophisticated account of health sector reform in the 1980s and 1990s in the US, Canada and Britain, Carolyn Tuohy (1999), a Canadian political scientist, reflected on why change occurred. She observed that 'particular windows of opportunity for change occur at certain times and not others, a pattern of timing that derived from factors in the broader political system not in the health care arena itself'. She argued that significant features of health systems arising from major reform were in fact accidents – byproducts of ideas in wider circulation at the time that a window of opportunity opened – and that decisions taken between the episodes of major reform were heavily influenced by the parameters or 'logic' that such major reforms put in place. These parameters were influenced by history, or the reforms that had gone before, the sequencing of reforms and rational (evidence-based) choice, as well as two other characteristics which she termed 'institutional mix' and 'structural balance'. By institutional mix she meant the balance of power between three main forms of social control: state hierarchy ('authority-based' control); professional collegiate institutions ('skill-based' control); and the market ('wealth-based' control). By structural balance she meant the balance of power between three main stakeholders: the state, healthcare professionals and private financial interests. Tuohy's argument was that reform of healthcare in different countries would most likely be incremental, and heavily bounded by the particular political system, social values, past history (including of major reforms) and the power of institutions and key groups. The resulting pathway of reform would be thus different across countries.

Tuohy also noted that there were few instances of significant changes in power between these stakeholders necessary to achieve episodes of very major reform in health care. Evans (2005) described the period when these episodes occur as 'punctuated equilibrium' and also noted that the 'punctuation marks may be wholly external to the system, even random – war or economic crisis . . . and their effects are unpredictable' as well as 'decidedly unpleasant'. This was echoed by US economist Victor Fuchs who ruefully noted in the 1990s that short of major change in the political climate that 'often accompanies a war, a depression, or large scale civil unrest' national health insurance in the US was unlikely (Fuchs 1991). However, between episodes of major reform Tuohy thought that the success of change would depend upon 'the "goodness of fit" between the strategy of change proposed and the internal logic of the system to which it is addressed', itself influenced by the structural balance and institutional mix. In turn she argued that these last two factors, in particular the role of the state, are heavily influenced by the ability for the prevailing political system in a country to exert authority over health systems, either directly (where the state was payer and possibly also the provider of care) – which is most effective – or less directly through regulation or through mobilisation of other key stakeholders – which is likely to be less effective, since it relies upon achieving consensus between different and powerful parties.

The dynamics of healthcare reform and the theory underpinning it, described by analysis of reform in three countries by Tuohy (1999), have also been identified and developed by many other writers, often political scientists (Hacker 2002; Hall and Taylor 1996). At present three theories appear to be mainly in play: historical institutionalism; rational choice institutionalism; and sociological institutionalism. Historical institutionalists believe that the power and mix of institutions is the main factor influencing the outcome of reform (Tuohy's institutional mix), and that 'institutions push policy along particular paths, where early choices and events play a crucial role in determining the subsequent development of institutions or policies', otherwise known as 'path dependency' (Oliver and Mossialos 2005). Rational choice institutionalists seek a further explanation as to the basis for the choices made by institutions, which is often rooted in welfare economics where institutions act to maximise benefits along the range of options they make available to key actors. Sociological institutionalists believe that the actions of institutions are not just informed by a welfare maximising logic, but also by culture or identity within institutions and that 'policy and institutional reforms will occur only if they are socially legitimate' (Oliver and Mossialos 2005) or chime in with a nation's culture.

In truth, as theorists grope towards better conceptual models which explain the dynamics of healthcare reform with more accuracy, in a subject as complex as health reform any single theory is likely to be inadequate. As Oliver and Mossialis (2005) put it with respect to healthcare reform in Europe, the answer to the question asked by Hollis (1994) 'does structure determine action, or action define structure?' is probably a bit of both.

Healthcare reforms across Europe

Regardless of the preferred theories of change, Evans (2005) suggested that the three most important questions driving health sector reform were:

- Who pays for care (and how much)?
- Who gets care (what kind, when, from whom)?
- Who gets paid how much, for doing what?

Evans suggested that conflict between major stakeholders revolves mainly around differences in viewpoints as to how these questions should be answered.

The extent to which government (or 'politics' as termed in the title of this chapter) is involved in healthcare depends heavily not just upon the extent to which political systems can consolidate authority, or upon the appearance of a window of opportunity for change, but on the extent to which government (national or local) is motivated to act. A primary factor to induce motivation must be the extent to which government pays for healthcare and thus seeks to control expenditure. Figure 2.1 shows that across OECD countries the government is a major payer even in countries such as the US, and thus is constantly seeking to reform healthcare.

In the face of rising health expenditures and pressures to spend more from providers, users and other supply-side stakeholders, all governments in Europe have been constantly active in attempting to reform healthcare. Analysing recent reforms across 11 European countries described in a special edition of the *Journal of Health Policy Politics and Law*, Evans (2005) notes a surprisingly similar story over the past 50 years – different reforms but 'parallel development' – in contrast to what might have been expected given the unique set of conditions (such as institutional mix as highlighted by Tuohy) in each country. He describes two distinct phases to reform. The first was the establishment of near universal and comprehensive systems of collective payment for healthcare (through taxation and/or compulsory social insurance) – major reform which in many European countries was prompted by significant political events in the case of northern and middle Europe linked to World War II, and in southern European states such as Greece, Spain and Portugal linked to the later overthrow of right-wing authoritarian regimes. The second phase (from the mid-1970s onwards) was essentially one of containing costs, which has been difficult since governments have been faced 'by highly intelligent and highly motivated opponents who are trying to drive them up' (Evans 2005: 287) such as the pharmaceutical industry and doctors. Modifying physicians' behaviour, Evans warns, has led to 'head-on conflict over professional organisation and autonomy' where the public are unsurprisingly likely to side with the professionals arguing for more funding rather than governments demanding parsimony. He also notes that while each country has a unique history and institutional mix, surprisingly reforms since the 1970s across European countries have focused on similar objectives and the pathway of reform has not been dissimilar.

Closer inspection of ongoing attempts at reform across Europe in the last two decades reveal some broad patterns, at least across middle and northern European countries (*Journal of Health Policy* 2005; *Health Economics* 2005). First, the main goals of reform have been similar: to control

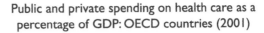

Public and private spending on health care as a
percentage of GDP: OECD countries (2001)

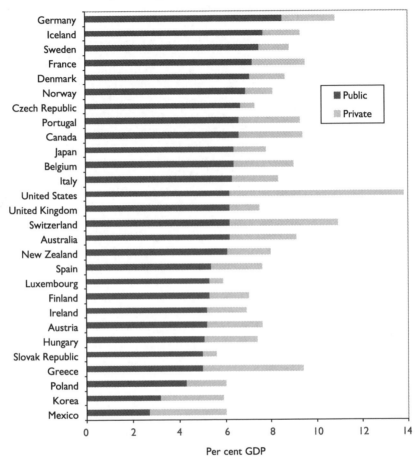

costs, improve cost effectiveness and access to care while protecting key
social or collective objectives such as equity of access to care and public
satisfaction. Second, incremental rather than radical change has generally
been the norm – change bounded in part by the institutional mix and
power both within the political and healthcare arena. Progress has been
limited in particular by, as Tuohy (1999) described, governments in some
countries needing to achieve consensus with other political parties or key
corporate bodies, such as in Germany and the Netherlands. Third, there
has been an emphasis in some countries of devolution of health reforms
to regions or other geographical areas and central frustration (and resulting central intervention) with lack of progress. Fourth, there has been
an emphasis in many countries such as Germany (Wortz and Busse 2005),

Holland (Schut and Van de Ven 2005) Austria (Stephan and Sommersguter-Reichmann 2005) and England (Oliver 2005) on reviewing the incentives operating on providers, with the tentative development of market-style incentives, such as competition and greater consumer choice underpinned by new methods of paying hospitals based case-mix based tariffs derived using diagnostic-related groups.

Maynard (2005) observed that the weak evidence base to many of the reforms in Europe had resulted in 'a lack of clarity in defining public policy goals, establishing trade-offs and aligning incentives with those objectives'. He also observed that many governments, such as in France and the US, had taken the 'wrongheaded' step of introducing reforms to curb the demand for care by increasing co-payments for users, a policy which tended to penalise those least well off and the needy as well as the worried well, rather than the more important priority of tackling providers over the more significant problem of supplier-induced demand. For example, he noted a failure across Europe of governments to act or be effective in addressing specific problems of: variations in use of care arising from variations in medical practice; the lack of evidence on the cost effectiveness of treatments; and specifically the management of people with chronic medical conditions. This observation is perhaps is understandable. It is far easier for governments to introduce co-payments than it is to tackle powerful suppliers about their behaviour.

The overall result in Europe over the past decade argues Evans (2005) has been mixed and tentative – drops in inpatient utilisation, continued escalation in the expenditure on pharmaceuticals, and the costs of physicians' services somewhere in the middle. He concludes by reflecting that 'effective coping depends both upon the resources of the state ... and upon the degree of democratic responsiveness of the state itself to broader public values' (Evans 2005: 291), but warns that the obvious political difficulty of the phase two agenda may strengthen the hand of those who seek to erode the phase one reforms in Europe. An additional warning might be that attempts to increase efficiency and quality of care using sharper market incentives might also lead to the undermining of social objectives, unless there is effective monitoring and regulation to counter it.

To a manager, the discussion so far may not make comfortable reading. If, on the one hand, major reforms are influenced heavily by factors in the wider political and institutional arena and are heavily bounded by history, then what hope is there to influence the shape of reform? On the other hand, if episodes between major reforms are influenced by the shifts in power between and probably within major stakeholders, among whom are the professionals running institutions, then there may be hope. Such high-level analysis might help those managing healthcare to understand and predict the pathway of reform and identify the features that may or may not be modifiable nationally or locally. In the next section the influence of politics on healthcare in the UK National Health Service (NHS) is focused upon. The objective is to help promote understanding of the pathway of reform in a specific system and predict what might happen in the short to medium term.

Reform in the UK NHS

The main objectives driving healthcare reform in Europe are also in play in the UK NHS. But there are particular features about the political system, and the healthcare system and the ideology of the government in power over the last decade, which are distinctive and help to explain the pathway of reform in the UK compared to Europe. These features are discussed briefly below.

The political system

A distinctive feature of the UK political system is a parliamentary system of government with a 'first past the post' method of electing Members of Parliament. On occasion this has allowed governments to be elected with sufficiently large majorities to create an 'elected autocracy', with little need to achieve consensus over policy with either other political parties or indeed key corporate and professional stakeholders. The landslide victory of the Labour government in 1997 and subsequently two further victories (albeit with smaller majorities) has allowed significant progress on reform in healthcare to be made relative to other European states. Within the UK, the Labour government in 1997 committed to greater devolution of political power. The immediate result was the creation in 1998 of an elected Parliament in Scotland, an elected Assembly in Wales and, until it was suspended in 2002, an elected Assembly in Northern Ireland (NI). While the specific powers of each political body are different, each has significant freedoms with respect to public policy including healthcare. The speed of public sector reform has been different across the UK, partly dependent upon the need to achieve a consensus among political parties in the devolved political bodies in different countries, the shape of the reform programme and the tools designed by governments to implement it. Up until the late 1990s, reforms to the NHS had been applied similarly across the four countries of the UK, and while the NHS was never exactly the same in each country, in practice the policy differences between the countries were marginal in comparison to the similarities.

This changed following devolution. In England, the emphasis has been on national targets to improve performance (particularly reducing waiting times), increasing capacity and more latterly sharper market-style incentives, described further below. In Scotland the 1990s 'quasi-market' has been abolished and steps taken to build a professionally led, integrated system based on concepts such as managed clinical networks. In Wales, the focus has been on improving the public health through partnership working between the local NHS, local government and communities. In Northern Ireland, developments have been largely stalled by political uncertainty.

It is still too early to assess the overall impact of these different reforms to healthcare across the UK. In an analysis of performance across a range of high-level indicators, such as health status, patient satisfaction, waiting times, activity rates and staffing levels, the main difference between the four UK countries since 1997 was the significant reduction in the time waited by NHS patients in England for treatment as shown in Table 2.1 (Alvarez-Rosete et al. 2005).

The reason for the improved relative performance in England has been because reducing waiting has been the policy with highest priority. Measurable and time-specific targets were set and monitored, investment was focused on achieving the target, non-NHS providers were allowed to supply capacity to help reduce waiting and strong performance management and sanctions for failure were applied to managers (Bevan and Hood in press). This approach, a combination of strong performance management from the centre and stronger market-style incentives, was not adopted in other UK countries – largely for political reasons. For example, in Scotland, while some targets have been set centrally (such as to reduce waiting times for elective care), there has been a strong move against using financial incentives to improve performance. Instead, the emphasis to NHS reform has been to merge commissioners and providers of care and develop professionally led integrated networks and pathways of care.

The healthcare system

A distinctive feature in the UK is the extent to which government pays the costs (compared to other countries in Europe) and the extent to which health services are state owned and run. In 2005–6, 8.3% of gross domestic product (GDP) was spent on healthcare in the UK, 7.1% of GDP on the NHS funded largely through general taxation. Unlike the case across most of Europe, in the UK the state not only funds most healthcare but also owns all of the commissioners of state-funded care (for example, all strategic health authorities and primary care trusts), many of the providers (for example, all NHS trusts and community health services), and contracts almost exclusively with independent providers of primary care (GPs) and semi-autonomous NHS bodies – NHS foundation trusts. The NHS has some unusual features compared to other enterprises; for example, its budget is cash limited and NHS organisations must either break even each year or not breach their annual funding limit; it provides comprehensive services which are (largely) free at the point of use; individuals cannot buy NHS care directly but have care bought on their behalf by commissioners (for example, primary care trusts); there are enormous information discrepancies between individuals and service providers, which means that individuals rely heavily on informed agents (for example, GPs) to help direct them to the most appropriate care; and service providers are formally accountable directly

Table 2.1 NHS waiting times across four UK countries, 1997 and 2003

	England 1996–97	England 2002–03	Scotland 1996–97	Scotland 2002–03	Wales 1996–97	Wales 2002–03	NI 1996–97	NI 2002–03
Inpatient and day case waiting list								
Inpatient and day case waiting (% waiting of total population)	2.3	1.9	N/A	N/A	2.2	2.5	2.7	3.3
Percentage waiting less than 6 months (% of the waiting list)	74.9	80.6	N/A	N/A	N/A	63	62.2	60.1
Percentage waiting more 6 months but less than 12 months (% of the waiting list)	22.4	19.4	N/A	N/A	N/A	21	20.6	18.4
Percentage waiting 12 months or longer (% of the waiting list)	2.7	0	N/A	N/A	9.9	15.9	17.1	22
Outpatient waiting list								
Outpatient waiting (% waiting of total population) at March 2003	N/A	N/A	N/A	N/A	3.5	7.4	3.7	8.4
Percentage waiting less than 3 months (% of the waiting list)	N/A	80	N/A	N/A	72	45.7	64.8	42.1
Percentage waiting less than 6 months (% of the waiting list)	N/A	100	N/A	N/A	94.1	67.6	80.7	61.4
Percentage waiting more than 6 months (% of the waiting list)	N/A	0	N/A	N/A	5.9	32.4	19.3	38.6

Source: Alvarez-Rosete et al. (2005).
N/A = data not available or not recorded in a comparable format

to the Secretary of State rather than to the patients treated or populations served (with the exception of foundation trusts).

Historically, the government largely left it to the professionals to provide a good quality service. As Rudolf Klein has noted, there was an implicit pact between the government and the profession whereby the former set the overall budget for the NHS and the latter largely spent it, provided each did not challenge the other (Klein 2000). By the 1980s this had changed and the government, through the Department of Health and local NHS bodies, took an increasingly direct role to improve the performance of NHS institutions, particularly providers of care. This was done through primary and secondary legislation, directives from the centre, and performance management locally, regionally, or sometimes nationally. Where the government was not able to act directly through operational directives and performance management, in particular with respect to GPs as independent contractors, it has attempted to shape the activities of GPs through legislation and the financial incentives of the national GP contract. The bulk of these efforts has been largely to improve the performance of institutions with respect to politically determined priorities, rather than the quality of care provided by professionals, which has more often been the preserve of the professional regulatory bodies such as the General Medical Council and the Royal Colleges.

The prevailing environment in the UK NHS, then, is one in which government has a very strong role in improving performance through reform. Bevan and Robinson (2005) argued that 'path dependency' does help us understand the path of reform in England and the underpinning political logics in the NHS are those of a 'state hierarchical system in which GPs and hospital doctors determine both demand and supply'.

Ideology

In the UK, particularly in England, apart from the fact of relatively large parliamentary majorities giving a significant democratic mandate for change, perhaps the most important feature shaping recent healthcare reform has been the ideology or 'mission' of successive New Labour governments led by Tony Blair. Upon election in 1997 there was much talk, as in Germany and the US, of finding a 'third way', a different mission which took politics to a new place 'beyond left and right' – beyond a spectrum with the free market at one end and nationalised state bureaucracies at the other. A mantra used by government in healthcare was 'what counts is what works'; in other words, the government was to implement reforms that were shown to achieve desired objectives regardless of the ideologically correct way of achieving them. Despite much analysis by academics (Giddens 1998, 2000), the 'third way' was not convincingly conceptualised or operationalised. Neither was 'what works' found, since that required significant investment in building an evidence base to reform in the public sector which would also take up much needed time when reform was pressing. Instead, what has seemed to be the main lodestar to New Labour governments since 1997 was the step taken in 1994 to scrap clause 4 – a clause in the constitution of the Labour Party:

> To secure for all the workers by hand or by brain the full fruits of their industry and the most equitable distribution thereof that may be possible *upon the basis of the common ownership of the means of production, distribution and exchange,* and the best obtainable system of popular administration and control of each industry of service. (My emphasis; http://www.cool-stuff.co.uk/LabourWatch/c4.html)

In scrapping the clause, a rubicon had been crossed that had taken a 60-year journey (since the big nationalisations of enterprise in the 1940s and 1950s). With respect to the UK's biggest nationalised industry, the NHS, the diagnosis made by core New Labourites was not dissimilar to that made by Margaret Thatcher a decade earlier – that the NHS was in-efficient, painfully slow to change, dominated by entrenched provider interest and insufficiently responsive to users, and too big to be run successfully from the centre. A stimulant needed was greater competition between suppliers, both institutions and professionals, to improve per-formance quality responsiveness and efficiency, while protecting equity of access to care as far as possible. In England a radical reform programme took shape, which because of devolution did not emerge in the three other UK countries.

Three broad phases to NHS reform in England since 1997 have been described: phase 1, central direction (national standards and directives); phase 2, financial investment and support (for example, the work of the Modernisation Agency); and, the most significant, phase 3, 'constructive discomfort' (Stevens 2004) or 'edgy instability' – the introduction since 2000 of market-style incentives to improve the quality and efficiency of care. This has been underpinned by policies such as patient choice (DH 2005a), encouraging private providers (secondary, community and pri-mary) to compete for NHS business through the letting of contracts (nationally by government as well as locally by commissioners) to non-NHS providers (DH 2006a), introducing a new system of prospective payment to hospitals payment by results (DH 2002), allowing NHS trusts to achieve foundation status with much greater freedom to operate independently of the state (for example, NHS foundation trusts are not subject to directives by the Secretary of State or performance manage-ment by the centre) (DH 2006b), and attempting to develop commission-ing by primary care trusts (DH 2005b). It is intended that all NHS trusts should achieve foundation status by 2008. These reforms are in the early stages of implementation and the market for provision, such as it is, is immature. There is no prospect of wholesale and overnight privatisa-tion as was the case with the denationalised utilities, rather a gradual development of market-style incentives, plurality of providers, a payment system for providers to support choice and competition underpinned by effective regulation (Dixon 2005).

It is clearer where this broad direction of travel may lead in theory than in practice. In theory it seems that the introduction of stronger market forces into healthcare is here to stay. In England, market-style incentives could well be extended beyond provision to commissioning bodies (all NHS owned and run at present), which could compete, like US managed care organisations, with each other for consumers. One aspect of reform that Labour has been consistent on has been to rule out alternative private sources of funding of healthcare, so that the bulk of care remains free at the point of use – a fundamental founding principle of the NHS. On this basis the national health *service* could indeed become national health *insurance*, with a plurality of organisations, state owned, voluntary and private, competing to provide services.

The introduction of market-style incentives in Scotland Wales and Northern Ireland will depend upon their impact in England, in particular on waiting times for elective care, and the contribution to progress of other reforms in these countries. But the likelihood is that across the UK, as elsewhere in Europe, there will be increasing recognition that a blend of levers to improve performance is needed, and that blend will appropriately include market-style incentives (such as competition between institutions and consumer choice). As has been demonstrated across Europe in the last two decades, how prominent these incentives will be in that blend will depend on a number of factors, including the ideological complexion of governments, the relative political power of other key stakeholders (such as the professions) and the extent to which there is convincing evidence that these incentives are helping to solve key local problems.

Again as demonstrated across Europe, the pathway of reform is unlikely to be linear and likely to be stalled by cautious implementation. For example, in the Netherlands in the late 1980s the Dekker Plan promoted radical reform – regulated competition to give more incentives to providers and insurers to improve performance (Schut and Van de Ven 2005). While the theory of how this would work appeared convincing, in practice implementation was very difficult, not so much because of political conflict in this case but because a number of technical aspects of the reforms had not been worked out or implemented to allow regulated competition to occur. In particular the following had not been determined (Schut and Van de Ven 2005): risk adjustment to reduce adverse selection by insurers; pricing and product classification for providers to reduce the temptation to skimp on care provided; a better system of outcome and quality measurement so that contract negotiations between insurer and provider would focus on these areas not just price; better information to promote choice among consumers; and an effective regulatory framework. While progress has been made on these in the intervening years, implementation is still in a very early stage.

In Sweden, the process of reform towards market-style reforms has proceeded crabwise, delayed perhaps less by technical problems as experienced in the Netherlands but more by the political process (Anell 2005). In Sweden healthcare is mostly funded and provided by the county councils, whereas overall goals and policies are set by national government. The county councils and national government may be of different political complexion; for example, between 1991 and 1994 when a non-socialist coalition government was in power and in favour of market-style incentives such as competition and consumer choice and national governments have varied in their willingness to devolve decision making locally. The lack of political stability between central and local government has contributed to difficulties in developing and implementing policies, resulting in delay.

In England, in practice though, the reform path is less clear in the short to medium term. Whether or not permission to continue to develop market-style incentives in the NHS is granted by parliamentarians is likely to be partly contingent upon the successful implementation of the current round of reforms, in particular the extent to which they improve efficiency and quality and critically while protecting equity of access – an objective which trumps all others according to many Labour parliamentarians. With respect to the progress of implementation, the signs so far are mixed. The most significant risks are financial management of hospitals (in part related to the implementation of Payment by Results (National Audit Office 2004) and managing the closures that will be necessary. There is likely to be a change in leadership of the Labour Party before the next election, and the extent to which the new leader will support the expansion of market forces in healthcare is unclear. Indeed, the extent to which a new leader will prioritise equity of access to care over and above efficiency and quality of care is unknown.

Influencing the dynamics of reform in the UK

In the discussion above, readers can be forgiven for concluding that in the UK, at least in England, government alone is responsible for influencing the path of healthcare reform. There seems to be little to counter the general current towards market-based reform in England. So much for the 'institutional mix' and 'structural balance' outlined earlier, one might think. In fact the government is overwhelmingly the most influential body shaping healthcare, but other bodies (apart from other political parties) do have influence, although perhaps less so than in other countries with more corporatist politics requiring consensus, such as in Germany or Holland. Other bodies with influence on healthcare reform in the UK include those shown in Box 2.1.

Across Europe, the bodies who have had the biggest effect in stalling reform have included professional groups and trade unions. But in the UK both groups in the last two decades have been weakened by a combination of external events, suboptimal leadership and erosion of their

Box 2.1   UK bodies with influence on the pathway of healthcare reform

- Professional bodies (e.g. General Medical Council, Royal Colleges)
- Other trade representative groups (e.g. the NHS Confederation, British Medical Association, Foundation Trust Network, Institute of Healthcare Management, NHS Alliance, National Association of Primary Care)
- Trade unions
- Regulatory bodies (e.g. Healthcare Commission, Monitor, Audit Commission, Commission for Social Care Inspection)
- NHS Ombudsman
- Research organisations (e.g. universities, think tanks)
- Private consultancy organisations
- Private industry (private providers and suppliers of goods and services, e.g. pharmaceutical industry, private hospitals) and private payers e.g. private insurance companies
- Legal system
- Media

powers by Parliament. The power of the medical profession in the UK was severely assaulted by public outrage over two significant events in the 1990s – the poor quality of heart surgery in a children's unit in Bristol Royal Infirmary (2001) and the case of Dr Harold Shipman, a GP convicted of murdering dozens of his patients (2005). Each case in its own way demonstrated the weakness of the medical profession in regulating itself, and an arrogance towards responding to public concern about the quality of care. The General Medical Council and to an extent the Royal Colleges have been preoccupied since then in improving the quality of care and regulation rather than developing a national stance over the shape of healthcare reform. In the case of the unions, their powers had been eroded in the 1980s by successive Conservative governments and they have faced declining membership. Together with some of the trade bodies (such as the British Medical Association) they have been active in lobbying for, or more often against, recent reforms. But while they may have strong links with the Labour government, in particular with back-bench MPs, their lack of an alternative vision for the future of healthcare (other than more of the past), which particularly promotes greater power for patients over providers, has limited their success.

The NHS Confederation (2005), arguably at present the strongest mouthpiece for managers in the UK, has largely been supportive of the general direction of healthcare reform although critical over problems with implementation. It is by this representative body, other than by individual and personal contacts with key policymakers, that at present managers working within the NHS can have their greatest impact on the shape of reform. There is understandable pressure in the NHS for managers not to be freely critical of current policy. In general, research institutions have been insufficiently mobilised and motivated to mount a comprehensive critique of policy based on evidence and follow it through with effective lobbying – arguably it is not their role. In the last decade a number of new independent regulators have been created by government, and their influence in the NHS is a prominent feature. But while having an 'arm's length' relationship with government and exerting a strong 'behind the scenes' influence on policy, the regulators must choose very carefully the issues on which to go public. The pharmaceutical industry is highly influential, not least because of the strong relationship it has with the Department of Health (DH) as its sponsor and chief government negotiator with the industry as to the prices the industry can charge for supplies to the NHS under the pharmaceutical price regulation scheme (DH 2005c). The media have had a strong role, but more in criticising policy and identifying perverse consequences locally rather than developing a constructive alternative vision.

The institutional mix and structural balance in the UK has thus been skewed heavily in the government's favour in the last two decades and resulted in a greater number and more radical healthcare reforms than have been possible elsewhere in Europe. With greater plurality of providers, particularly with new powerful private suppliers entering the healthcare market in England at least, corporate interests may be more influential in future including the power to stall certain reforms. But for as long as government remains the major payer of healthcare in the UK, there is a workable majority in Parliament, and the professional bodies and trade unions remain on the back foot, further major reforms are likely. The door to greater market forces is likely to remain open, given the apparent broad political consensus that these incentives have a role in improving system performance. The conflicts in the UK and Europe will revolve around how strong these incentives should be (ideologically and in the light of evidence of their impact) and most fundamentally to what extent social objectives can be traded off against the universally desired objective of improving efficiency.

Conclusion

This chapter has outlined a few of the theories that might underpin the dynamics of change in the health sector internationally. It has examined briefly the broad pattern of reforms in the healthcare sector across Europe, showing that reforms have been designed with similar objectives, that reform has been incremental, and much focused on altering the behaviour of patients rather than the suppliers of care. More radical reform has been stalled chiefly though conflicts over fundamental questions relating to who pays, who gets care, and who gets paid; conflicts which have been played out mainly between government, powerful professional and private interests and unions. Then, using the example of the National Health Service in England, it has described the direction of travel of policies now being developed and how and why government has been able to design and begin to implement more radical reform relative to other European countries. It suggests that the institutional mix in England at least has broadly favoured the government's agenda, and suggests that the power of managers to shape reforms in the short to medium term future will be limited. In other countries, that power may be greater given the different structural balance and institutional mix, the political processes in play and the more unpredictable windows of opportunity often created by events external to the health arena.

Summary box

- Governments across the developed world are constantly active in reforming healthcare, chiefly because of the extent to which governments pay healthcare costs.
- Incremental reform has been the norm, radical change is usually influenced by external political or economic events unrelated to healthcare. Incremental reform is highly influenced by the balance of power of key professional and corporate institutions present in each country and the system of government.
- Conflicts between key stakeholders tend to revolve around who pays, who gets care, who gets paid, and how much.
- In Europe over the past decade, reforms have been designed with similar objectives, but much has focused on 'demand-side' rather than 'supply-side' issues.
- In the English NHS, radical reform has been more possible because of the Westminster system of Parliament, the significant democratic mandates given to governments in power, and the relative weakness of other professional, trade and corporate stakeholders.
- The reforms in England, as in many other countries in Europe, have introduced market-style incentives into healthcare. This is likely to continue and a prevailing conflict will be the extent to which social objectives such as equity of access to care are traded off with efforts to improve efficiency using these incentives.

Self-test exercises

1 What has been the broad thrust of healthcare reform in your country over the last decade?
2 What are, and are intended to be, the main levers to improve performance in the health sector? For example:

- control from central government, regional or local government
- market-style incentives (such as competition between providers, insurers/commissioners, consumer choice)
- the local democratic voice of the population (such as through local councils, citizens' juries)

- third-party regulation
- other.

3 What has delayed the progress of reform? For example:

- technical considerations (e.g. setting accurate prices, adequate risk adjustment for insurers, information for consumers, information on quality and outcomes for insurers/commissioners)
- political considerations (e.g. inability of coalition governments to agree on a clear path, conflict between central and local government, frequent change of government, conflict between major stakeholders)
- economic considerations (e.g. lack of investment)
- other.

4 How might progress be accelerated?
5 How has the broad approach to health sector reform affected your institution?
6 How could barriers to progress be best overcome locally?
7 How influential have you been in helping to shape health sector reforms at local or a national level?
8 How might you be be more influential in future?

References and further reading

Alvarez-Rosete, A., Bevan, G., Mays, N. and Dixon, J. (2005) Effect of diverging policy across the NHS. *British Medical Journal*, 331: 946–50.

Anell, A. (2005) Swedish healthcare under pressure. *Health Economics*, 14: 237–54.

Bevan, G. and Hood, C. (in press) What's measured is what matters: Targets and gaming in the English public health care system. *Public Administration*.

Bevan, R.G. and Robinson, R. (2005) The interplay between economic and political logics. *Journal of Health Policy Politics and Law. Special Issue: Legacies and Latitude in European Health Policy*, 30(1–2): 53–78.

Bristol Royal Infirmary (2001) *The Bristol Royal Infirmary Inquiry. Final Report July 2001. http://www.bristol-inquiry.org.uk/final_report/* (accessed 1 January 2006).

Department of Health (DH, 2002) *Reforming NHS Financial Flows. Introducing Payment by Results*. London: Department of Health. *http://www.dh.gov.uk/ assetRoot/04/06/04/76/04060476.pdf* (accessed 1 November 2005).

Department of Health (DH, 2005a) Patient Choice. *http://www.dh.gov.uk/ PolicyAndGuidance/PatientChoice/fs/en* (accessed 1 November 2005).

Department of Health (DH, 2005b) Commissioning a Patient-led NHS. *http:// www.dh.gov.uk/PublicationsAndStatistics/Publications/PublicationsPolicyAnd-Guidance/PublicationsPolicyAndGuidanceArticle/fs/en?CONTEN-T_ID=4116716&chk=/%2Bb2QD* (accessed 10 November 2005).

Department of Health (DH, 2005c) The 2005 Pharmaceutical Price and

Regulation Scheme. *http://www.dh.gov.uk/PolicyAndGuidance/MedicinesPharmacyAndIndustry/PharmaceuticalPriceRegulationScheme/ThePPRSScheme/fs/en* (accessed 1 January 2006).

Department of Health (DH, 2006a) DH Commercial Directorate. Aims and Objectives. *http://www.dh.gov.uk/AboutUs/HowDHWorks/DHOrganisation-Structure/DHStructureArticle/fs/en?CONTENT_ID*=4110133&chk=yF4Vfi (accessed 1 January 2006).

Department of Health (DH, 2006b) NHS Foundation Trusts. *http://www.dh.gov.uk/PolicyAndGuidance/OrganisationPolicy/SecondaryCare/NHS-FoundationTrust/fs/en* (accessed 1 January 2006).

Dixon, J. (2005) *Regulating Health Care. The Way Forward.* London: King's Fund.

Evans, R.G. (2005) Fellow travellers on a contested path: Power purpose and the evolution of European health care systems. *Journal of Health Policy Politics and Law. Special Issue: Legacies and Latitude in European Health Policy*, 30(1–2): 277–93.

Fuchs, V.R. (1991) National health insurance revisited. *Health Affairs*, 10: 7–17.

Giddens, A. (1998) *The Third Way: Renewal of Social Democracy.* Bristol: The Polity Press.

Giddens, A. (2000) *The Third Way and its Critics.* Bristol: The Polity Press.

Hacker, J.S. (2002) *The Divided Welfare State.* Cambridge: Cambridge University Press.

Hall, P.A. and Taylor, R.C.R. (1996) Political science and the three new institutionalisms. *Political Studies*, 44: 936–57.

Health Economics (2005), 14.

Hollis, M. (1994) *The Philosophy of Social Science: An Introduction.* Cambridge: Cambridge University Press.

Journal of Health Policy Politics and Law (2005) *Special Issue: Legacies and Latitude in European Health Policy*, 30(1–2): 1–309.

Klein, R. (2000) *The New Politics of the NHS.* London: Prentice Hall.

Maynard, A. (2005) European health policy challenges. *Health Economics*, 14: 255–63.

Metcalf, D. (1990) Union presence and labour productivity in British manufacturing industry: a reply to Nolan and Marginson. *British Journal of Industrial Relations*, 28(2): 249–66.

National Audit Office, Audit Commission (2004) *Financial Management in the NHS. NHS (England) Summarised Accounts 2003–4.* London: The Stationery Office.

NHS Confederation (2005) http://www.nhsconfed.org/ (accessed 1 January 2005).

Oliver, A. (2005) The English National Health Service: 1979–2005. *Health Economics*, 14: S75–S99.

Oliver, A. and Mossialos, E. (2005) European health systems reforms: Looking backward to see forward? *Journal of Health Policy Politics and Law. Special Issue: Legacies and Latitude in European Health Policy*, 30(1–2): 7–28.

Schut, F.T. and Van de Ven, W.P.M.M. (2005) Rationing and competition in the Dutch health-care system. *Health Economics*, 14: S59–S74.

Shipman Inquiry (2005) *The Shipman Inquiry. Final Report January 2005. http://www.the-shipman-inquiry.org.uk/home.asp* (accessed 1 January 2006).

Stephan, A. and Sommersguter-Reichmann, M. (2005) Monitoring political decision-making and its impact in Austria. *Health Economics*, 14: S7–S23.

Stevens, S. (2004) Reform strategies for the English NHS. *Health Affairs*, 23: 37–44.

Tuohy, C. H. (1999) *Accidental Logics. The Dynamics of Change in the Health Care Arena in the United States, Britain and Canada.* Oxford: Oxford University Press.

Wortz, M. and Busse, R. (2005) Analysing the impact of health system change in the EU member states – Germany. *Health Economics*, 14: S133–S149.

Websites and resources

Organisation for Economic Co-operation and Development (OECD). Contains an analysis of international health policies, and also key data on health and healthcare for all OECD countries: *http://www.oecd.org/home/ 0,2987,en_2649_201185_1_1_1_1_1,00.html*

World Health Organisation Regional Office for Europe. Contains information about a range of health issues and health policies across Europe: *http:// www.euro.who.int/programmesprojects*

Commonwealth Fund. Contains an up-to-date analysis of the state of healthcare and reform in the USA and some international issues: *http:// www.cmwf.org/*

King's Fund. Contains analysis of health sector reform in England: *www.kingsfund.org.uk*

European Observatory on Health Systems and Policies. For up-to-date description and analysis of health sector reform in Europe: http:// www.lse.ac.uk/collections/LSEHealthAndSocialCare/ europeanObservatoryOnHealthCareSystems.htm

Department of Health. Contains a full description of policies in the English NHS and useful sources of data: http://www.dh.gov.uk/Home/fs/en

Scottish Office. Contains a description of policies in the Scottish NHS and useful sources of data: *http://www.scotland.gov.uk/Home*

National Assembly for Wales. Contains information about healthcare policies and relevant data: *http://www.wales.gov.uk/subihealth/index.htm*

Northern Ireland Executive. Contains information about health policy in Northern Ireland: *http://www.northernireland.gov.uk/az2.htm*

Health Affairs. A journal covering health sector reform in the USA but also some European countries: *http://www.healthaffairs.org/*

Journal of Health Policy Politics and Law. A journal covering the political science aspects of health reform in the Americas and Europe: http://jhppl. yale.edu/

3 Financing healthcare: funding systems and healthcare costs

Suzanne Robinson

Introduction

Healthcare funding in developed countries accounts for a large percentage of gross domestic product (GDP) and is usually the largest single industry in most countries. Increased demand and technological advances mean that healthcare expenditure continues to grow, whilst on the supply side there is a constant pressure because resources are scarce. Policymakers face tough decisions in this regard. Do they increase funding, contain costs, or both? Whilst this debate continues in the literature (Mossialos et al. 2002; Dixon et al. 2004), policymakers and managers alike need to balance the books and thus find enough revenue to meet healthcare expenditure. With public sector borrowing becoming a less attractive economic policy option in developed countries, policymakers are increasingly looking towards the structure and organisation of healthcare systems – including revenue collection (demand side) and organisation of service provision (supply side) – as a means to manage ever-increasing pressures on health expenditure.

This chapter explores four areas relevant to the financing of healthcare in developed countries:

- The first section draws on the work of Mossialos et al. (2002) and Murray and Frenk (2000) to provide a framework by which to facilitate understanding and analysis of healthcare funding.
- The second section draws on data from the Organisation for Economic Co-operation and Development (OECD) and Office of Health Economics (OHE) to explore the levels of healthcare expenditure in selected OECD countries.
- The third section looks at the examples of how money is distributed through healthcare systems.
- The fourth section identifies some of the pressures on healthcare costs and expenditure.

Healthcare funding: an analytical framework

The financing and provision of healthcare is simply a transaction between the providers who transfer resources to patients, and the patients or third party who transfer resources to the providers (Mossialos and Dixon 2002). This has been described by Reinhardt (1990) as the healthcare triangle, as set out in Figure 3.1.

Whilst countries have different funding systems in operation the underlying logic is the same. The simplest transaction occurs when direct payments are made between the patient and the provider of the health-care service. The uncertainty which surrounds ill health and the need for expensive healthcare means that most healthcare systems have a third party element; that is a body that collects resource from individuals and makes decisions as to how to allocate that resource to providers, this third party being either public or private. This third party element offers financial protection against the risk of becoming ill and allows that risk to be shared amongst the protected population. Third party provision may cover part or all of a country's population, for once the revenue has been collected it can then be used to reimburse either the patient or provider of the service. Therefore, the healthcare funding system is simply a way in which funds are collected, either via primary (patient) or secondary (third party) sources, and hence distributed to providers.

The functional components of healthcare financing

The functional components of healthcare financing can be subdivided into the following three categories: revenue collection; fund pooling; and purchasing (Murray and Frenk 2000). These functions often vary between countries with many combinations being in operation. Figure

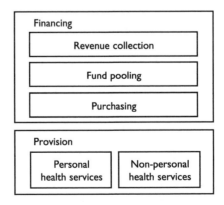

Figure 3.1   Healthcare triangle
Source: Mossialos et al. (2002)

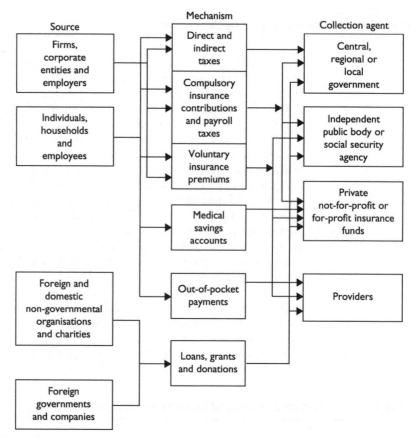

Figure 3.2   Funding sources, contribution mechanisms and collection agents
Source: Mossialos et al. (2002)

3.2 illustrates the various funding sources, mechanisms and collection agents that operate in healthcare systems.

Revenue collection refers to the way money is moved around the system and is concerned with the source of funding (examples include the individual or the employer), the mechanism of funding (examples include direct or indirect taxes and voluntary insurance), and the collection agent (examples include central or regional government). The main mechanisms of revenue collection are through taxation, social insurance contributions, voluntary insurance premiums and out-of-pocket payments.

Taxes can be levied on individuals, households and businesses through direct taxes, and they can also be applied to transactions and commodities in the form of indirect taxes, such as taxes on fuel and alcohol. Direct and indirect taxes can be collected nationally, regionally and locally, with variation occurring between countries. Social insurance contributions are income related and generally shared between employees and

employers, with contributions usually collected by an independent public body. Private insurance contributions are paid independently by the
individual, as part of an employment package, with the employer paying
all or part of the insurance. Patients may incur out-of-pocket payments
for some or all of their healthcare.

Murray and Frenk (2000) suggest that the strategic design of revenue
collection can affect the performance of a health system. A key aspect
cited is around the structural arrangements and the governance of performance, this being largely concerned with issues of public and private
participation. Fund pooling is when a population's healthcare revenues
are accumulated, with financial risk being shared between the population.
Fund pooling is distinct from revenue collection, for not all mechanisms
of collection, such as medical savings accounts (which currently operate
in the US and are a tax-free savings account for medical expenses) and
out-of-pocket payments enable risk pooling. Factors associated with this
approach that may affect performance include the separation of fund
pools for different population groups and subsidisation across different
risk groups (Murray and Frenk 2000).

Purchasing is the allocation of fund pools to healthcare providers.
There is a wide range of purchasing activities which may involve the
government acting as both the collection agent (raising revenue through
general taxation), and the purchaser of services, for example, specific
healthcare programmes. A number of countries have some form of activity that involves governments (local or regional) acting as both the collection agent and the purchaser of services. These include the UK, Finland
and Denmark (Ervik 1998; Hurst and Siciliani 2003).

There are also more complex systems which involve a separate agent
who allocates resources to purchasers. For example, in France revenue is
collected by local agencies who then transfer to a central agency which
allocates the money to the relevant social security departments who then
transfer funds to the relevant purchasing agents (Evans 2002). Strategic
issues include decisions around what is to be purchased, including the
selection criteria for interventions. Other aspects include how to make a
choice of providers and what mechanisms to use for purchasing. There is
further discussion of this in Chapter 12. A large number of purchasers
may lead to competition between purchasers and increased demands on
providers (Murray and Frenk 2000).

There are policy issues which relate to all of these categories. The
main policy decisions tend to focus on the equity and efficiency of
healthcare systems. Equity of financing will depend on both the level
and distribution of contributions, for example, how much money is
needed and who should contribute. Equity of access relates to the accessibility of services and to issues around informal payments and user
charges (Dixon et al. 2004). Efficiency is largely concerned with the
management and distribution of resources and can be influenced by pooling and purchasing mechanisms (see Dixon et al. 2004 for a more detailed
discussion).

Funding healthcare

Figure 3.3 presents figures on the total health spending in 2002 for a selection of OECD countries. The OECD median total spend for those countries listed in Figure 3.3 was $2607 in 2002. The United States had the highest healthcare spend per capita ($5287) of all the countries assessed, with its per capita spend being 45% higher then Switzerland ($3649), which is the country with the next highest spend, with Spain having the lowest OECD spend per head at $1728.

Table 3.1 presents the share of expenditure as a proportion of GDP for a selection of OECD countries. The figures show a rise in healthcare

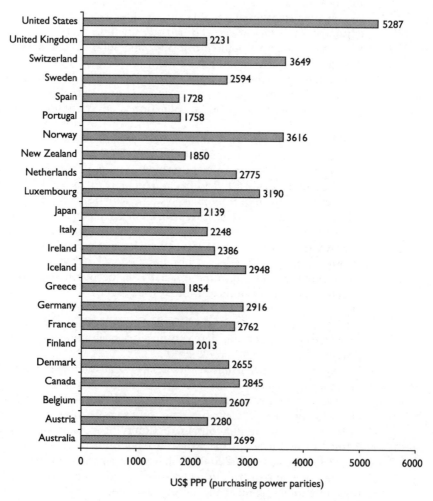

Figure 3.3   Total health expenditure per capita (US$ PPP, 2002)
Source: OECD Health Data (2005), copyright OECD (2005)

Table 3.1 Total expenditure on health as a percentage of GDP in selected OECD countries, 1960–2002

	1960	1970	1980	1990	1995	1996	1997	1998	1999	2000	2001	2002
Australia	4.1	4.3	7.0	7.8	8.3	8.4	8.5	8.6	8.7	9.0	9.1	9.3
Austria	4.3	5.1	7.4	7.0	8.0	8.2	7.5	7.6	7.7	7.6	7.5	7.6
Belgium	3.4	4.0	6.4	7.4	8.4	8.5	8.4	8.5	8.6	8.7	8.8	9.1
Canada	5.4	7.0	7.1	9.0	9.2	9.0	8.9	9.2	9.0	8.9	9.4	9.6
Denmark	3.6	5.9	9.1	8.5	8.2	8.3	8.2	8.4	8.5	8.4	8.6	8.8
Finland	3.8	5.6	6.4	7.8	7.5	7.6	7.3	6.9	6.9	6.7	6.9	7.2
France	3.8	5.4	7.1	8.6	9.5	9.5	9.4	9.3	9.3	9.3	9.4	9.7
Germany	4.7	6.2	8.7	8.5	10.6	10.9	10.7	10.6	10.6	10.6	10.8	10.9
Greece	3.6	6.1	6.6	7.4	9.6	9.6	9.4	9.4	9.6	9.9	10.2	9.8
Iceland	3.0	4.7	6.2	8.0	8.4	8.4	8.3	8.7	9.4	9.3	9.3	10.0
Ireland	3.7	5.1	8.4	6.1	6.8	6.6	6.4	6.2	6.3	6.3	6.9	7.3
Italy	3.6	5.1	7.0	7.9	7.3	7.4	7.7	7.7	7.7	8.1	8.2	8.4
Japan	3.0	4.5	6.5	5.9	6.8	7.0	6.9	7.2	7.4	7.6	7.8	7.9
Luxembourg	0.0	3.6	5.9	6.1	6.4	6.4	5.9	5.8	6.2	5.5	5.9	6.1
Netherlands		5.7	7.5	8.0	8.4	8.3	8.2	8.2	8.4	8.3	8.7	9.3
New Zealand	4.3	5.1	5.9	6.9	7.2	7.2	7.4	7.8	7.7	7.8	7.9	8.2
Norway	2.9	4.4	7.0	7.7	7.9	7.9	7.8	8.5	8.5	7.7	8.9	9.9
Portugal		2.6	5.6	6.2	8.2	8.4	8.5	8.4	8.7	9.2	9.4	9.3
Spain	1.5	3.6	5.4	6.7	7.6	7.6	7.5	7.5	7.5	7.4	7.5	7.6
Sweden	4.4	6.9	9.1	8.4	8.1	8.4	8.2	8.3	8.4	8.4	8.8	9.2
Switzerland	4.9	5.5	7.4	8.3	9.7	10.1	10.2	10.3	10.5	10.4	10.9	11.1
United Kingdom	3.9	4.5	5.6	6.0	7.0	7.0	6.8	6.9	7.2	7.3	7.5	7.7
United States	5.0	6.9	8.7	11.9	13.3	13.2	13.0	13.0	13.0	13.1	13.8	14.6

Source: OECD Health Data (2005), copyright OECD (2005)

expenditure in all countries over the last 40 years. The greatest increases have been in the United States, Netherlands and Portugal. Even in the UK, where increases in healthcare spending have tended to be less than most other OECD countries, there has been an increase in healthcare expenditure. Allowing for inflation, the UK National Health Service (NHS) in 2002 cost seven times more than in 1949, with the average cost per person rising nearly six times above the 1949 level (Office of Health Economics 2004).

The rise in healthcare expenditure across OECD countries is due to a number of factors such as increased pay and price inflation, population growth, expansion of services and increase in technological advances. The fact that the healthcare sector is one of the major employers in almost all economies means that the pay bill is the single largest component of many healthcare budgets. In the UK NHS, 62% of total revenue (i.e. non-capital) expenditure in 2001–02 was for wages and salaries (Office of Health Economics 2004). Whitfield et al. (2005: 16) suggest that nearly half of the recent increases in NHS funding in England (since 2003) have gone towards 'increased pay, new terms and conditions for GPs, consultants and other NHS staff'.

Various explanations are put forward to explain the differences in healthcare expenditure between countries. Ginsburg and Nichols (2003) suggest that prices are crucial drivers in cross-national differences in health spending. For example, in the United States where health expenditure is high, salaries, medical equipment, pharmaceutical and other supplies tend to be more costly than other OECD countries (OECD 2005). The fact that markets, including labour markets, do not satisfy the conditions necessary in the perfect competitive market (Donaldson and Gerard 2005; McPake et al. 2002), leads to varying degrees of monopoly power on the supply side of the market and varying degrees of monopsony power (that is when the product or service of a number of sellers is only demanded by one buyer) on the demand side (Ginsburg and Nichols 2003). Thus, the functional components of healthcare financing do have an effect on healthcare expenditure, with the bargaining power of both providers and payers of services differing between countries. Further discussion of the different methods of revenue collection and their effects on healthcare costs is set out below.

Figure 2.1 (p. 17) presents the public and private healthcare expenditure as a percentage of total healthcare expenditure for a selection of OECD countries. All countries have a mix of both public and private health expenditure with Denmark, Japan, Luxemburg, Norway, Sweden and the UK all having over 80% health expenditure incurred through public funds. Public funds include state, regional and local government bodies and social security schemes. Even in the United States, which has the largest private expenditure on healthcare (55%), public healthcare expenditure still accounts for 45% of total health expenditure.

Revenue generation

This section will provide detail about the various methods of revenue generation used in Europe and other OECD countries such as the United States, Canada, New Zealand and Australia, analysing the main advantages and disadvantages of each method. The different forms of revenue generation include:

1 private insurance
2 taxation

- different sources of taxation – direct or indirect
- different types – general or hypothecated
- different levels – national/local

3 social health insurance
4 charges and co-payments.

Most countries operate through a mixed funding system, which usually includes some element of taxation. Ervik (1998: 5) describes taxation as a 'normative and political component that expresses what a society understands as a reasonable tax burden and an equitable distribution of the tax burden'. Direct taxation is often seen as a progressive means of raising revenue, with studies showing that poorer households pay a higher percentage of gross income in direct taxes (see Glennerster 1997; Manning et al. 1989). From a health perspective, it could be argued that indirect taxes on things like cigarettes and alcohol are justifiable as they can lead to a reduction in the consumption of these products. Nonetheless, the fact that in many OECD countries a higher number of low income groups tend to consume such products means that indirect taxes are regressive. Most countries have some form of indirect taxation on certain goods and services. However, it is difficult to ascertain how much of this revenue is used to fund healthcare.

General taxation

The UK is an example of a healthcare system that is funded predominantly through general taxation (see Table 3.1). The UK Treasury sets out what budget will be spent on healthcare, and once that is set the resource is distributed to the purchasers or commissioners of care, with the majority of services being free to users at the point of provision. Other countries that use general taxation as a mechanism to fund healthcare include Denmark, Finland, New Zealand and Spain.

Funding healthcare through general (direct) taxation is seen as a progressive way of raising revenue. In most countries, tax is proportional to income, with those on higher incomes paying more tax than those on lower incomes, thus allowing for redistribution of resources from the wealthy to the poor, from the healthy to the sick, and from those of working age to the young and old. In addition, the financing of services is divorced from the provision of services, which is important for equitable access. Advocates of a universal tax-based model, such as the NHS in the UK, suggest that the fact that income is not tied to an individual's financial contribution means that provision is more likely to be based on clinical need rather than ability to pay (Wagstaff et al. 1999). This claim is however somewhat disputed with suggestions that the UK operates a multi-tier service with access to care being affected by age, gender, education, wealth and race (for further discussion see Health Policy Consensus Group 2005). Further advantages of this form of revenue collection are that it is relatively efficient to administer, this being due to the collection of funds through the existing taxation system, and not incurring additional costs for the health sector. The fact that government is the main payer for and purchaser of healthcare in a tax-funded system allows general taxation to act as a mechanism to control costs, with providers not easily being able to increase revenue by raising prices or premiums, as in private insurance and social insurance (Baggott 2004).

The major disadvantages of a system based on general taxation include the fact that health services are closely tied to the economy and government taxation policies. In times of economic recession, reductions in tax revenues can have major effects on the health budget. The fact that all public services need to compete for limited tax revenues means there will always be winners and losers. Health budgets may suffer if government gives high priority to public services other than health and/or to low taxation rather than public services. It can be difficult to raise revenue because an increase in the health budget means that the budget to other services may need to be cut, or tax increased, both of which can prove unpopular with electorates. It is suggested that tax raises might be more popular if the government were explicit about their spending intentions, that is, with taxes earmarked for health (Wilkinson 1994; Jones and Duncan 1995; Baggott 2004). The fact that taxes are not hypothecated in countries such as the UK means that the population of these countries is unable to judge the fiscal viability (i.e. affordability) of health services. A general taxation system of funding healthcare also means that taxpayers and patients have little or no notion of the cost of services and therefore cannot make judgements about value for money of services received. Furthermore, the rising demand for services in the UK since the establishment of the NHS in 1948 suggests that funding through general taxation has been an inefficient way of balancing the expectations of patients with the capacity of the system (Health Policy Consensus Group 2005). However, the rising demand for healthcare services is evident in all countries regardless of the system of funding mechanism.

Hypothecated taxation

Hypothecation or earmarking tax revenues for healthcare purposes, is suggested by some as a useful means of securing support for tax increases (Jones and Duncan 1995; Le Grand and Bennett 2000). Australia has a percentage of its healthcare funding financed by hypothecated tax – the Medicare Levy (Health Policy Consensus Group 2005).

Those in favour of hypothecated taxes argue that it allows citizens to make a more direct connection with the purpose of taxation and have more understanding of the associated costs and benefits. There is some evidence to suggest that people are more comfortable with rises in taxation to pay for healthcare in comparison with increases targeted at non-health services. There is however no evidence to suggest there would be continued support for such an approach if a number of tax increases were needed in relatively quick succession. Studies looking at the potential effects of adapting a hypothecated tax approach for health services in the UK suggest that a move to hypothecated taxes is unlikely to provide any advantages over the current system (Wilkinson 1994; Jones and Duncan 1995).

One of the disadvantages of hypothecated taxation is the negative effect on the less popular but no less vital services which are important to a welfare state (Le Grand and Bennet 2000; Baggott 2004). For example, other services such as education, housing and transport, which often have important implications for health, could be disadvantaged by hypothecation of funding for health. Furthermore, hypothecation could lead to the 'benefit' principle of taxation; that is, people believing that they should only pay taxes for services for which they are going to benefit (see Le Grand and Bennett 2000). Hypothecating taxes for health could similarly lead those with private insurance to argue that they should not pay all or part of the health tax because they have no capacity to benefit.

Local taxation

Denmark's healthcare is predominantly funded through taxation, but unlike the UK its main source of funding is from local (county and municipal) taxation, although these local taxes are supplemented by state (national) taxes. Analysis has shown that local taxes are generally less progressive than national taxes (i.e. local taxes often take a larger proportion of tax from people whose income is low), as is demonstrated by the experience of Denmark and other countries such as Finland, Sweden and Switzerland, who also have a high proportion of revenue generated by local taxation (see Wagstaff et al. 1999; Health Policy Consensus Group 2005). In the absence of a national system of redistribution, local taxation could therefore create regional inequity. For example, if local tax rates vary by region this could lead to horizontal inequities (i.e. equal treatment for equal need, irrespective of any other characteristic such as income, sex, race, etc., Mossialos et al. 2002). Variations in local tax rates for both Denmark and Sweden suggest that horizontal inequities are evident when such mechanisms of revenue collection are used (Mossialos et al. 2002). There are suggestions that local taxations could lead to inefficient resource allocation and priority setting (Mossialos et al. 2002).

The decentralisation of local tax funding is seen as a major advantage over national taxation for the clear link between revenue raised and local spending allows for potentially much greater transparency. There is also greater direct political accountability for healthcare funding and expenditure, for local politicians are likely to be closer to the electorate than their national counterparts. A further advantage is that healthcare is separated from national priorities with this mechanism of decentralisation allowing for local needs to be more easily met. The Health Policy Consensus Group suggests that local taxation combined with local electoral accountability of hospitals is a factor that adds to the high rate of patient satisfaction reported in Denmark (Health Policy Consensus Group 2005).

Social insurance

In France, all residents are covered by social insurance, with the population having no choice to opt out of the national system. Under this system resources are levied (as a social insurance contribution) from employees and employers and, as with general taxation, these contributions are generally set as a proportion of income regardless of health need. The main difference between social insurance and income tax is that the revenue raised is earmarked for health, thus allowing, in theory, for greater transparency. In some systems such as Germany individuals earning over a certain threshold have the option to opt out of the social insurance scheme: 'As a result in 1999 there were 7.4 million with comprehensive private health insurance' (Dixon and Mossialos 2002: 48). Collection bodies in a social insurance system are non-profit agencies, separate from government. Health systems vary in the way they administer a social insurance approach; for example, in France people usually pay for ambulatory doctors' bills at the point of use and then apply for and receive reimbursement from the insurance agency at a later date. This means that patients are more conscious of the cost of certain health procedures. In Germany, however, patients receive services free at the point of use, with physicians obtaining reimbursements from the social insurance sickness funds (Dixon and Mossialos 2001).

Private insurance

Private healthcare insurance markets have tended to develop around public health systems and in many countries private insurance plays a residual role in terms of healthcare funding; for example, in systems such as UK where private insurance provides supplementary coverage to the public system and can enable faster access to certain services such as elective hospital care or, as in the case of France, 'provide reimbursement for co-payments required by the public system' (Buchmueller and Couffinhal 2004: 4). Even in the Unites States, where the level of expenditure on private insurance is high (around 35% of total healthcare expenditure in 2000), public expenditure accounts for a higher share of health financing (around 44% of total healthcare expenditure in 2000). In the United States, the elderly (those over 65 years) and qualified disabled persons are eligible for Medicare, and some of the poor are allowed Medicaid or state Children's Health Insurance Programme (Colombo and Tapay 2004). Medicare and Medicaid are public insurance programmes which provide coverage for the elderly (Medicare), the military, veterans, and for some of the poor and disabled (Medicaid).

Private insurance can be classified into the following categories: substitutive, supplementary or complementary (Mossialos et al. 2002). In Germany, individuals earning higher incomes can opt out of the public funding system and purchase private health insurance, thus substituting for state funding of healthcare. This form of substitutive insurance undermines the redistribution effect of taxation or social insurance and leads to a regressive system of funding. Furthermore, as income is related to risk of ill health (the poorer you are, the more likely you are to fall ill), substitutive insurance means that those with the poorest health or at greatest risk are left in the public system, which reduces the overall pooling and risk-sharing mechanism in the health system, and those with the lowest income could potentially end up paying the higher premiums.

There have been real concerns in both Germany and the Netherlands about the effects and fairness of a having two-tiered system of health insurance (Health Policy Consensus Group 2005). A study by Wagstaff et al. (1999) showed that differences in access to care tend to be based on a person's insurance status, leading to a tendency towards pro-rich distribution of healthcare use in Ireland, France and the United States. Systems that rely heavily on private insurance are often criticised due to their inequitable nature; that is, these systems are based on a person's ability to pay for care rather than on clinical need (Wagstaff et al. 1999). The National Coalition on Health Care (2004) suggests that around 16% of Americans had no health insurance coverage in 2003, with the majority of the uninsured being those on the lowest incomes.

In an attempt to reduce the effects of a two-tiered system, the Netherlands introduced a new Health Insurance Act (January 2006). The new Act means a move to a mandatory universal healthcare insurance system. The only parties who will be exempt are military personnel in active service and conscientious objectors to insurance. Insurance will be provided through private providers and individuals are able to choose their insurance provider. Insurers are legally bound to accept all applicants and therefore cannot restrict or charge higher premiums for the elderly or sick or exclude someone on the basis of wealth or health.

By law all residents in the Netherlands should have some basic health insurance coverage (which may vary between insurance providers); supplemental health insurance will also be available on an individual basis or collectively via employers or similar group schemes. The idea of the Health Insurance Act is to increase market forces through the expansion of the private insurance sector, allowing for individual choice (in terms of insurer and packages available). This in turn (it is hoped) will increase efficiency and quality of care. The intention is that government intervention through regulation of private insurers will allow for more equitable coverage. The new system is seen as a 'private health insurance system with social conditions' (Ministry of Health Welfare and Sport 2006).

In countries such as the UK, Australia, New Zealand and Spain, private health insurance plays a supplementary role, with this being an additional option to add to public insurance for those who desire and can afford it. One of the advantages of supplementary insurance is that it can allow quicker access to services for people holding private insurance, especially in systems such as the UK and New Zealand which traditionally experience significant waiting times for diagnostic tests or elective treatments.

Whilst private insurance may allow for quicker access to services, there is no evidence to suggest this may lead to higher quality services (Baggott 2004) and it could also lead to inequity of access to care, with those who are privately insured accessing services which for others are almost impossible to acquire either via public insurance or paying direct. For example, the lack of UK NHS dentists is limiting access for certain people who cannot afford to pay direct payments or take out private insurance (Kamel Boulos and Picton Phillipps 2004).

The function of private insurance in France is to act as a complementary insurance system which 'tops up' reimbursements made to people by the public system. Some argue that the advantage of this form of complementary insurance is its ability to free up capacity in the public system by allowing those who can afford to pay to receive treatment in the private sector. In contrast, those who oppose a system of supplementary private insurance claim that it encourages a two-tier system that allows quicker access to services for those who can afford to pay and thus should not be allowed on overall equity grounds.

Countries like the United States which have a relatively high percentage of private insurance have the greatest difficulty in controlling healthcare costs and tend to have the biggest healthcare spend per head of population. Private insurance reduces the cost of treatment at the point of consumption and makes 'illness' a less undesired state. However, there is some evidence to suggest that supplier-induced demand is taking place in countries that have private health insurance. For example, Savage and Wright (2003) suggest that moral hazard (i.e. the influence of being insured leading to over-provision or accessing of services), is taking place in the Australian private health insurance system, with evidence of an increase in the expected length of hospital stay of people who are privately insured. A study by Robertson and Richardson (2000) conducted in Australia demonstrated that procedure rates after heart attack were around two to three times higher for patients who were privately insured than those who are publicly insured.

Private insurance systems tend to incur higher administrative costs per insured person than public health coverage systems. In the United States for example, the average administrative cost (12% in 1999) of private insurers exceeded that of public programmes – Medicare (5%) and Medicaid (6.8%) (Woolhandler et al. 2003). The higher administrative costs of private insurers tend to be ascribed to marketing, underwriting and other costs such as billing, provision of care and product innovation (Colombo and Tapay 2004).

Out-of-pocket payments and charges for healthcare

Out-of-pocket payments and charges make up a proportion of healthcare spending in all health systems. This is the only mechanism that allows for price consciousness; that is, for patients to have a true notion of the costs of service and thus be able to make judgements around the price and (possibly) value for money of care received. Charges are often seen as a way of raising additional revenue, as indicated by this extract from research conducted by the British Medical Association:

> BMA calculated that £1.25 billion could be raised by a £40 fee for food and accommodation in hospital, while a £10 fee to see a GP could raise £3.3 billion (or £2 billion with exemptions for elderly and children). (BMA 2002: 28–9)

Even in a publicly funded system such as the UK, charges have been levied on things like prescriptions almost since the early days of the NHS. Other countries that impose charges include Sweden, New Zealand and Portugal which charge many people for visiting their family doctor, and Germany, France and Belgium which charge for an element of hospital stays (Baggott 2004). As patients demand better quality services, including non-clinical services such as bedside computers, phones and televisions, the question arises as to where charges should stop. Nutritious food and pleasant surroundings are commonly considered to be essential components of good quality care, but each system has to make a judgement as to the point at which services are deemed to require an additional payment from users, and if this payment is to be levied on all or just some people according to their ability to pay. Charges and co-payments are therefore criticised for being a regressive means of raising revenue, limiting access to services and discriminating against those on low incomes.

Patient fee-for-service payments is used in a number of countries including New Zealand, Australia and the US. Studies have shown that patients may be deterred from accessing services when they have to direct payment at the point of use (Carrin and Hanvoravongchai 2003; Schoen et al. 2004). A study by Schoen et al. (2004) demonstrates that in countries like New Zealand and the US where fees for general practitioners' services have historically been levied, cost-related access problems were much higher than in the UK and Canada where services tend to be free at the point of use (Schoen et al. 2004). Recent policy reforms in New Zealand have tried to alleviate this problem by moving from fee-for-service payments to GPs to capitation funding of primary health organisations, although this only acts as a subsidy and fee-for-service activity still forms part of the payment mechanism for many patients (Malcolm 2004; Ashton 2005; McAvoy and Coster 2005).

Whilst patient charges are often seen as a method to curtail costs, there is a suggestion that they actually provide incentives to increase healthcare activity (see Greenfield et al. 1992; Feldstein 1999; Carrin and Hanvoravongchai 2003). For example, 'fee-for-service funding for general practice has a built-in "perverse incentive" that is the more you see and the quicker you see them the more you earn' (Bollen 1996: 214).

Patients are often reluctant to pay for elements of their care at the point of delivery, and appropriate systems have to be developed to collect charges. However, such systems can often be costly to administer and are not always cost effective, especially when charges are small (Carrin and Hanvoravongchai 2003).

Ways of distributing funding

Structural, political and historical factors all affect the ways in which money flows around healthcare systems. In all systems, there is some mix of public and private provision. For example, since the development of the UK NHS in 1948, the majority of funding and provision in the system has been provided in the public sector, although some private sector activity has occurred on both the demand and supply side. However, recent government policy has seen the development of a market approach to reforming the health system in England, although this is not the first attempt to have an internal market in the UK system (see Le Grand et al. 1998 discussion on the internal market of the Thatcher government). In 2002, the English Department of Health published *Reforming NHS Financial Flows: Introducing Payment by Results* (DoH 2002), the aim of this policy being to incentivise the NHS to behave more like a private sector business organisation in how it accounts for funding and activity. Payment by Results means that hospitals are moving away from having block contracts as a way of funding activity. Block contracts have been seen as a cause of considerable local variation in prices paid for procedures that give little incentive for extra productivity since higher activity means no change in revenue (Siciliani and Hurst 2003). The new Payment by Results system is based on a national tariff for clinical procedures and hospitals will only be paid on a fee-for-service basis for procedures that they have undertaken, thus providing incentives for higher productivity, that is, the more you do, the more you get paid (see Dixon 2005 for more discussion on Payment by Results).

A number of other countries such as Australia, Belgium, Denmark, Norway and Sweden have moved towards a system that involves some activity-based funding However, the extent of this activity varies between countries (Rodrigues et al. 2002; Hurst and Siciliani 2003). An OECD study comparing waiting times found that they are less of a problem in countries which rely mainly on activity-based funding than those that have mainly fixed budgets. Results from these countries suggest a rise in activity that leads to shorter waiting times and shorter lengths of stay in hospital (Hurst and Siciliani 2003; Siciliani and Hurst 2003). In this way, patients, and indeed taxpayers, should have more transparency with regard to how their money is being spent in the health system (Dixon 2005). Critics have warned that such methods reward volume, not quality, of service and that there is a real possibility of hospitals developing cost-cutting strategies that could compromise the quality of services. For example, in the United States there is evidence that activity-funding incentives have led to an increase in patient mortality in the period following hospital discharge (King's Fund 2005).

The NHS (in England not across the wider UK) is actively encouraging more plurality of providers of healthcare, including the independent sector (both for-profit and not-for-profit providers). Examples include independent sector treatment centres to provide services such as cataract removal and hip replacement for NHS patients funded directly from the public purse. The idea of developing a stronger market in healthcare is to increase competition and, it is hoped, to lead in turn to greater efficiency and an increase in the quality of service provision (Timmins 2005). If these government policies prove to be effective this could lead to a major change in the way the money flows around the English system and lead to a fundamental shift that entails the divorcing of funding from the provision of services. One thing for sure is that the 'UK government believes that the use of private providers does not undermine the principles of the NHS if care is provided free to patients' (Timmins 2005: 1195). However, it is too early to speculate about the effects of increased competition and changes to the financial flows through payment by results in the English context.

In an effort to increase efficiency, equity and quality of healthcare services, other countries as part of a wider health system reform are attempting to alter the way resources are allocated around the system. For example, New Zealand's Primary Health Care Strategy is aimed at reducing health disparities and improving health outcomes by 'reducing co-payments, moving from fee-for-service to capitation, promoting population health management and developing a not-for-profit infrastructure with community involvement to deliver primary care' (Hefford et al. 2005: 9). Howell (2005) questions the cost effectiveness of the reforms and suggests that 'limited competition and governance requirements mean that current institutional arrangements are unlikely to facilitate efficacy improvements' (Howell 2005: 2).

Pressures on healthcare costs/spending

> The following is a government health warning: just when you thought your health spending was under control, the cost pressures are likely to start rising again. (OECD 2003)

A common feature of all healthcare systems is the scarcity of resources necessary to meet the continually growing demand. Health expenditure continues to rise year on year in all OECD countries (Office of Health Economics 2004). The two major factors often cited for these increases in expenditure are the rise of new technology and the ageing population, plus other factors such as the increase in incidence of chronic illness (including cardiovascular disease, cancer and diabetes), rising levels of obesity, the growth in consumerism and the impact of infectious diseases such as the SARS outbreak in South East Asia in 2003.

The proportion of the world's people classified as older (defined as those over 65 years of age) is expected to rise from around 6.9% of the total population to 15.6% over the next 50 years (Mahal and Berman 2001). This demographic change results from a combination of increased life expectancy, a decline in mortality rates and subsequent declines in fertility rates. Projecting over the next decade, Cotis (2005: 1) suggests that the 'implications of these demographic developments mean that the number of elderly will rise significantly relative to the number of working age. By the mid-century there will be only two people of working age to support one person of 65 or more.' This is a challenge for policy-makers and the healthcare system, having implications for the cost and provision of healthcare.

Conclusion

This chapter has explored the systems of funding used in the field of healthcare. All healthcare systems have some mix of public and private financing, and the former usually consists of some element of taxation. Whilst the funding sources, mechanisms and collection agents vary between countries, all countries feel the pressure of increasing expenditure, scarce resources and the need to provide both an efficient and equitable healthcare service.

The last decade has seen the expanding use of expensive new technology such as cardiovascular equipment, dialysis machines and telemedicine. These advances, along with ongoing and more sophisticated developments in pharmaceuticals, have all had an impact on the range and quality of care provided to patients, yet are very costly to administer and place increasing pressure on overall healthcare spending (OECD 2003). The last 20 years have likewise seen a rise in consumerism as societies gain greater access to health information extending across regional and country borders, and users of healthcare systems increasingly see themselves as 'consumers'. Patients demand access to the latest technology that can assist in their care and expect to receive high quality services that offer good access and a degree of choice (Cotis 2005).

The increase in demands and the limitation of resources mean that governments are forced to look at the way in which the funding systems operate. This can lead to changes in the way resources are collected and distributed around the health system. As part of a wider health system reform a number of countries are currently adopting activity-based financing. The idea is that this more market-based approach will allow for greater transparency in terms of funding and activity and provide more market-like incentives (i.e. money follows activity), which in turn will lead to the provision of more efficient and high quality services.

Summary box

- Healthcare funding in developed countries accounts for a large percentage of gross domestic product (GDP).
- Country variations exist between the amounts of healthcare expenditure both in terms of total healthcare spending and healthcare expenditure as a percentage of GDP.
- The United States has the largest percentage of private health activity and the highest healthcare expenditure in the world.
- All healthcare systems have some mix of public and private financing, and the former usually consists of some element of taxation.
- The funding source, mechanism and collection agent vary greatly between countries.
- Growing demands for healthcare place increasing pressures on expenditure, with these increases being due to: technological advances; an ageing population; an expansion in the incidence of chronic disease; and rises in consumerism and patients' expectations.
- Increased demands and limited resources are likely to lead policymakers to look at the funding of healthcare structures as a mechanism to improve efficiency and quality of services.

Self-test exercises

1 What are the main factors that have influenced the rise in healthcare expenditure over the last 20 years? To what extent is this having an impact within your own country's healthcare system, and in what ways can that impact be seen?
2 Thinking of your own country's funding contribution mechanisms, what are the major disadvantages evident in your system? How do these relate to other OECD countries?
3 Again thinking of your own country's funding contribution mechanisms of healthcare funding, what are the major advantages evident in your system? How do these relate to the experience of other OECD countries?

References and further reading

Ashton, T. (2005) Recent developments in the funding and organisation of health services in New Zealand. *Australia and New Zealand Health Policy*, 2(9).
Baggott, R. (2004) *Health and Health Care in Britain* (3rd edn). Basingstoke: Macmillan.

Bollen, M.D. (1996) Recent changes in Australian general practice. *Medical Journal of Australia*, 164: 212–15.

British Medical Association (BMA, 2002) *Healthcare Funding Review*. London: British Medical Association.

Buchmueller, T.C. and Couffinhal, A. (2004) *Private Health Insurance in France*. OECD Working Paper 12. Paris: Organisation for Economic Co-operation and Development.

Carrin, G. and Hanvoravongchai, P. (2003) Provider payments and patient charges as policy tools for cost-containment: How successful are they in high-income countries? *Human Resources for Health*, 1(1): 6.

Colombo, F. and Tapay, N. (2004) *Private Health Insurance in OECD Countries: The Benefits and Costs for Individuals and Health Systems*. OECD Working Paper 15. Paris: Organisation for Economic Co-operation and Development.

Cotis, J. (2005) *Challenges of Demographics*. Paris: Organisation for Economic Co-operation and Development.

Department of Health (DoH, 2002) *Reforming NHS Financial Flows: Introducing Payment by Results*. London: Department of Health.

Dixon, J. (2005) Payment by results – new financial flows in the NHS. *British Medical Journal*, 328: 967–8.

Dixon, A. and Mossialos, E. (2001) Funding health care in Europe: Recent experiences. In T. Harrison and J. Appleby *Health Care UK*. London: King's Fund, pp. 66–77.

Dixon, A. and Mossialos, E. (eds) (2002) *Health Care Systems in Eight Countries: Trends and Challenges*. Geneva: World Health Organization. European Observatory on Health Care Systems.

Dixon, A., Langenbrunner, L. and Mossialos, E. (2004) Facing the challenges of health care financing. In J. Figueras, M. McKee., J. Cain and S. Lessof *Health Systems in Transition: Learning from Experience*. Geneva: World Health Organisation. European Observatory on Health Systems and Policies

Donaldson, C. and Gerard, K. (2005) *Economics of Health Care Financing: The Invisible Hand*. London: Palgrave Macmillan.

Ervik, R. (1998) *The Redistribution Aim of Social Policy: A Comparative Analysis of Taxes, Tax Expenditure Transfers and Direct Transfers in Eight Countries*. New York: Syracuse University Press.

Evans, R.G. (2002) Financing health care: Taxation and the alternatives. In E. Mossialos, A. Dixon, J. Figueras and J. Kutzin (eds) *Funding Healthcare: Options for Europe*. Maidenhead: Open University Press.

Feldstein, P. (1999) *Health Care Economics*. Albany: Delmar.

Ginsburg, P.B. and Nichols, L.M. (2003) *The Health Care Cost-Coverage Conundrum Annual Essay*. Washington, DC: Centre for Studying Health System Change.

Glennerster, H. (1997) *Paying for Welfare: Towards 2000*, 3rd edn. Englewood Cliffs, NJ: Prentice-Hall.

Greenfield, S., Nelson, E.C., Zubkoff, M., Manning, W., Rogers, W., Kravitz, R.L., Keller, A., Tarlov, A.R. and Ware, J.E. (1992) Variations in resource utilization among medical specialties and systems of care. Results from the medical outcomes study. *Journal of American Medical Association*, 267(12): 1624–30.

Health Policy Consensus Group (2005) *Options for Healthcare Funding*. London: Institute for the Study of Civil Society.

Hefford, M., Crampton, P. and Foley, J. (2005) Reducing health disparities through primary care reform: The New Zealand experiment. *Health Policy*, 72: 9–23.

Howell, B. (2005) Restructuring Primary Health Care Markets in New Zealand:

from Welfare Benefits to Insurance Markets; *Australia and New Zealand Health Policy*, 2: 20.

Hurst, J. and Siciliani, L. (2003) Tackling excessive waiting times for elective surgery: A comparison of policies in twelve OECD countries. OECD Working Papers. Paris: Organisation for Economic Co-operation and Development.

Jones, A. and Duncan, A. (1995) *Hypothecated Health Taxes: An Evaluation of Recent Proposals.* London: Office of Health Economics.

Kamel Boulos, M.N. and Picton Phillipps, G. (2004) Is NHS dentistry in crisis? 'Traffic light' maps of dentists distribution in England and Wales. *International Journal of Health Geographics*, 3: 10.

King's Fund (2005) *Payment by Results. www.kingsfund.org.uk/news/briefings/payment_by.html* (accessed 19 December 2005).

Le Grand, J. and Bennett, F. (2000) Should the NHS to be funded by a hypothecated tax? *Fabian Review*, Winter, 1–9.

Le Grand, J., Mays, N. and Mulligan, J. (eds) (1998) *Learning from the Internal Market: A Review of the Evidence.* London: King's Fund.

McAvoy, B.R. and Coster, G.D. (2005) General practice and the New Zealand health reforms – lessons for Australia? *Australia and New Zealand Health Policy*, 2: 26.

McPake, B., Kumaranayake, L. and Normand, C. (2002) *Health Economics: An International Perspective.* London: Routledge.

Mahal, A. and Berman, P. (2001) *Health Expenditure and the Elderly: A Survey of Issues in Forecasting, Methods Used and Relevance for Developing Countries.* Harvard: Burden of Disease Unit.

Malcolm, L.A. (2004) How general practice is funded in New Zealand. *Medical Journal of Australia*, 181(2): 106–7.

Manning, W.G., Keeler, E.B., Newhouse, J.P., Sloss, E.M. and Wasserman, J. (1989) The taxes of sin. Do smokers and drinkers pay their way? *Journal of the American Medical Association*, 261(11): 1604–9.

Ministry of Health Welfare and Sport (2006) *www.denieuwezorgverzekering.nl* (accessed 28 January 2006).

Mossialos, E., Dixon, A., Figueras, J. and Kutzin, J. (eds) (2002) *Funding Healthcare: Options for Europe.* Maidenhead: Open University Press.

Murray, J. L. and Frenk, J. (2000) A framework for assessing the performance of health systems. *Bulletin of the World Health Organisation*, 78(6): 717–31.

National Coalition on Health Care (2004) *Health Insurance Coverage. www.nchc.org* (accessed 19 December 2005)

OECD (2003) Making health systems fitter. *OECD Observer*, 238(4). *www.oecdobserver.org/news/fullstory.php/aid/1021/Making_health_systems_fitter.html* (accessed 19 December 2005).

OECD (2005) *OECD Health Data 2005: Statistics and Indicators for 30 countries.* Paris: Organisation for Economic Co-operation and Development.

Office of Health Economics (2004) *Compendium of Health Statistics 2003–2004.* London: Office of Health Economics.

Reinhardt, U.E. (1990) OECD *Health Care Systems in Transition: The Search for Efficiency.* Paris: Organisation for Economic Co-operation and Development.

Robertson, I. and Richardson, J. (2000) Coronary angiography and coronary artery revascularisation rates in public and private hospital patients after acute myocardial infarction. *Medical Journal of Australia*, 173: 291–5.

Rodrigues, J.M., Paviot, B.T. and Martin, C. (2002) DRG information system, healthcare reforms and innovation of management in the western countries during the 90s: Where are the key success factors? *Casemix*, 4(1):16–21.

Savage, E. and Wright, D. (2003) Moral hazard and adverse selection in Australian private hospitals: 1989–1990. *Journal of Health Economics*, 22(3): 331–59.

Schoen, C., Osborn, R., Trang Huynh, P., Doty, M., Davis, K., Zapert, K. and Peugh, J. (2004) Primary care and care system performance: Adults' experiences in five countries. *Health Affairs Web Exclusive. http://content.health-affairs.org/cgi/content/full/hlthaff.w4.487/DC1* (accessed 19 December 2005).

Siciliani, L. and Hurst, J. (2003) *Explaining Waiting Times Variations for Elective Surgery across OECD Countries.* OECD Working Papers. Paris: Organisation for Economic Co-operation and Development.

Timmins, N. (2005) Use of private sector health care in the NHS. *British Medical Journal*, 331: 1141–2.

Wagstaff, A., van Doorslaer, E., van der Burg, H., Calonge, S., Christiansen, T., Citoni, G., Cerdtham, U., Gerfin, G., Gross, M. and Hakinnen, L. (1999) Equity in the finance of health care: Some further international comparisons. *Journal of Health Economics*, 18: 283–90.

Whitfield, L., Pritchard, M.J. and Latchmore, L. (eds) (2005) *An Independent Audit of the NHS under Labour (1997–2005).* London: King's Fund.

Wilkinson, M. (1994) Paying for public spending: Is there a role for earmarked taxes? *Fiscal Studies*, 15: 119–35.

Woolhandler, S., Campbell, T. and Himmelstein, D. (2003) Cost of health care administration in the United States and Canada. *New England Journal of Medicine*, 349(8): 768–75.

Websites and resources

Australian Institute of Health and Welfare (AIHW). *http://www.aihw.gov.au/*

Department of Health, England. Contains full description of policies and useful data sources: *http://www.dh.gov.uk/Home/fs/en*

Department of Health and Social Services Northern Ireland. *http://www.dhsspsni.gov.uk/*

European Observatory on Health Systems and Policies. Provides details of funding and healthcare system information: *http://www.euro.who.int/observatory*

Health of Wales. *http://www.wales.nhs.uk/*

Ministry of Health Welfare and Sport. Provides details of the recent changes to the Netherlands funding system: *www.denieuwezorgverzekering.nl*

New Zealand Ministry of Health. *www.moh.govt.nz/moh.nsf*

NHS Scotland. *http://www.show.scot.nhs.uk/*

Office of Health Economics. Provides detail on economic issues including information and data on healthcare funding: *http://www.ohe.org/*

Organisation for Economic Co-operation and Development (OECD). Key source for healthcare funding data and relevant publication from 30 OECD countries: *http://www.oecd.org/about/0,2337,en_2649_201185_1_1_1_1_1,00.html*

World Health Organisation (WHO). Provides international information on healthcare expenditure, including country data and publications: *http://www.who.int/en/*

National and local government websites also provide information relating to health funding and expenditure.

4 Healthcare systems: an overview of health service provision and service delivery

Lawrence Benson

Introduction

This chapter is concerned with the organisation of healthcare systems, healthcare provision and service delivery. In this context, it also explores the different forms of ownership and control of healthcare organisations, and the impact of ownership and control on system design and service delivery.

Healthcare services are often delivered within systems and organisations comprised of three distinct but increasingly overlapping and fluid subsystems – primary, secondary and tertiary care. In this chapter a model of an overall healthcare system and these three components is introduced, and an example of a healthcare organisation from each of these three subsystems is described, though it is recognised that healthcare organisations increasingly cut across the boundaries of primary, secondary and tertiary care and such vertical integration may provide opportunities for improving overall system performance.

The chapter also outlines a range of different models of ownership and control for healthcare organisations – ranging from for-profit commercial companies, through independent not-for-profit entities, to government-funded and controlled agencies. Examples from a range of different healthcare systems are used to explore the effects of ownership and control on healthcare system performance.

Healthcare systems: a typology

The provision of healthcare services within a regional or national healthcare system can be usefully categorised and analysed through the classification of three main subsystems or sectors – primary, secondary and tertiary care (see Figure 4.1). Each of these sectors can be modelled as a subsystem of the whole healthcare system, though in many countries the

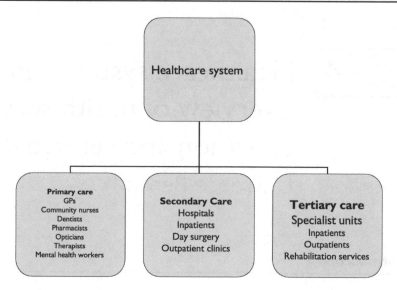

Figure 4.1   Sectors of healthcare within a healthcare system

boundaries between these sectors are often ambiguous or blurred, and frequently shift as health services provision moves from one sector to another. The three sectors overlap and while a patient can be expected to follow a linear journey across the three sectors, it is frequently true that an individual patient may be in receipt of services provided within more than one sector at the same time. A typical patient journey would start with contact with primary care for an initial diagnostic consultation, and might then involve the patient being referred to secondary care for more specialised diagnosis and treatment. In some cases, with complex or highly specialised diseases or treatments, the patient may then also need to be referred on to tertiary services for more specialised or follow-up care. The patient's journey will often be cyclical, with a return to secondary care and then discharge back to primary care for longer term support and monitoring.

Increasingly the boundaries between the three sectors and the subsystems they create have become blurred. For instance, it is common to see services once delivered predominantly at local or regional hospitals being now being delivered in primary care settings closer to where the patient lives or within the patient's home (a trend that is discussed in more detail in Chapter 8). In part, this may be a result of technological progress, like the provision of diagnostic testing equipment in primary care settings or of the increasing capacity and expertise of primary care practitioners. It means that conditions once managed in secondary care (like diabetes, heart disease, or common mental health problems) are increasingly dealt with in primary care. It may also be a result of deliberate policy initiatives, motivated both by a belief that primary care based services will be more cost effective than those based in secondary care, and by a desire to see services located closer to patients and in community settings which are more convenient and easier to access.

Definitions of primary care abound with considerable debate on this issue in the literature (Lewis 1999; Summerton 1999; Peckham and Exworthy 2003). However, for the purpose of this chapter the World Health Organisation (WHO) definition is cited as 'the first level of contact of individuals, the family and the community with the national health system bringing health care as close as possible to where people live and work, and constitutes the first element of a continuing health care process' (WHO 1978).

Primary healthcare is delivered through a wide range of different health professionals including family physicians, dentists, pharmacists, opticians, nurses and therapists (Boerma 2006). These professionals are either geographically based in the local community or provide an outreach service from a secondary or even tertiary centre. In some healthcare systems (e.g. the UK) the general practitioner (also known as the family physician) serves as the gatekeeper to other professionals within primary care or refers patients on to secondary or tertiary services. In many other healthcare systems, for example, France, Germany and the USA, the patient has direct access to more specialist consultation and care by obstetricians, paediatricians, cardiologists and others. In some countries, primary care physicians are organised into medical groups or practices which are often the focus for the provision of a range of other community-based health services, and may also be involved in the provision of social care, diagnostic services, and in providing some semi-acute care and even in commissioning secondary care services for their patient population. In other countries, primary care physicians are more likely to be in solo or small group practice, working independently from office premises. In these cases, primary care services are likely to be rather more fragmented, and less well connected to secondary care.

Secondary or acute care services (the terms are often used interchangeably though they are different) have been predominantly hospital based in most developed countries, although this is now starting to change as there is greater flexibility in where some services can be physically sited and provided (McKee and Healy 2002). However, secondary care can be described as episodic treatment provided for an illness or health problem and generally seen as curative in nature and will typically consist of inpatient, day case and outpatient services. Secondary care services receive the great majority of their patient referrals from family physicians but will also see patients admitted directly from their emergency departments. Here one can see an overlap of primary and secondary care as the emergency department may often be used as the primary care provider by patients but be situated in the physical and organisational setting of a general hospital providing secondary healthcare services.

The patient may then require more specialised care which cannot be given at most secondary care providers and therefore be referred to a tertiary care centre which serves the larger population of a region or country.

Across a healthcare system the number of patient contacts and episodes decreases as one moves from primary care through to secondary and tertiary care and needs are addressed in the first two sectors – most patients are seen, diagnosed and treated in primary care. However, conversely there is an increase in costs as patients move through the sectors, with the costs of secondary and tertiary care often being much higher than those in primary care. This can be visualised (Peckham and Exworthy 2003) in the model in Figure 4.2. It is not surprising therefore that there is constant pressure to address increasing healthcare costs by attempting to develop the capacity of primary care providers and indeed to facilitate the ability of the patient to provide self-care.

Heathcare systems: examples of typical healthcare organisations

Making generalisations about the structure of healthcare services or healthcare organisations across primary, secondary and tertiary care is invidious, because there are many different ways of organising service delivery and considerable variation is found both within national healthcare systems and internationally between countries. But understanding the relationships between primary, secondary and tertiary care is made easier if we use some practical examples. Below, we describe a 'typical' primary care organisation – a family practice with 9000 patients; a common secondary care organisation – an acute hospital serving a population of around 200,000 people; and a tertiary service – a regional cancer centre serving a region of 3.2 million.

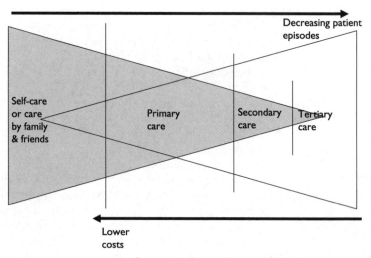

Figure 4.2   Relationships between healthcare expenditure and levels of care
Source: Adapted from Peckham and Exworthy (2003).

Primary care organisation – a group family practice with a practice list of 9000+ patients

The practice has three full-time and four part-time general practitioners who are the family physicians to their patients and also individually offer areas of specialty to the patients registered with the practice such as minor surgery, contraception, maternity and child health surveillance. The practice is supported by a range of other healthcare professionals either directly employed by the practice (for example, practice nurses and healthcare assistants) or provided by another primary care organisation and also secondary care providers (for example, community nurses, mid-wives, school nurses, community psychiatric nurses, podiatrists, physio-therapists, dieticians and psychologists). The services provided in addition to a standard medical consultation with one of the doctors include:

- family planning
- maternity care
- child health surveillance
- immunisations against disease for adults and children
- screening for disease, e.g. cervical cancer, coronary heart disease, diabetes and hypertension – done through targeted programmes and clinics, e.g. for people over 75, well women and well people clinics
- monitoring and management of chronic diseases, e.g. asthma, diabetes, hypertension
- mental health services, e.g. counselling and therapies.

Secondary care organisation – a general acute hospital serving a district of 200,000 people

The hospital employs 2500 staff. It has 420 inpatient beds and across a year will receive 5000 elective admissions, 21,500 emergency admissions, 18,000 day cases, 63,000 visits to its emergency department and 230,000 outpatient visits from patients.

Its clinical services are organised within five directorates or divisions – surgery and anaesthetics, children's and women's services, general medicine and older people, diagnostics and therapeutics, and clinical therapy and rehabilitation. The specific services within these five directorates are detailed in Table 4.1

Tertiary care organisation – a specialist cancer services centre serving a regional population of 3.2 million people

The tertiary hospital specialises in the treatment of cancer services and serves a region of around 3.2 million people. The services provided include specialist surgery, chemotherapy, radiotherapy, adult leukaemia, palliative and supportive care services for young people with cancer, and

Table 4.1   Clinical services at a district general acute hospital

Clinical directorate	Services
Surgery and anaesthetics	Accident and Emergency General Surgery Trauma and Orthopaedics Ear, Nose and Throat Oral Surgery Intensive Care
Children's and women	Maternity Gynaecology
Medicine and older people	General Medicine Dermatology Diabetes Haematology Oncology Neurology
Diagnostics and therapeutics	Radiology Pharmacy Pathology
Clinical therapy and rehabilitation	Community Rehabilitation Physiotherapy Dietetics Occupational Therapy Podiatry Speech and Language Therapy

endocrinology. The centre has 250 inpatient beds and sees 11,000 new patients each year, most as referrals from secondary care providers, though some patients are referred directly to the tertiary hospital from primary care. There are 14 secondary care providers in the region served by the tertiary hospital and who refer to it, but it also receives some referrals from other regions in the country. It employs nearly 2000 staff.

The service for diabetes in the UK is used as an example to demonstrate how care is managed and delivered across the primary, secondary and tertiary care sectors. Historically there has been a wide variety in the pattern of care for the management of patients with diabetes, particularly in respect to primary and secondary care. In some areas the local secondary care provider/hospital has taken the greater proportion of diabetic patients for their routine monitoring and management of the disease and yet in other localities the majority of patients are cared for in primary care either by GP or other clinicians in this community setting (practice nurses, community nurses, opticians, podiatrists). A review in 2000 across England and Wales of diabetes highlighted these differing patterns of care (Audit Commission 2000) and outlined existing patterns of care for patients making routine demands on healthcare services (see Figure 4.3). Examples of this ranged from large GP practices (with over 20,000

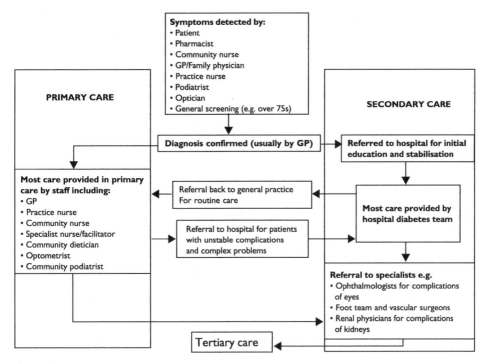

Figure 4.3 Patterns of care for people with diabetes
Source: Adapted from Audit Commission (2000).

patients) in rural settings contracting with secondary providers for monthly clinical sessions from a hospital consultant from a diabetes centre to advise GPs, to a diabetes centre within a large hospital serving a large population and having on site both secondary and specialist tertiary services. A systematic review of the diabetes care delivered in primary or secondary care settings concluded that there was little evidence to support that the setting in itself was a determinant for the effectiveness of the routine care to the patient (Griffin and Kinmonth 1997) as much depended on individual clinicians, patients and locally available models of care.

However, the increasing incidence in diabetes in the UK population has been addressed by government policy (DOH 2001) requiring minimum standards of service to be followed which cover the routine care of stable diabetes. This has concentrated the attention of primary and secondary care organisations in more effectively coordinating services for diabetes across a locality. These services are increasingly delivered in primary care settings through a more specialised workforce of GPs, practice and community nurses, podiatrists and opticians with particular training in the management of diabetes. However, this has not meant a detailed prescribed model of care insistent on a particular pattern of care across sectors. There has also been a growth in services of hospital based diabetes centres advising primary care professionals on the management of diabetes and the better coordination of services for patients with complications from their condition. Typically in the UK there are a growing number of professionals who work regularly both in primary and secondary care settings including diabetes specialist nurses, dietitians and retinal screening staff (Watkins 2003).

If there is to be a greater shift in the pattern of care across secondary and primary settings in a locality, then the respective strengths typically exhibited by primary and secondary care together with patient preferences need to be recognised. The strengths often offered by each sector are summarised (Audit Commission 2000) in Table 4.2.

Patient journeys and the healthcare system

It is helpful to illustrate the relationships between primary care, secondary care and tertiary care by using a patient's journey through the healthcare system. In Figure 4.4 the patient journey of a woman diagnosed with ovarian cancer is mapped across the healthcare system and illustrates how the patient moves across primary, secondary and tertiary healthcare provision. This example shows that there are many opportunities to redesign this care pathway to reduce the number of contacts to the different parts of the system (GP practice, local general hospital and regional specialist centre), to minimise the number of handovers or referrals and to make appropriate use of each sector.

Table 4.2   Strengths of primary and secondary care settings for diabetes care

Strengths of primary care teams	Strengths of hospital diabetes teams
Continuity of care to the patient	Specialist care with complications or special groups (such as children and pregnant women)
Knowledge of the patient, their family and comorbidities	Second-line treatment for patients with poor diabetes control
Expertise in managing chronic condition	Expert support and training for all staff in the locality caring for people with diabetes (including practice nurses, GPs, community podiatrists and dietitians)
Services often delivered to the home by the patient	Specialist patient education for a critical mass of patients including those with special needs (such as ethnic minority groups) and providing input from a range of disciplines
May be preferred by patients for routine care	A focus for diabetes care in the hospital including training, guidelines and links with specialist teams in secondary and tertiary organisations including ophthalmology, vascular surgery and nephrology

Source: Adapted from Audit Commission (2000).

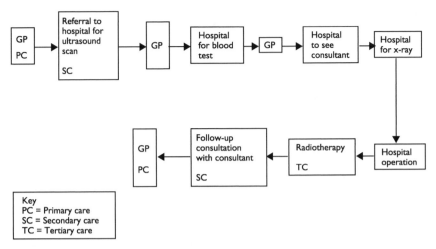

Figure 4.4 Patient journey – diagnosis and treatment of ovarian cancer
Source: Adapted from Modernisation Agency (2005).

A redesigned care pathway like this could be more efficient in its use of resources, more effective in maximising the long-term health outcomes for the patient, and more patient-centred in terms of reducing patient contacts and visits to multiple healthcare providers. In this case there are opportunities to place more of the diagnostic services into primary care, to ensure that as many diagnostic tests are made at one point on the patient's journey as possible to speed and rationalise diagnosis, and more radically to move some services between sectors (see Figure 4.5).

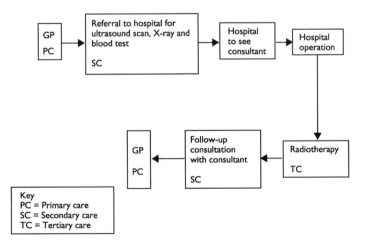

Figure 4.5 Redesigned patient journey – diagnosis and treatment of ovarian cancer
Source: Adapted from Modernisation Agency (2005).

Healthcare systems and models of ownership and control for healthcare organisation

There is a wide range of models of ownership of healthcare organisations seen in use across different healthcare systems, but they can usefully be grouped into four main forms (Preker and Harding 2003):

- commercial, for-profit organisations – companies, etc.
- independent not-for-profit organisations – charities or public benefit corporations
- publicly owned organisations independent of or at arms length from government
- publicly owned and government controlled organisations – state agencies.

These different types of healthcare organisations operate within health-care systems that vary enormously in terms of the extent of government involvement in both funding and provision, and it is difficult to make sense of one or other model of ownership without understanding the wider system or funding context. To explore these differences we will describe the USA and UK (more specifically the English) healthcare systems and draw from each of them some examples of each of these four models.

US healthcare system

The US healthcare system is funded through a complex mix of private and governmental insurance and health services are provided by health-care organisations based on all four models in our typology above (Flood 2000; Kovner and Knickman 2005). The US healthcare system is often portrayed as being primarily private both in funding and provision – with a reliance on employer-sponsored health insurance, a limited government role in the direct funding and provision of healthcare services, and a much greater reliance on the mechanisms of the market, including com-petition and contracting, than would be found in other developed coun-tries (Blank and Burau 2004). In reality, government at both the state and federal level still plays a hugely important role in shaping health policy, funding health services, and regulating healthcare provision (Woolhan-dler and Himmelstein 2002; Sparer 2005).

The independent not-for-profit hospital is the most common model of ownership for secondary care services in the USA with 60% of com-munity hospitals being so owned contrasted to 23% owned by state and local government and just 17% owned by for-profit entities (AHA 2005). But there are large multi-hospital for-profit groups such as Tenet Health-care Corporation (a commercial organisation) which owns 73 hospitals and manages more on behalf of their owners across 13 states (Tenet Healthcare Corporation 2005) and large not-for-profit integrated healthcare systems such as Kaiser Permanente.

The UK and the NHS in England

The UK healthcare system is predominantly based upon a 'national health service' model which essentially means that government plays a dominant role in funding and providing health services (Deber 2002; Blank and Burau 2004). Funding for the healthcare system comes largely from general taxation and every UK citizen has universal coverage for clinically needed health services. This healthcare system has parallels in many other countries, including Finland, New Zealand and Sweden (OECD 2004). The use made of private medical insurance is limited, and private healthcare providers traditionally play a rather peripheral role in service provision. Since the introduction of devolution to Northern Ireland, Scotland and Wales in the late 1990s, health policy has been the responsibility of the devolved administrations and this has resulted in some divergence in arrangements for healthcare funding and delivery (Baggott 2004; Ham 2004). In England, there are some significant moves away from the dominant role of government in healthcare provision, with the gradual introduction of more independent publicly owned providers (foundation hospitals) and the greater use made of independent for-profit healthcare organisations mainly to address demand for elective surgery at independent treatment centres and diagnostic centres (Baggott 2004; Lewis and Dixon 2005).

For-profit healthcare companies in the USA

US for-profit healthcare organisations were originally predominantly physician owned and run (Williams 2005). This has now become increasingly rare and they are often run by investor-owned commercial companies. Companies can either be privately owned or registered as public companies – for the latter, their shares are tradeable on stock exchanges and they are accountable to their shareholders as their owners. For-profit healthcare organisations have as their primary operating goal making a profit for their shareholders and this may result in more direct pressure on services to increase efficiency or reduce costs, and to focus on 'profitable' areas of business. This often raises concerns that an overconcentration on profit can detract from these healthcare organisations' focus on quality of care, or make them less likely to serve wider community needs (Deber 2002; Woolhandler and Himmelstein 2004). However, the counter-argument is that the provision of high quality care for patients will increase satisfaction and may win these companies market share, and that they can only grow and prosper by serving their communities efficiently and effectively. There is much dispute within the US literature as regards the relative merits of different forms of ownership and particularly between for-profit and not-for-profit organisations (Cutler 2000; Devereaux et al. 2004; Williams 2005).

Not-for-profit healthcare organisations in the USA

Not-for-profit healthcare organisations are still trading entities and they can still make an operating surplus or loss – but the crucial difference is that when they make a surplus that income is reinvested in the healthcare organisation and its services and is not distributed to shareholders (Deber 2002; Raffel et al. 2002).

The origins of not-for-profit healthcare organisations are often rooted in philanthropic and charitable concerns. Church-affiliated hospitals are probably still the most readily recognised not-for-profit healthcare organisations in the USA (Raffel et al. 2002). They are largely community based but also include many large university teaching hospitals, which are often owned by academic institutions which are themselves not-for-profit. Their not-for-profit status often means that they have some exemptions from income and other taxes. They can raise capital through borrowing against assets from commercial lenders (such as banks) and also from donations and fundraising in their communities.

Kaiser Permanente is an example of a huge scale not-for-profit healthcare system that brings together (in a single integrated healthcare system) prepaid insurance, physician group practice, preventive medicine and the organised delivery of secondary and tertiary services. It tries to deliver as many services as possible within its system and where patients can go to a single medical centre for all their medical care so further blurring the lines between primary, secondary and tertiary care. It was one of the first health maintenance organisations in the USA (a type of managed care organisation) and has 8.2 million members, with 136,511 non-physician employees, 11,000 doctors, 30 hospitals, 431 medical office buildings and operating revenues of $22.5 billion in 2002 (Kaiser Permanente 2005).

Publicly owned and government controlled healthcare providers in England

NHS trusts were established in the UK from 1991 (DOH 1989; Merry 2003) and they are still the main form of secondary and tertiary healthcare provider. They are statutory bodies, owned and controlled by the Department of Health and the Secretary of State for Health who has extensive legal powers of direction over all aspects of their work. NHS trusts have a statutory legal duty to remain solvent and also to deliver quality services in line with national targets set by government and to act in partnership with local agencies. Each NHS trust has a board consisting of non-executive and executive directors charged with the governance of the organisation. The non-executive directors are appointed through a national appointments commission. NHS trusts are accountable to the Secretary of State for Health and have a direct line of accountability to central government. They are performance managed by their strategic health authority (a regional body) and engage with their local purchasing bodies – primary care trusts. NHS trusts are also regulated by the Healthcare Commission and required to work within nationally set targets and standard (Dixon 2005).

When they were first established in the early 1990s, NHS trusts were perceived by many as being an important attempt to depart from what was then a healthcare system run largely by command and control from central government. However, the promised freedom and autonomy of NHS trusts did not materialise and in some ways they became more closely controlled by government than other parts of the NHS (Ham 2003). Now, all NHS hospital trusts in England are to be given the opportunity to become foundation trusts, which are described below.

Publicly owned healthcare providers independent of government in England

Foundation hospital trusts were established in England from April 2004 (DOH 2002) as independent legal entities which, although still within the NHS and publicly owned, are outside the general powers of direction of the Secretary of State for Health. Formally, they are public benefit corporations, controlled by a membership made up of local people and members of staff, with an elected board of governors (Walshe 2003). Initially, only high performing NHS trusts could apply for foundation status but the intent is that all NHS trusts will be able to become foundation organisations eventually. It seems that one intention of the foundation model is to distance NHS providers further from national politicians and government and to develop closer links with the local stakeholders of patients, the local community (whether or not as service users) and employees.

The model of governance adopted by foundation hospitals is based upon a local membership drawn from patients, the wider community, employees and representatives of local organisations (Lewis 2005). The members of the foundation trust elect a board of governors whose role it is to appoint and oversee the board of directors and represent the interests of the local community in the management and stewardship of the local community (DOH 2002). Governors who are public members can be elected to become non-executive directors of the board of directors. The board of governors appoints executive and non-executive directors who then operationally run the organisation. Unlike NHS trusts, there is no direct line of accountability between the foundation trust and the Secretary of State for Health.

Local NHS commissioning bodies remain the main payers for services provided by foundation trusts, as is the case for NHS trusts. The mechanisms to involve patients and the public are similar to those used by NHS trusts. However, the model governance adopted by foundation trusts presents a clear opportunity to involve these stakeholders even further.

Although foundation trusts have arguably a governance model based on greater local ownership and control, they are regulated by the independent regulator for foundation trusts (which is called Monitor).

Monitor has wide-ranging powers over foundation trusts, including approving their initial application for foundation trust status, issuing their operating licence, and being able to step in and take control if they fail to perform adequately. Foundation trusts are also required to work within system-wide principles and targets and are subject to review of the quality of services they provide by the Healthcare Commission, the industry regulator (Healthcare Commission 2005).

Healthcare systems and organisations: does ownership and control matter?

Public sector healthcare organisations have often been viewed as inflexible and less able to innovate and therefore meet the needs and wants of their patients (Deber 2002). In systems where the public sector dominates, these organisations have been accused of developing complacent attitudes protected often by being in a monopolistic position and being given few clear incentives to improve performance. The outcomes can be poor access to healthcare and little choice available to the consumer. They are also often judged as being poor at working in the interests of patients across organisational boundaries in health and social care boundaries and thereby being accused of operating in silos (DOH 1997; Glendinning and Rummery 1998). They are more bound by 'red tape' or bureaucratic policy, rules and constraints within a command and control environment at the behest of diktat from national/regional government policymakers. There is therefore the danger of quashing any autonomy felt by the organisation and the maintenance of highly centralised decision making. In some healthcare systems there may have been an underinvestment in such organisations resulting in antiquated technology. Governance of these organisations has been criticised often as poor with the disadvantage of having multiple, over-ambitious and sometimes contradictory objectives set by government, weak supervisory structures within the organisation and an information-poor environment (Harding and Preker 2003).

In the defence of public sector healthcare, organisations that have undergone reform and significant investment can be said to be more committed and responsive to policy designed to improve the quality of healthcare, for example, through the adoption of clinical governance (Sheaff et al. 2006). In some healthcare systems, public sector organisations can be attributed as having lower costs, particularly administrative costs, than in the private sector and particularly for-profit organisations.

The case for for-profit organisations is that they are nimble and quick to meet a market demand and adopt innovation more readily as they are not cluttered by many objectives but one primary driver, the maximisation of profit (Deber 2002). They may be less bound by red tape from government although not escape the state in its role as regulator. They can develop and exercise economies of scale as they grow and work across jurisdictional boundaries (e.g. geographically across a country) far more easily than a public sector organisation which might serve one locality. They will invest in the latest technologies to gain market share and also customers might be attracted by an integration of services through the provision of primary, secondary and tertiary care and therefore assert a competitive advantage over rivals.

However, the dominant driver of profit maximisation may result in higher costs passed on to the consumer, and poor quality of clinical outcome for both morbidity and mortality (Deber 2002). The for-profit organisation may not burden itself with activities such as training of clinicians, research and ties with the local community which may often be key aims of public and not-for-profit organisations. The increasing dominance of the for-profit healthcare organisation may also result in 'cream skimming' of patients where those with complex needs are not sought as being of high risk and potentially costly to the organisation/ company and the public sector is then left as a safety net for these patients (Deber 2002). The pursuit of societal goals such as the reduction of health inequalities across a population is more easily coordinated where there is less diversity in providers of healthcare and where there is not a fundamental clash of values between the pursuit of profit and the maximisation of health for all.

Many healthcare systems across the world are engaged in moving the purchase and delivery of healthcare increasingly from the direct command and control of government and away from the centre or core of the public sector (Preker and Harding 2003; Sheaff et al. 2006). This has resulted in services being delivered by healthcare organisations which are in the broader public sector (for example, NHS self-governing trusts and perhaps more radically English NHS foundation hospital trusts) or private sector (populated by not-for-profit and for-profit organisations). Although services may be publicly funded, the accountability of these organisations is increasingly exercised through public to private or public to public contracts and regulatory systems (Harding and Preker 2003). There is a trend in many systems towards a greater diversity of ownership by government, shareholders, local residents and consumers of health services.

The main argument for delivering healthcare further from the core of the public sector is that more efficient production of healthcare across the system will result (Harding and Preker 2003) prompted by greater contestability and competition within the system. However, this continues to be an area of heated debate and contention and the arguments for encouraging the growth of organisations either publicly owned (although perhaps not under the direct control of government) or privately owned but having a not-for-profit model are perhaps most vociferously voiced in the US when this system is analysed (Deber 2002; Devereaux et al. 2004; Woolhandler and Himmelstein 2004). Here evidence is presented supporting claims that for-profit healthcare organisations are not only more costly (and this includes hospitals and managed care organisations) but provide poorer quality of care in respect to morbidity and even mortality (Deber 2002; Himmelstein et al. 1999;

Devereaux et al. 2002). In this system at least it could be said that the form of ownership does matter in respect to access to effective healthcare.

Conclusion

It has been seen that healthcare systems have been traditionally modelled or described in terms of three main subsystems – the primary, secondary and tertiary sectors. This model is useful to a point when describing healthcare systems but it remains under constant challenge as the boundaries between sectors become increasingly blurred and shifted. One important driver for this is the redesign of the patient's journey to ensure services are delivered more effectively and in places of greater convenience to the patient. There are powerful arguments for the delivery of more services within primary care, not only because it may be more efficient and less costly than providing the same services in the secondary or tertiary sectors.

The examples that have been given above of different forms of healthcare organisation ownership and control may mean that the approaches taken to construct logical and well-coordinated patient journeys may be different in different healthcare systems. For example, in government owned or heavily influenced healthcare organisations a great deal may be achieved through command and control, with government issuing national standards or performance targets and monitoring healthcare providers against them. However, in a more diverse, plural and decentralised healthcare system, access to a well-integrated healthcare system may represent a competitive advantage when attracting customers and building market share, and competition and contestability between providers or systems may drive improvements in performance.

It is perhaps safest to conclude that simplistic assumptions about the organisation and delivery of health services are likely to be wrong as often as they are right. No ideal model for service delivery and organisation emerges – rather, we identify a range of competing and sometimes paradoxical drivers and constraints. For example, integrating primary and secondary care services in a single organisation may avoid some of the unhelpful boundaries and handovers in patient journeys, but could also tend to draw resources into secondary care at the expense of primary care services. Using a model of ownership which gives greater autonomy to healthcare providers may promote innovation and competitive pressures may drive improvements in performance, but it may also make system wide planning and coordination much more difficult. Moving services from secondary to primary care may reduce unit costs of provision, but can also affect the quality of care and lower referral thresholds in ways that would increase costs elsewhere in the healthcare system. Healthcare systems are complex systems, and the likely effects of policy initiatives and system reforms should be both examined prospectively and studied and evaluated properly if we are to learn what works.

> **Summary box**
>
> - Healthcare systems have been traditionally modelled on the basis of primary, secondary and tertiary sectors.
> - Family practitioners and particularly physicians often act as gatekeepers to the secondary and tertiary healthcare systems.
> - This traditional model is constantly being challenged and boundaries between primary, secondary and tertiary sectors are becoming blurred.
> - Healthcare expenditure per patient episode increases from primary, to secondary and to tertiary care whilst levels of patient activity and numbers of visits are greatest in primary care.
> - Mapping the patient's journey through a healthcare system identifies opportunities for this journey to be more centred on the needs of the patient.
> - A range of different models of ownership of healthcare organisations exists within healthcare systems which have different mixes of private and public funding and provision of healthcare.

Self-test exercises

1 Develop an existing patient journey that crosses the three sectors of primary, secondary and tertiary care and involves your healthcare organisation. How could this be improved and how could you ensure that improvements are made? How could you involve the patient in the redesign of this journey?

2 Identify the model of ownership for your healthcare organisation and identify both the advantages and disadvantages that this model brings?

3 How does your healthcare organisation identify the views of its patients/service users? What are the current concerns of your patients and how do these match with patient concerns from across your healthcare system?

References and further reading

American Hospitals Association (AHA, 2005) *Fast Facts on U.S. Hospitals from AHA Hospital.* http://www.aha.org/aha/resource_center/fastfacts/fast_facts_US_hospitals.html (accessed 14 December 2005).

Audit Commission (2000) *Testing Times – A Review of Diabetes Services in England and Wales.* London: Audit Commission.

Baggott, R. (2004) *Health and Healthcare in Britain*, 4th edn. Basingstoke: Palgrave Macmillan.

Blank, R.H. and Burau, V. (2004) *Comparative Health Policy.* Basingstoke: Palgrave Macmillan.

Boerma, W.G.W. (2006) Coordination and integration in European primary care. In R.B. Saltman, A. Rico and W. Boerma (eds) *Primary Care in the Driver's Seat?* Maidenhead: Open University Press.

Cutler, D.M. (2000) *The Changing Hospital Industry: Comparing Not-for-Profit and For-Profit Institutions*, Chicago: University of Chicago Press.

Deber, R.B. (2002) *Delivering Health Care Services: Public, Not-for-Profit, or Private?* Ottowa: Commission on the Future of Health Care in Canada.

Department of Health (DOH, 1989) *Working for Patients*. London: DOH.

Department of Health (DOH, 1997) *The New NHS Modern, Dependable*. London: DOH.

Department of Health (DOH, 2001) *National Service Framework for Diabetes*. London: DOH.

Department of Health (DOH, 2002) A *Guide to NHS Foundation Trusts*. London: DOH.

Devereaux, P.J., Choi, P.T., Lacchetti, C. et al. (2002) A systematic review and meta-analysis of studies comparing mortality rates of private for-profit and private not-for-profit hospitals. *Canadian Medical Association Journal*, 166(11): 1399–1406.

Devereaux, P.J., Heels-Andsell, D. and Lacchetti, C. (2004) Payments for care at private for-profit and private not-for-profit hospitals: A systematic review and meta-analysis. *Canadian Medical Association Journal*, 170(12): 1817–23.

Dixon, J. (2005) *Regulating Health Care – The Way Forward*. London: King's Fund.

Flood, C.M. (2000) *International Health Care Reform*. London: Routledge.

Glendinning, C. and Rummery, K. (1998) A duty of partnership: Bringing health and social care together. *British Journal of Health Care Management*, 4(6): 294–7.

Griffin, S. and Kinmonth, A.L. (1997) Diabetes care: The effectiveness of systems for routine surveillance for people with diabetes. *Cochrane Systematic Reviews*, 4: 1–13.

Ham, C. (2003) Autonomization and centralization of UK hospitals. In A.S. Preker and A. Harding (eds) *Innovations in Health Service Delivery: The Corporatization of Public Hospitals*. Washington, DC: World Bank.

Ham, C. (2004) *Health Policy in Britain*, 5th edn. Basingstoke: Palgrave Macmillan.

Harding, A. and Preker, A.S. (2003) A conceptual framework for the organisational reform of hospitals. In A.S. Preker and A. Harding (eds) *Innovations in Health Service Delivery: The Corporatization of Public Hospitals*. Washington, DC: World Bank.

Healthcare Commission (2005) *The Healthcare Commission's Review of Foundation Trusts*. London: Healthcare Commission.

Himmelstein, D.U., Woolhandler, S., Hellander, I. and Wolfe, S.M. (1999) Quality of care in investor-owned vs not-for-profit HMOs. *Journal of the American Medical Association*, 282(2): 159–63.

Kaiser Permanente (2005) *https://newsmedia.kaiserpermanente.org/* (accessed 13 December 2005).

Kovner, A.R. and Knickman, J.R. (eds) (2005) *Jonas and Kovner's, Health Care Delivery in the United States*, 8th edn. New York: Springer.

Lewis, J. (1999) The concepts of community care and primary care in the UK: The 1960s to the 1990s. *Health and Social Care in the Community*, 7(5): 333–41.

Lewis, R. (2005) *Governing Foundation Trusts – A New Era for Public Accountability*. London: King's Fund.

Lewis, R. and Dixon, J. (2005) *NHS Market Futures – Exploring the Impact of Health Service Market Reforms*. London: King's Fund.

McKee, M. and Healy, J. (2002) *Hospitals in a Changing Europe*. Maidenhead: Open University Press.

Merry, P. (2003) *The NHS in England 2003/04*. London: NHS Confederation.

Modernisation Agency (2005) *Process Mapping, Analysis and Redesign – Improvement Leader's Guide*. London: Department of Health.

OECD (2004) *Towards High-Performing Health Systems*. Paris: Organisation for Economic Co-operation and Development.

Peckham, S. and Exworthy, M. (2003) *Primary Care in the UK*. Basingstoke: Palgrave Macmillan.

Preker, A.S. and Harding, A. (eds) (2003) *Innovations in Health Service Delivery: The Corporatization of Public Hospitals*. Washington, DC: World Bank.

Raffel, M.W., Raffel, N.K. and Barsukiewicz, C.K. (2002) *The U.S. Health System – Origins and Functions*, 5th edn. New York: Delmar–Thomson Learning.

Sheaff, R., Gene-Badia, J., Marshall, M. and Svab, I. (2006) The evolving public–private mix. In R.B. Saltman, A. Rico and W. Boerma (eds) *Primary Care in the Driver's Seat?* Maidenhead: Open University Press.

Sparer, M.S. (2005) The role of government in U.S. health care. In A.R. Kovner and J.R. Knickman (eds) *Jonas and Kovner's, Health Care Delivery in the United States*, 8th edn. New York: Springer.

Summerton, N. (1999) Accrediting research practices. *British Journal of General Practice*, 49(438): 63–4.

Tenet Healthcare Corporation (2005) http://www.tenethealth.com/ TenetHealth (accessed 13 December 2005).

Walshe, K. (2003) Foundation hospitals: A new direction for NHS reform? *Journal of the Royal Society of Medicine*, 96: 106–10.

Watkins, P.J. (2003) *ABC of Diabetes*. London: British Medical Journal Books.

Williams, S. (2005) *Essential of Health Services*, 3rd edn. New York: Delmar–Thomas Learning.

Woolhandler, S. and Himmelstein, D.U. (2002) Pay for national health insurance and not getting it: Taxes pay for a larger share of US health care than most Americans think they should do. *Health Affairs*, 21(4): 88–98.

Woolhandler, S. and Himmelstein, D.U. (2004) The high costs of for-profit care. *Canadian Medical Association Journal*, 170(12): 1814–15.

World Health Organisation (WHO, 1978) *Declaration of Alma-Ata, International Conference on Primary Health Care*, Alma-Ata, USSR, 6–12 September.

Websites and resources

American Hospitals Association. National organization that represents and serves many thousands and types of hospitals, health care networks in the US, and their patients and communities: *http://www.hospitalconnect.com/aha/about/*

European Health Management Association. A network of health organisations throughout Europe with the aim of improving health through better management: *http://www.ehma.org*

European Health Observatory. Provides a very useful outline and review of European healthcare systems: *http://www.euro.who.int/observatory*

Foundation Trust Network. Represents all existing foundation trusts in the English NHS as well as many of those aspiring to foundation trust status: *http://www.foundationtrustnetwork.org/*

Healthcare Commission. English healthcare regulator established in 2004: *http://www.healthcarecommission.org.uk/Homepage/fs/en*

King's Fund. An independent charitable institution which researches and evaluates health and social care policy: *http://www.kingsfund.org.uk/*

NHS Confederation. The main membership body for UK NHS organisations: *http://www.nhsconfed.org/*

Organisation for Economic Co-operation and Development (OECD). Provides a review and analysis of healthcare systems from across the developed world: *http://www.oecd.org/home/*

Picker Institute Europe. Promotes understanding of the patient's perspective at all levels of healthcare policy and practice. Captures patient satisfaction feedback from European countries: *http://www.pickereurope.org/*

5 Managing healthcare technologies and innovation

Ruth McDonald and Tom Walley

Introduction and overview

In recent decades health technology assessment (HTA) has been of increasing interest to health policymakers and researchers. Health technologies have the potential to prolong life or enhance quality of life for patients. However, in modern health systems, which face a gap between demand for care and available resources, such technologies also present challenges. Governments have responded to these challenges by seeking to 'manage' access to new and existing health technologies in a proactive fashion, rather than merely reacting to their development. This means that health services managers are increasingly expected to play a proactive role in the process.

This chapter provides an introduction and overview to the subject of HTA and explains why this is an important issue for those charged with managing health services. The first section describes what is meant by HTA before briefly examining its role in relationship to priority setting. We then outline the various stakeholders involved in HTA processes and consider the challenges posed by attempts to incorporate competing stakeholder perspectives. Following this we discuss HTA in theory and practice, drawing on examples from various countries to illustrate the influence of contextual factors on the development of HTA and the extent to which its outputs influence decision making. We then examine the role of managers with regard to HTA and consider the challenges faced by managers in the context of applying HTA findings. In the next section we present other challenges which face the HTA process and discuss ways in which HTA needs to adapt to the changing nature of healthcare provision and demand in the twenty-first century. The chapter concludes with a brief summary of key points.

What is HTA?

Health technologies, assessment and appraisal

The International Network of Agencies of HTA (INAHTA) describes the process as 'a multi-disciplinary field of policy analysis, which studies the medical, social, ethical and economic implications of development, diffusion and use of health technology'. The term 'health technology' does not just refer to medical technology. It covers a wide range of methods of intervening to promote health, including the prevention, diagnosis or treatment of disease, the rehabilitation or long-term care of patients, as well as drugs, devices, clinical procedures and healthcare settings. However, in practice HTA tends to concentrate on a fairly narrow range of technologies (i.e. drugs, devices and procedures) rather than service delivery issues (where should care be provided and by whom?) and public health interventions (Holland 2004). HTA processes seek to assess existing technologies and to engage in horizon scanning to identify emerging technologies which may be candidates for assessment.

Some commentators distinguish between technology *assessment* and *appraisal*. HTA is described as an analytical process of gathering and summarising information about health technologies. Appraisal is seen as a political process of making a decision about health technologies taking into account assessment information and values and other factors (Stevens and Milne 2004). However, an alternative view is that HTA is also value laden and a political process. HTA approaches vary between countries, but in general much of the focus of HTA methods is concerned with evaluating the costs and benefits of technologies. Decisions about which technologies to evaluate and which costs and benefits to include reflect value judgements. In this sense, the distinction between HTA as a 'neutral' process and appraisal as a political one is open to challenge (Ten Have 2004). This becomes increasingly important as many countries are moving away from merely identifying health technologies of doubtful effectiveness towards assessment of cost effectiveness. The implications of this are that HTA processes will be used to inform the setting of healthcare priorities, ruling out some technologies and ruling in others. Both the HTA process and the application of its outputs might be seen as highly political processes therefore (Webster 2004).

Box 5.1 provides an example based on a recent appraisal undertaken by the National Institute for Health and Clinical Excellence (NICE).

HTA processes and stakeholder interests

There are many stakeholders to be considered in relation to HTA processes. Often these stakeholders encompass different views and competing interests. In addition to government, third party payers, clinicians, organisations that provide and manufacture healthcare and health

Box 5.1 Statins for the prevention of cardiovascular events

The technology – statins

Raised cholesterol is one of a numbers of risk factors associated with the development of cardiovascular disease (CVD). Statins are drugs developed to lower cholesterol levels and hence reduce the risk of coronary events.

NICE appraisal

In addition to receiving evidence from interested parties, NICE commissions an independent academic centre (an 'Assessment Group') to review the published evidence on the relevant technology when developing technology appraisals guidance. In the case of statins a team at Sheffield University reviewed the evidence from clinical trials and economic studies and also developed a model to estimate the costs and health outcomes associated with a lifetime of statin treatment using an NHS perspective (i.e. what would be the health benefits and what would be the costs to the NHS?).*

Estimating costs and benefits

The Assessment Group used data from UK epidemiological studies to estimate cardiovascular event rates. The effect of statins on the reduction of events was based on the results of clinical trials. Health-related utility or quality of life was based on data from a large UK population-based survey. The costs associated with treating cardiovascular events were taken from published UK sources, supplemented by expert opinion where data from published sources were unavailable.

Findings

Secondary prevention (i.e. patients with disease)

The cost per quality adjusted life year (QALY) was estimated to vary between £10,000 and £16,000 for patients between age 45 and 85, with little difference in the results for men and women. For people with diabetes and a history of cardiovascular disease, the cost per QALY was estimated to be below £9000 for all age groups since they are at a relatively high risk of coronary events.

Primary prevention (people who do not have cardiovascular disease)

The estimated cost per QALY varied substantially according to risk level and age of treatment initiation. It was lower at higher levels of risk and in younger age cohorts. The lower costs per QALY associated with commencing treatment at a younger age reflect the greater potential to prevent events, and thus the higher benefits accrued from remaining in the event-free health state. At an annual risk of a cardiovascular event ranging from 3% to 0.5%, the ranges of cost per QALY gained were £10,000 to £31,000 at age 45 years to £37,000 to £111,000 at age 85 years. The costs per QALY were lower for people with diabetes. On the basis of these findings, NICE defined a risk cut-off point which means that relatively low risk patients should not receive statins.

NICE guidance published in November 2005 states:

'Statin therapy is recommended for adults with clinical evidence of CVD.

Statin therapy is recommended as part of the management strategy for the primary prevention of CVD for adults who have a 20% or greater 10-year risk of developing CVD.'

* NICE operates from an NHS perspective which means its focus with regard to costs, is on costs to the NHS budget as opposed to any costs which may be incurred by individuals. In general NICE aspires to extend its remit to other costs involving the public purse such as social services expenditure, but finds this difficult.

technologies, the importance of patient and public views as contributing to the process is widely recognised. However, the nature of HTA processes, and in particular their emphasis on economic evaluation and evidence-based medicine, has implications for the ways in which these different groups can make their views heard in the HTA process.

Whilst the INAHTA definition of HTA describes it as a broad and multi-faceted process, in practice the focus is on clinical effectiveness and increasingly on economic evaluation. Furthermore, the major proportion of HTA investment concerns pharmaceuticals, despite the fact that these account for between 10% and 15% of total expenditure on health services in most modern health systems (Lothgren and Ratcliffe 2004). These factors contribute to a situation in which patient and public views, both in terms of contributing to and using HTA processes are peripheral (Coulter 2004). HTA processes draw on evidence from 'scientific' studies and expert knowledge, using a hierarchy of evidence where the gold standard is the randomised controlled trial and expert opinion is towards the bottom of the hierarchy. Lay perspectives do not feature in the hierarchy, which implies that these may not be seen as valid forms of knowledge. However, the framing of HTA in terms of clinical outcomes risks ignoring other outcomes which are important to patients. Evidence suggests that lay opinion may be at odds with the views of researchers or clinicians with regard to the relative importance of outcomes (Ham and Coulter 2001), but currently HTA processes tend to reflect the latter rather than incorporating the former. A further problem is that HTA processes tend to start with a technology or technologies and assess whether or not these are cost effective. Patients may start with different questions, such as 'What are the characteristics of the diagnosis/disorder/ disease and what are the different ways in which it can be treated?' (Coulter 2004). As Angela Coulter (2004: 95) writes:

> What is needed is a better synthesis between the different ways of deciding on priorities, with explicit principles publicly debated and agreed at the macro-level, greater transparency and more public involvement at the meso- or organizational level, and sufficient flexibility at the micro-level to avoid the rigidities of the 'one-size-fits-all' approach to treatment decision-making, which tends to downplay the importance of clinicians' experience and patients' values and preferences.

Box 5.2 The NICE Citizens' Council

The Citizens' Council was established in 2002 to help provide advice about the broad social values that NICE should take into account when preparing its guidance. The 30 members of the Council reflect the age range, gender, socio-economic status, disability, geographical location and ethnicity of adults in England and Wales. The Council's first report discussed clinical need and was concerned with identifying areas where the Council's views would be most useful and relevant to NICE and its advisory committees. Subsequent reports have included the subjects of age discrimination and treatments for very rare diseases.

Are there circumstances when age should be taken into account when NICE is making a decision about how treatments should be used in the NHS? The Council concluded that:
- health should not be valued more highly in some age groups than others
- social roles at different ages should not influence considerations of cost effectiveness (i.e. people with children or with special professional responsibilities should not be given priority)
- where age is an indicator of benefit or risk, discrimination is appropriate.

Should the NHS be prepared to pay premium prices for drugs to treat very rare (so-called 'ultra orphan') diseases? The majority of the Citizens' Council concluded that the NHS should be prepared to pay premium prices but that:
- the disease should be severe or life threatening
- the treatment should produce real and demonstrable improvements in health
- some limit has to be placed on the amount that the health service should be asked to pay for these treatments in the future.

The NICE Citizens' Council established in England and Wales is an attempt to incorporate public views into the HTA process. Box 5.2 provides more information about this process.

The pharmaceutical industry is also an important stakeholder in the HTA process. Whilst governments want to obtain new medicines at as low a cost as possible, they are also keen to maintain a viable and competitive pharmaceutical industry. Denying new drugs to patients on grounds of cost is likely to result in an unfavourable response from the public and the pharmaceutical industry. In the UK, for example, when NICE refused to sanction the use of the anti-influenza drug Relenza, the chairman of Glaxo Wellcome, the drug's manufacturer, warned that leading drugs companies would consider pulling out of Britain if the government adopted an 'antagonistic' attitude towards the pharmaceutical industry. In Australia, HTA findings have been used in drug pricing and reimbursement decisions since 1993. Whilst Australia's domestic pharmaceutical industry is much smaller than its UK counterpart, government policy attempts to strike a balance between the desire to obtain drugs at the lowest possible cost and the aim of encouraging the growth of a domestic pharmaceutical industry with its associated benefits (i.e. research capacity development, export earnings, employment, and so on). Maintaining this balance is not always easy. Once governments become involved in regulating the pharmaceutical industry in terms of the safety, efficacy and more recently cost effectiveness of its products, the industry becomes a political actor, eager to shape the process by which it is to be regulated (Abraham 2002). The phrase 'regulatory capture' describes a regulatory regime in which the regulator acts to protect the regulated and not the general public interest. There are a number of ways in which 'capture' can be facilitated including the so-called revolving door. This involves regulatory staff moving from industry and then moving back there, with the result that regulatory agencies are much friendlier to the industry and its lobbying mechanisms than may be good for the nation's health.

HTA and priority-setting processes

Theory and practice

The extent to which HTA processes feed directly into policy varies between countries. HTA processes may have been created to respond to a perceived policy gap, but they were not created in a vacuum. Rather they reflect the context of the countries in which they were developed. In France the main HTA agency, the National Agency for Accreditation and Evaluation in Health (ANAES), provides reports to a variety of different customers. These include national health insurance funds, academic societies, healthcare institutions and professionals. However, ANAES acts in a purely advisory capacity and its reports have no formal status (Orvain et al. 2004).

In contrast, in England, the National Institute for Health and Clinical Excellence (NICE) issues guidance in the form of technology appraisals and NHS bodies must make funding available for implementation within three months of an appraisal's publication (DH 2002). One of NICE's key objectives is to promote equitable access to treatments of proven clinical and cost effectiveness. However, in less centralised systems local decision making means that achieving equity at a national level is less of a priority.

In Sweden, for example, which has a well-established government body and local organisations for HTA, county councils are free to take decisions regardless of HTA reports. Rather than collaborating, councils have tended to compete to offer new prestigious technologies. HTA in Dutch healthcare dates from the 1980s and its development was linked to the notion that HTA could be of major importance in government priority setting. The intention was that new technologies should be subject to HTA before coverage in the health benefits package could be considered. However, there is no formal requirement for this to take place. Furthermore, unlike, for example, the centralised English model, the Dutch system is characterised by a plurality of stakeholders and a concept of 'self-governance', which means that whatever can be undertaken by the private sector should not be undertaken by government. A situation of mutual dependence between key stakeholders (government, providers and insurers) means that HTA outputs cannot be imposed from above. Instead, whilst at the national (macro) level government is supportive of the HTA process, the focus of policy is on the meso and micro levels of the system with healthcare insurers, providers and health professionals being encouraged to promote the appropriate use of scarce healthcare resources. In practice, however, it is not clear that these HTA processes are working in the ways intended.

Whilst HTA systems reflect the particular context of the countries in which they have developed, there are a number of common themes which can be observed with regard to many of these systems. These include an increasing tendency towards a narrow definition of HTA as economic evaluation and, with a small number of exceptions, the lack of any direct mechanism for ensuring that HTA outputs feed into policy. These factors may explain why HTA outputs have often been ignored in many countries despite the development of elaborate processes for assessing the costs and benefits of healthcare technologies (Oliver et al. 2004).

Some commentators highlight the lack of expertise amongst health services managers in interpreting and using HTA information as presenting barriers to the adoption and use of HTA outputs. Here the suggestion is that a greater involvement in the HTA cycle of those responsible for making resource allocation decisions will lead to increased use of HTA outputs and enhanced efficiency in healthcare systems (Rutten 2004). However, even in the English context, where NHS institutions are required to implement NICE guidance, recent evidence suggests that implementation 'has not always been timely or comprehensive' (Audit Commission 2005: 23). Much of the problem regarding implementation, it is suggested, is due to deficient management practices. In the next section we examine why HTA is such an important issue for managers and then consider the challenges which the 'management' of health technologies and innovation poses for managers.

HTA – what role for management?

As discussed in the introduction to this chapter, in modern health systems, which face a gap between demand for care and available resources, health technologies have come to be regarded as a challenge to be proactively managed. As we noted above, inadequate knowledge, a lack of involvement in HTA processes and deficient management practices have all been cited as barriers to the effective management of health technologies.

However, it is not clear that managers share this analysis of the problem. In a recent survey of NHS senior managers in England, affordability was identified as the major barrier, with 85% of survey respondents stating that the funds available to implement NICE guidance were insufficient (Audit Commission 2005). Other barriers to implementation included lack of access to necessary resources (e.g. staff, equipment, space), managerial overload (a high volume of work generally and many other changes requiring managerial capacity happening simultaneously), resistance to change and a lack of knowledge about the existence of NICE guidance. The report identified that where robust implementation systems were in place, however, funding was not the biggest barrier and clinician resistance tended to be more significant (on this point see also Sheldon et al. 2004). Clear weaknesses in the financial management arrangements underpinning the implementation of NICE guidance were identified and the report presents recommendations for strengthening these in order to improve guidance implementation.

Figure 5.1 illustrates the steps that should be followed by NHS bodies. Insofar as these components represent a proactive process for the management of health technologies, they might be conceived as having broader application beyond NHS settings. This model, which conceptualises implementation as a management problem to be resolved by technical fixes, is in keeping with the view of HTA as a technical, 'rational' process. The focus on better planning, the preparation of business cases and improved costing arrangements ignores issues such as clinician resistance and affordability. If managers choose not to implement NICE guidance due to lack of resources, they are required to record this in the organisation's risk register and to 'manage' this risk. However, failure to implement NICE guidance is likely to attract criticism since implementation forms part of core standards against which the organisational (and in particular management) performance is assessed.

Alternatively, managers may be placed in the position of having to divert resources from other services in order to fund the implementation of NICE guidance. Only a small percentage of health technologies are subject to formal HTA processes and managers are often faced with having to make difficult decisions about the allocation of scarce resources. Where proposed health service developments have not been subjected to formal HTA processes, denying requests for additional resources is likely to be easier. This may not be the best decision for patients in the long run, but where the costs and benefits of developments are vague or uncertain, the pressure to allocate resources can be more easily resisted.

Our research amongst local health managers responsible for managing the entry of new drugs in the local health economy suggests that the absence of information on costs and benefits may help managers refuse requests for funding (McDonald et al. 2001). We found that since the licensing of new drugs placed managers in a difficult position, the managers we interviewed conceptualised new health technologies as problems whose diffusion (and hence cost) was to be contained. Their energies were expended on limiting the spread of costly drugs, with success being defined in terms of cost containment. At the same time, managers described their aims as ensuring that cost-effective medicines were available for local populations. This reflects, in part, the fact that managers may have certain aims and values to which they aspire, but these are often compromised by the harsh realities of life in a cash-strapped system. In addition, managers often face multiple and competing objectives and may resort to informal resource allocation mechanisms.

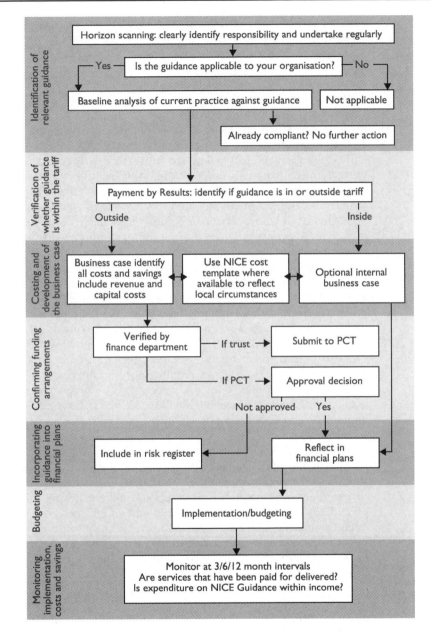

Figure 5.1   Implementing NICE guidance – recommended good financial management model

Source: Audit Commission (2005) © Audit Commission *Managing the Financial Implications of NICE Guidance.* (2005).

Notes: Payment by Results refers to a tariff-based payment system for health services provided in England. PCT refers to primary care trust, the local NHS funding & commissioning agency in England.

These provide a means by which resources can be rationed, thereby achieving some compromise with regard to these competing objectives. These informal priority-setting processes may avoid drawing attention to the fact that access to health technologies is being restricted. However, such processes tend to result in inequalities in access to care and a blurring of accountability to the public who fund the system.

Managers lack legitimacy with regard to informal rationing decisions. In the public's eyes rationing by health service managers may be viewed as inappropriate with clinicians much better qualified to make such choices (Dolan et al. 1999). This explains why managers have difficulty in persuading clinicians to comply with NICE guidance. It also explains why various attempts have been made at formal priority-setting processes which are designed to take account of the evidence on costs and benefits and provide a more transparent and equitable means of allocating resources. Attempts to adopt a more 'rational' approach to priority setting are not unproblematic, however. In particular, where resources are limited and managers have little or no legitimacy for engaging in explicit rationing, attempts to introduce 'rational' processes may flounder due to affordability issues (see Box 5.3 case study, for example).

Alternatively, in a Canadian context, others have reported how agreement has been reached when faced with difficult choices on new cancer drugs (Martin et al. 2001). In this example a committee was established in Ontario that included managers, clinicians and members of the public. Whilst formal HTA processes emphasise the importance of deciding in advance the criteria by which evidence is to be judged (e.g. only good quality randomised control trials will be included), these decision makers were uncertain about the criteria and started to make decisions anyway. In this way, they 'discovered' clusters of factors implicit in their priority-setting rationales. These factors included benefit, harm, evidence, need, cost, availability of alternatives, precedent, convenience, budget constraint, total patient population affected, total cost to the system, access to treatment, pressure from physician and patient groups and historical precedent. Rationales also changed as costs increased. For example, the decision makers agreed to fund an expensive drug for myeloma patients but not for patients with breast cancer. The evidence of benefit of the drug in the two diseases was very similar, but the larger number of breast cancer patients meant that total costs were higher for this group.

The fact that this committee achieved some success may be partly because it included members of the public, but it was also due to additional resources being made available by the Ministry of Health to fund new drugs, which dramatically reduced the need to deny cancer patients access to these drugs. This example also lends support to the notion that such decisions reflect political judgements rather than an 'objective' assessment of costs and benefits. Such instances of formal priority setting are the exception rather than the rule, with resource allocation much more likely to be the result of less transparent processes. This state of affairs reflects irreconcilable tensions faced by managers in a system which promotes 'rational' priority setting and at the same time frowns

Box 5.3   Case study: Prioritising new cancer drugs

Context and setting

The North West of England. A specialist cancer hospital collaborated with a consortium of six health authorities to appraise drug developments and draw up priorities for 1997–8.

Key points

- Providers and commissioners of healthcare were under pressure to introduce new and expensive cancer drugs within limited budgets.
- Evidence of benefits and cost estimates were presented for various new drugs in accordance with the original aim of prioritising drugs according to formal criteria and processes.
- In the context of insufficient funds, commissioning managers sought to contain expenditure and to raise the threshold for funding new drugs. In contrast, doctors sought to move the threshold down to reflect their special interests and the expectations of their patients.
- Stakeholders disagreed on the value to be placed on trial outcomes (for example, although studies reported tumour response rates, which suggest clinical progress, they do not necessarily correlate with better survival or quality of life.)
- The variation in available resources and other service priorities between the six commissioning organisations (health authorities) made it impossible to agree a common approach to funding for these drugs.

Authors' conclusions

Commissioning managers face 'a dichotomy of political rhetoric on setting priorities. They are expected to divorce competing budgetary pressures from the objective assessment of new interventions and set priorities by assessing needs. . . . Ideally, commissioning decisions would be made with sound knowledge of the effectiveness of interventions. However, in practice, evidence based commissioning is hindered by a limited evidence base and influenced by political and financial pressures' (Foy et al. 1999).

The authors subsequently reported repeating the exercise in the 1998–99 and 1999–2000 contracting rounds: 'However, most available growth monies have been absorbed by large increases in activity and pay awards. Little money has been left for new expensive cancer drugs, despite strong evidence of their cost effectiveness' (So et al. 2000).

on explicit rationing processes which are likely to be politically unpopular.

Presenting a set of rules for what managers should do about HTA is difficult, since the role depends on the system in which managers are operating. Where formal processes exist, the role of managers may be outlined in detail (as in the Audit Commission document set out in Figure 5.1). Alternatively, where decisions are made informally and largely by clinicians, managers may have little or no role with regard to the implementation of HTA outputs. In the Netherlands, for example, insurers' payouts are based on established clinical practice rather than evidence of clinical or cost effectiveness (Berg et al. 2004). Whilst there is a trend towards attempts to use guidelines to influence clinical decision making, managers have no control over clinical decision making. Furthermore, HTA outputs, which typically start with a clear diagnosis as opposed to a collection of symptoms, do not reflect the sorts of questions that doctors encounter in everyday practice. Providing managers with more training to enable them to understand HTA processes is unlikely to improve their ability to influence decisions in such contexts.

Challenges for the future

If HTA findings are to be incorporated into decision making more widely, there are a number of challenges to be addressed. There are some difficult technical issues to do with the design and methodologies used in HTA. There is a need to adapt HTA to the demands of a changing healthcare system in which chronic and complex care needs are increasingly the norm. There is also a need to broaden the range of stakeholders and perspectives represented in HTA.

Technical issues

These relate to issues such as speeding up the process, reaching agreement on a common approach to the choice of comparator (e.g. placebo or other) and further exploring the potential for pooling of resources across international boundaries to conduct HTAs (Sampietro-Colom et al. 2002). Classifying these issues as 'technical', however, does not mean that they can be resolved easily. For example, a review of 326 submissions made to the Australian Pharmaceutical Benefits Scheme found significant problems with 67% of these, with the vast majority of problems concerning uncertainty about comparative clinical efficacy (Schubert 2002). Whilst pharmaceutical industry estimates of efficacy are usually derived from placebo-controlled clinical trials, HTA agencies prefer comparisons with existing treatments. This means that drug manufacturers construct models estimating the likely costs and benefits of their drug when compared with other treatments, even though they do not have any trial data on direct comparisons on which to base these comparisons.

Demographic and system changes

The redesign of health systems to reflect the needs of an ageing population and a change to the traditional ways of providing care is high on the agenda of health policymakers in the developed world. Health systems of the future are likely to reflect moves away from services geared to acute episodes of care and towards self-care and the co-production of health.

Staff costs represent the majority of healthcare expenditures and in a context where health professionals are an increasingly scarce resource the roles and responsibilities of health professionals are already undergoing changes in most healthcare systems. Health systems of the future are likely to be characterised by a redistribution of work and the creation of new types of healthcare workers. This means that HTA processes in the future will need to be able to produce outputs which relate to these new models of care, rather than the rather narrow definitions of 'technology' on which almost all HTA programmes are currently focused.

Incorporating other perspectives – broadening out HTA

As we have outlined, there is often a tension between 'lay' and scientific knowledge, with HTA processes tending to privilege the latter. A major challenge for HTA concerns the incorporation of societal values into what is, for the most part, a process of economic evaluation. Broadening out HTA beyond economic evaluation in terms of other non-economic (e.g. ethical) dimensions and other spheres of activity (e.g. public health related interventions) and perspectives (e.g. starting with disease which may be of interest to patients and clinicians, as opposed to HTA being skewed to high-cost technologies) represents a significant challenge. Whilst it may be possible, at least in theory, to devote additional resources to HTA processes in order to examine additional spheres of activity and clinical perspectives, incorporating ethical dimensions may be more difficult. As the example from Ontario illustrates, priority setting often involves making decisions first and then 'discovering' rationales afterwards. These rationales also change according to the context. This suggests that the tensions inherent in attempting to combine competing rationales (e.g. economics versus ethics) or forms of knowledge (lay versus 'scientific') are unlikely to be resolved by providing additional HTA resources or attempting to make management processes more efficient.

Conclusion

In this chapter we have presented an introduction to HTA and described why it is an important issue for managers to understand what HTA involves. We do not provide any simple advice or words of help to outline the appropriate course of action for managers to take with regard to HTA processes and outputs. Certainly managers should be aware of such processes, but the role of managers will largely depend on the organisational and health system context in which they are operating. In many countries, there are no formal requirements for managers to make use of HTA outputs. Even in the English NHS where managers face clear guidelines concerning appropriate action, the existence of competing objectives, resource scarcity and limited legitimacy make it difficult to comply with these guidelines. This reflects the fact that HTA and priority setting are complex political processes whose problems are not amenable to resolution by technical fixes or the application of more systematised ways of working.

Summary box

- Health technologies present opportunities for health gain, but they are now seen as processes to be carefully managed since they also present potential threats.
- Health technology assessment (HTA) is an analytical process of gathering and summarising information about health technologies
- HTA is also a highly politicised process involving multiple groups of stakeholders and often competing interests.
- There are tensions between decontextualised HTA assessments dealing with statistical lives and the real world context, which involves named patients and mitigating factors.
- The HTA process is evolving – key challenges include the incorporation of societal values into what are largely economic calculations and the broadening out of HTA beyond its current narrow focus.
- In resource-constrained and highly politicised healthcare systems, applying HTA outputs in practice will always be a challenge.

Self-test exercises

1 What knowledge do you have about the HTA processes which relate to the health system you work in? Do you agree with the way in which these processes are undertaken? Would more knowledge in this area improve your ability to apply HTA outputs?

2 How much input should members of the public have in HTA processes? If public opinion suggests a new and expensive drug should be funded, where should the money come from to fund this? Is this left to managers to resolve?

3 Have you been involved in making decisions about resource allocation? If so, how have these been taken? If not, who takes these decisions and on what basis? What part do managers' own values play in the process and can they put them to one side? How accountable and transparent are these processes?

References and further reading

Abraham, J. (2002) The pharmaceutical industry as a political player. *The Lancet*, 360: 1498–1502.

Audit Commission (2005) *Managing the Financial Implications of NICE Guidance*. London: Audit Commission.

Berg, M., van der Grinten, T. and Klazinga, N. (2004) Technology assessment, priority setting, and appropriate care in Dutch health care. *International Journal of Technology Assessment in Health Care*, 20(1): 35–43.

Burls, A., Austin, D. and Moore, D. (2005) Commissioning for rare diseases: View from the frontline. *British Medical Journal*, 331(7523): 1019–21.

Coulter, A. (2004) Perspectives on health technology assessment: Response from the patient's perspective. *International Journal of Technology Assessment in Health Care*, 20(1): 92–6.

Department of Health (DH, 2002) *Directions to Primary Care Trusts and NHS Trusts in England Concerning Arrangements for the Funding of Technology Appraisal Guidance from NICE*. London: Department of Health.

Dolan, P., Cookson, R. and Ferguson, B. (1999) Effect of group discussion and deliberation on the public's views of priority setting in health care: focus group study. *British Medical Journal*, 318: 916–19.

Foy, R., So, J., Rous, E. and Scarffe, J. H. (1999) Perspectives of commissioners and cancer specialists in prioritising new cancer drugs: impact of the evidence threshold. *British Medical Journal*, 318: 456–9.

Ham, C. and Coulter, A. (2001) Explicit and implicit rationing: Taking responsibility and avoiding blame for health care choices. *Journal of Health Services Research and Policy* 6: 163–9.

Hill, S., Garrattini, S., van Loenhout, J., O'Brien, B. and de Joncheere, K. (2003) Technology appraisal programme of the National Institute for Clinical Excellence. A review by WHO. World Health Organization Europe. Available at *http://www.nice.org.uk/pdf/boardmeeting/brdsep03itemtabled.pdf*

Holland, W.W. (2004) Health technology assessment and public health: A commentary. *International Journal of Technology Assessment in Health Care*, 20: 77–80.

Lothgren, M. and Ratcliffe, M. (2004) Pharmaceutical industry's perspective on health technology assessment. *International Journal of Technology Assessment in Health Care* 20: 97–101.

McCabe, C., Claxton, K. and Tsuchiya, A. (2005) Orphan drugs and the NHS: Should we value rarity? *British Medical Journal*, 331(7523): 1016–19.

McDonald, R. (2002) *Using Health Economics in Health Services, Rationing Rationally?* Maidenhead: Open University Press.

McDonald, R., Burrill, P. and Walley, T. (2001) Managing the entry of new medicines in the National Health Service: Health authority experiences and prospects for primary care groups and trusts. *Health and Social Care in the Community*, 9(6): 341–47.

Martin, D., Pater, J. and Singer, P. (2001). Priority setting decisions for new cancer drugs: A qualitative case study. *Lancet*, 358: 1676–81.

Mayor, S. (2005) NICE to issue faster guidance on use of drugs by NHS. *British Medical Journal*, 331: 1101.

Oliver, A., Mossialos, E. and Robinson, R. (2004) Health technology assessment and its influence on health-care priority setting. *International Journal of Technology Assessment in Health Care*, 20(1): 1–10.

Orvain, J., Xerri, B. and Matillon, Y. (2004) Overview of health technology assessment in France. *International Journal of Technology Assessment in Health Care*, 20(1): 25–34.

Rutten, F. (2004) Health technology assessment and policy from the economic perspective. *International Journal of Technology Assessment in Health Care*, 20(1): 71–6.

Sampietro-Colom, L., Semberg, V., Estrada, D., Asplund, K., Barrington, R., Faisst, K. et al. (2002) European joint assessments and coordination of findings and resources. *International Journal of Technology Assessment in Health Care*, 18(2): 321–60.

Schubert, F. (2002) Health technology assessment – the pharmaceutical industry perspective. *International Journal of Technology Assessment in Health Care*, 18(2): 184–91.

Sheldon, T.A., Cullum, N., Dawson, D., Lankshear, A., Lowson, K., Watt, I., West, P., Wright, D. and Wright, J. (2004) What's the evidence that NICE guidance has been implemented? Results from a national evaluation using time series analysis, audit of patients' notes, and interviews. *British Medical Journal*, 329(7473): 999–1003.

So, J., Scarffe, J. H., Rous, E. and Foy, R. (2000) Lack of funding will inhibit evidence-based commissioning of cancer treatments. *British Medical Journal*, 320: 54.

Stevens, A. and Milne, R. (2004) Health technology assessment in England and Wales. *International Journal of Technology Assessment in Health Care*, 20(1): 11–24.

Ten Have, (2004) Ethical perspectives on health technology assessment. *International Journal of Technology Assessment in Health Care*, 20(1): 71–6.

Webster, A. (2004) Health technology assessment: A sociological commentary on reflexive innovation. *International Journal of Technology Assessment in Health Care*, 20(1): 1–6.

Websites and resources

Canadian Coordinating Office for Health Technology Assessment (CCOHTA). A primary source for unbiased, evidence-based information on drugs, devices, healthcare systems and best practices. CCOHTA is funded by Canadian federal, provincial and territorial governments. Provides access to free HTA reports and provides a history of CCOHTA as well as information on its processes. Sites from many other countries can be easily found by visiting the INAHTA website: *https://www.ccohta.ca/entry_e.html*

National Institute for Health and Clinical Excellence (NICE). The independent organisation responsible for providing national guidance on the promotion of good health and the prevention and treatment of ill health: Provides details of technology appraisals, clinical guidance, the NICE Citizens' Council and minutes of NICE committee and board meetings amongst other things: *http://www.nice.org.uk/*

NHS Health Technology Assessment Programme. Aims to ensure that high quality research information on the costs, effectiveness and broader impact of health technologies is produced in the most effective way for those who use, manage and provide care in the NHS. HTA reports can be downloaded free from its website: *http://www.ncchta.org/*

International Network of Agencies for Health Technology Assessment (INAHTA). Its mission is to provide a forum for the identification and pursuit of interests common to health technology assessment agencies. Membership since 1993 has grown to 41 member agencies from 21 countries. The network stretches from North and Latin America to Europe, Australia, and New Zealand and its website provides links to member websites around the world: *http://www.inahta.org/inahta_web/index.asp*

6 Health and well-being: the wider context for healthcare management

Ann Mahon

Introduction

This chapter looks at the social and cultural context within which health and illness are defined and experienced by people in different cultures and countries around the world. It also considers what strategies to improve health and prevent or treat illness and disease have been developed and implemented. It begins with an exploration of how health, illness and disease are defined and how such definitions influence health and illness behaviours. Patterns of health and illness across different countries and between different socio-economic groups are described and explanations for the existence of inequalities in health are also explored. The contribution of formalised systems of healthcare is thus set in context and the implications of this for public policy now and in the future are discussed. The final section of this chapter summarises some of the implications of the issues raised for the role of healthcare managers.

Definitions of health and illness

Health is an elusive concept. There is no single, definitive and objective definition of health and well-being. In recent decades there has been increasing recognition that definitions of health, illness and disease are constructed and experienced within the social, cultural, political and economic contexts within which people live their daily lives. Dubos, for example, argues:

> Health and disease cannot be defined merely in terms of anatomical, physiological or mental attributes. Their real measure is the ability of the individual to function in a manner acceptable to himself and to the group of which he is part. (Dubos 1987: 261)

This social or 'holistic' perspective contrasts with what has come to be known as the 'medical model', whereby medical knowledge is seen as based on a universal and generalisable science. This is in contrast to lay knowledge derived from 'unscientific' folk knowledge or individual experience. Mildred Blaxter argues that this dichotomy, set between biomedical, scientific models of healthcare and looser more holistic models – sometimes referred to as 'medical' and 'non-medical' perspectives – does not reflect reality and in practice an intermixing is inevitable. First, lay people have been taught to think in biomedical terms and second 'holistic' concepts are also a part of medical philosophy (Blaxter 1990). Cecil Helman (2001), an anthropologist and a general practitioner in the UK, looked at the relationship between medical and lay or folk beliefs surrounding health and illness. His focus was on the impact of health education, television programmes and increased access to healthcare on folk beliefs. His findings suggested that folk beliefs about illness and healthcare not only survive the impact of scientific medicine but in some cases may even be perpetuated by this contact. He argues that doctors do not or cannot differentiate between bacteria and viruses and so neither do their patients. The distinction is reinforced through, for example, overprescribing of antibiotics in general and particularly for viral illnesses. It strengthens the lay view that all germs are bad and similar in nature. Helman concludes that in the UK free access to health and medicine does not seem to have altered some of the traditional folk beliefs about health and illness – medical concepts like the germ theory of disease whilst being widely known to the lay public may be understood in an entirely different way and often in terms of a much older folk view of illness (Helman 2001).

Kleinman (1985) identified three sectors found in any modern healthcare system. These are the professional sector, the folk sector and the popular sector. The professional sector consists of professional scientific 'western' medicine and also professionalised indigenous healing traditions such as chiropractic and acupuncture. The folk sector represents non-professionalised healing specialists. The popular or lay sector comprises wellness activities performed in the family and community context. Given that most illness in all countries and cultures is managed (at least in the early stages) outside of formalised systems of healthcare (Kleinman's professional sector), conceptions of health and illness and how people manage their health and illnesses are of particular significance. For decades numerous epidemiological enquiries have estimated the proportion of symptoms presented to the professional sector (Wadsworth et al. 1971; Dunnell and Cartwright 1972). More recently Hughner and Kleine cite evidence that suggests between 70% and 90% of sickness is managed solely within in the lay domain in western society (Hughner and Kleine 2004).

Blaxter's (1990) work describes how the way in which health is conceived differs over the life course. Young men tend to speak of health in terms of physical strength and fitness. Young women think in terms of energy, vitality and the ability to cope. In middle age concepts of health become more complex with older people thinking in terms of function as well as ideas about contentment and happiness.

It is common for the terms 'illness' and 'disease' to be used interchangeably and for health to be viewed in simple terms as the absence of illness or disease. By looking more closely at how terms are defined we gain greater understanding of the social context of health and illness. The way lay people think about health and wellness influences their health and wellness-related behaviours – in other words what we do or do not do to become or remain healthy and how we interpret and respond to symptoms of illness. There has been a lot of research into lay people's understanding of health – most of it in the 1970s and 1980s and much of it based in the UK and USA. Typically these studies have looked at how health and illness are defined according to age, gender, specific disease categories, social class and ethnicity. Hughner and Kleine (2004) attempted to integrate and synthesise this research and identified 18 themes (set out in Table 6.1) that fall into four categories. The four categories are definitions of health (themes 1–5), explanations for health (themes 6–13), external and/or uncontrollable factors impinging on health (themes 14–16) and the place health occupies in people's lives (themes 17–18). Hughner and Kleine (2004: 397) conclude that popular worldviews about health and wellness are 'complex interweavings of information drawn from different sources including lay knowledge, folk beliefs, experiences, religious and spiritual practices and philosophy'.

More recently, particularly in those countries with indigenous populations such as New Zealand, Australia, Canada, India and others, there has been an increased recognition and acceptance of how indigenous peoples define health. For example, the 1999 Declaration on the Health and Survival of Indigenous Peoples proposed the following definition of indigenous health:

> Indigenous peoples' concept of health and survival is both a collective and an individual inter-generational continuum encompassing a holistic perspective incorporating four distinct shared dimensions of life. These dimensions are the spiritual, the intellectual, physical and emotional. Linking these four fundamental dimensions, health and survival manifests itself on multiple levels where the past, present and future co-exists simultaneously. (Durie 2003a: 510)

Healthcare changes and develops at an increasingly fast pace. The rise in 'alternative' therapies, changes in technological interventions and access to information about health and health-related issues, particularly through the internet, are inter alia likely to be having an impact on health and illness beliefs and behaviours. How these and other changes are influencing definitions and experiences of health and illness provide a fertile area for future research.

It is outside the scope of this chapter to give a comprehensive and critical account of studies conducted in different countries and cultures. Nevertheless it can be argued from this perspective that the 'medical model' is severely limited. Health is more than the absence of disease. Our

Table 6.1 Lay views of health: themes and associated statements

Theme	Example statement
Definitions of health	
1 Health is the absence of illness	'If I am not sick (for example, running a fever). I generally consider myself healthy.'
2 Health is functional ability	'As long as I am able to carry out my daily functions (e.g. going to work, taking care of the household) I consider myself healthy.'
3 Health is equilibrium	'The mind, body and spirit are all connected; all need to be in sync for good health.'
4 Health is freedom	'Good health is freedom; with it comes the ability to do what I want to do, to live how I want to live.'
5 Health is constraining	'Good health is constraining; with it individuals have to conform to the demands of society.'
Explanations for health	
6 Health through meditation or prayer	'Health and wellness can be maintained through meditation or prayer.'
7 Health is dependent upon mental attitude	'The power of a positive outlook or attitude can prevent sickness.'
8 Health through working	'As long as I keep going, I tend not to get sick – keeping busy doesn't allow one to have the time to get sick.'
9 Religious and supernatural explanations	'God works in mysterious ways; health and sickness is part of the divine plan.'
10 Health maintained through rituals	'The use of certain rituals is helpful in the maintenance of health (for example, reciting a prayer or psalm).'
11 Health is a moral responsibility	'I have a responsibility to my family to maintain my health.'
12 Health is maintained through internal monitoring	'I believe visiting a medical doctor for regular check-ups is important to maintain good health.'
13 Self-blame	'Many people suffer illnesses caused by their own bad habits.'
External uncontrollable factors	
14 Health as policy and institutions	'I believe good health is in part the product of governmental institutions that ensure the health of citizens.'
15 Modern way of life	'Many diseases of modern life result from the stressful and polluted environment in which we live.'
16 Health is genetics	'Often getting sick just happens and little can be done about it.'
Place of health in life	
17 The value and priority placed on health	'I have more important goals in my life than the pursuit of optimal health.'
18 Disparity between health beliefs and behaviours	'I know a lot about how to keep healthy (e.g. which type of eating and activity behaviours are considered healthy); however I often do not practice this health knowledge.'

Source: Hughner and Kleine (2004: 419).

beliefs about what causes our health influence our beliefs about how to behave when ill. Health beliefs interact with health behaviours, which has major implications for the relationship between health and healthcare organisations. The implications of the findings from studies of health and illness behaviour suggest that we need to rethink aspects of healthcare delivery, health education and health promotion and the role of not-for-profit organisations and communities.

Patterns of health and illness

There are both similarities and differences in the patterns of health, illness and disease across different countries and between different socio-economic and cultural groups within countries. Typically, health and illness are measured by three main indicators: those that measure life expectancy, mortality and morbidity. Tables 6.2 to 6.7 present a range of health and illness indicators for 15 World Health Organisation (WHO) member states. Life expectancy and the probability of dying under the age of 5 and between the ages of 15 and 60 are presented in Table 6.2. Death rates for all causes of death and then broken down to three major causal categories – communicable diseases, non-communicable diseases and injuries – are given in Table 6.3. A more detailed breakdown of death rates relating to each major causal category is given in Tables 6.4, 6.5 and 6.6. Finally, Table 6.7 presents data on performance relating to the achievement of WHO millennium development goals for each of the 15 selected countries.

The data shown in the tables illustrate the following:

1 Health inequalities between countries exist for all measures and disease categories.
2 There are considerable differences between countries in life expect-ancy at birth ranging from 50.7 years for South Africans to 80.4 years for Australians. A child born in a western European country or the USA is ten times less likely to die before the age of 5 years than a child born in India.
3 Across all countries women live longer than men, although the gap between men and women is smaller for some countries than for others.
4 The stage of economic, social and political development in countries is reflected in their patterns of health and illness. The populations of poor countries and those in political conflict have lower life expectancy and greater probability of dying prematurely.
5 The relative burden of the three major diseases categories varies con-siderably between different countries. Poorer developing countries continue to suffer high death rates from infectious diseases whilst richer countries have experienced the epidemiological transition from infectious diseases to the non-communicable chronic diseases.

Whilst these data illustrate the patterns of health and illness between

Table 6.2 Basic indicators for a selection of WHO member states, 2002

Member state and population (000)	Life expectancy at birth (years, both sexes)	Life expectancy at birth (males)	Life expectancy at birth (females)	Probability of dying (per 1000) under 5 years of age (males)	Probability of dying (per 1000) under 5 years of age (females)	Probability of dying (per 1000) 15–60 years of age (males)	Probability of dying (per 1000) 15–60 years of age (females)
Australia (19,544)	80.4	77.9	83	6	5	91	52
China (1,302,307)	71.1	69.6	72.7	31	41	165	104
Cuba (11,271)	77.1	75	79.3	8	7	138	89
France (59,850)	79.8	76	83.6	6	4	135	60
Germany (82,414)	78.7	75.6	81.6	5	4	118	60
Guatemala (12,036)	65.9	63.1	69	57	50	283	162
India (1,049,549)	61	60.1	62	87	95	291	220
Indonesia (217,131)	66.4	64.9	67.9	45	36	244	208
Netherlands (16,067)	78.6	76	81.1	6	5	94	65
New Zealand (3,846)	78.9	76.6	81.2	7	6	98	63
Papua New Guinea (5,586)	59.8	58.4	61.5	98	92	311	249
South Africa (44,759)	50.7	48.8	52.6	86	81	598	482
Sweden (8,867)	80.4	78	82.6	4	3	83	53
UK (59,068)	78.2	75.8	80.5	7	6	107	67
USA (291,038)	77.3	74.6	79.8	9	7	140	83

Source: Data drawn from *www.who.int/* healthcare info/ World Health Organisation health statistics and health information systems: death and DALY estimates for 2002 by cause for WHO member states.

Table 6.3   Estimated deaths per 100,000 by cause of death for selected WHO member states, 2002

Member state and population (000)	All causes of death	Communicable diseases[1]	Non-communicable diseases[2]	Injuries[3]
Australia (19,544)	647.6	28.1	578.7	40.7
China (1,302,307)	701.5	83.7	541.4	76.3
Cuba (11,271)	680.5	71.9	546.3	62.3
France (59,850)	833.8	52.9	712.2	68.7
Germany (82,414)	989.4	42.5	907.7	39.1
Guatemala (12,036)	680.7	338.8	271.0	71
India (1,049,549)	988.8	401.9	486.9	100
Indonesia (217,131)	748.9	219.5	453.9	75.4
Netherlands (16,067)	867.5	66.5	770.3	30.6
New Zealand (3,846)	710.7	23.5	647.4	39.9
Papua New Guinea (5,586)	836.5	435.9	321.4	79.1
South Africa (44,759)	1518.8	987.9	424.2	106.7
Sweden (8,867)	1027.2	51.2	929.4	46.5
UK (59,068)	1014.7	123.3	858.4	33
USA (291,038)	831.7	50.9	728.3	52.5

[1] See Table 6.4 for a more detailed breakdown of disease categories/death rates within the communicable diseases category.
[2] See Table 6.5 for a more detailed breakdown of disease categories/death rates within the non-communicable diseases category.
[3] See Table 6.6 for a more detailed breakdown of disease categories/death rates within the injuries category.
Source: Data drawn from *www.who.int/* healthcare info/ World Health Organisation health statistics and health information systems: death and DALY estimates for 2002 by cause for WHO member states.

different countries, they conceal the considerable inequalities between different socio-economic, cultural and ethnic groups within countries. This is well documented in the UK and other European countries in terms of social class or social status where it has become common to talk about the 'social gradient' present in health and illness data where the

Table 6.4 Estimated deaths per 100,000 by communicable, maternal, perinatal and nutritional causes for a selection of WHO member states, 2002

Member state and population (000)	Infectious and parasitic diseases	Respiratory infections	Maternal conditions	Peri-natal condition	Nutritional deficiencies	All communicable, maternal, peri-natal and nutritional conditions
Australia (19,544)	9.2	14.3	0.1	3.4	1.2	28.1
China (1,302,307)	39	22.4	0.8	20.9	0.6	83.7
Cuba (11,271)	7.9	59.2	0.5	3.6	0.7	71.9
France (59,850)	13	32.5	0.1	2.8	4.5	52.9
Germany (82,414)	14.3	25.4	0.1	2.0	0.9	42.5
Guatemala (12,036)	230.8	48.9	7.3	34.8	16.9	338.8
India (1,049,549)	197.3	107.0	12.7	72.6	12.3	401.9
Indonesia (217,131)	122	49	4.8	33.7	10.1	219.5
Netherlands (16,067)	11.8	50.2	0.1	2.7	1.8	66.5
New Zealand (3,846)	4.2	15.3	0.1	3.3	0.6	23.5
Papua New Guinea (5,586)	248.7	64.5	8.6	84.6	29.6	435.9
South Africa (44,759)	898.5[1]	53.5	5.6	18.2	12.6	987.9
Sweden (8,867)	12.4	35.4	0.0	1.2	2.1	51.2
UK (59,068)	8.2	110.8	0.1	3.4	0.8	123.3
USA (291,038)	22.1	20.6	0.2	5.5	2.5	50.9

[1] HIV/AIDS accounts for 794 of the 898.5 deaths in this category in South Africa.
Source: Data drawn from *www.who.int/* healthcare info/ World Health Organisation health statistics and health information systems: death and DALY estimates for 2002 by cause for WHO member states.

poorest and most deprived groups experience the poorest health while the more affluent members of society experience both better social and environmental conditions and better health status on a range of indicators.

In New Zealand, Australia, India, Canada and other countries with indigenous populations, national data conceal the poorer health status of

Table 6.5 Estimated deaths per 100,000 by non-communicable diseases for a selection of WHO member states, 2002

Member state and population (000)	Malignant and other neoplasms	Diabetes mellitus and endocrine disorders	Neuro-psychiatric Disorder	Sense organ disease	Cardiovascular and respiratory	Other	All non-communicable diseases
Australia (19,544)	190.6	23.6	38.1	0.0	281.3	45	578.7
China (1,302,307)	134.7	12	8.0	0	340.5	46.2	541.4
Cuba (11,271)	159.9	16	24.9	0.1	304.7	40.9	546.3
France (59,850)	247.5	32.9	62.1	0.1	300	69.5	712.2
Germany (82,414)	271	29.7	29.9	0.0	508.9	68.1	907.7
Guatemala (12,036)	44.1	21.9	17.0	0.2	141.7	46	271.0
India (1,049,549)	72.2	16.4	17.4	0.1	325.8	55.1	486.9
Indonesia (217,131)	87.7	26.2	16.3	0.1	266.4	57.2	453.9
Netherlands (16,067)	255.5	29.6	53.9	0.0	365.1	66.2	770.3
New Zealand (3,846)	198.4	30.5	41.2	0.0	338.4	38.8	647.4
Papua New Guinea (5,586)	50.9	15.4	9.9	0.1	188.8	56.4	321.4
South Africa (44,759)	87.1	32	15.3	0	243.8	45.9	424.2
Sweden (8,867)	248	27.6	77.9	0	514.4	61.7	929.4
UK (59,068)	260.6	17.6	45.2	0	459.7	75.4	858.4
USA (291,038)	197.1	37	53	0	379.7	61.3	728.3

Source: Data drawn from *www.who.int/* healthcare info/World Health Organisation health statistics and health information systems: death and DALY estimates for 2002 by cause for WHO member states.

Table 6.6 Estimated deaths per 100,000 by injuries for a selection of WHO member states, 2002

Member state and population (000)	Road traffic accidents	Other non-intentional injuries	Self-inflicted injuries	Violence	War	All causes of injuries
Australia (19,544)	8.6	19.3	11.3	1.5	0	40.7
China (1,302,307)	19.2	33.1	20.9	3.0	0	76.3
Cuba (11,271)	13.1	28.7	15.2	5.3	0	62.3
France (59,850)	13.9	38.2	15.9	0.7	0	68.7
Germany (82,414)	8.6	15.9	13.9	0.7	0	39.1
Guatemala (12,036)	6.5	24.9	2.3	37.1	0	71.0
India (1,049,549)	18	58.2	17.4	5.5	0.5	100
Indonesia (217,131)	23.9	26.7	11.3	9.4	3.8	75.4
Netherlands (16,067)	6.4	14.2	8.9	1.1	0	30.6
New Zealand (3,846)	12.7	13.8	12.2	1.2	0	39.9
Papua New Guinea (5,586)	15.3	37.8	10	15.6	0	79.1
South Africa (44,759)	30.3	22.7	10.5	43.2	0	106.7
Sweden (8,867)	6.3	26.4	12.8	1.0	0	46.5
UK (59,068)	6.5	17	8.5	1.1	0	33.0
USA (291,038)	15.5	21.1	10.3	5.4	0	52.5

Source: Data drawn from *www.who.int/* healthcare info/ World Health Organisation health statistics and health information systems: death and DALY estimates for 2002 by cause for WHO member states.

their indigenous people. There are 350 million indigenous people representing over 5000 cultures in 70 countries on every continent (Smith 2003). The gap in life expectancy between indigenous and non-indigenous populations is estimated to be a staggering 19 to 21 years in Australia, 8 years in New Zealand, 5 to 7 years in Canada and 4 to 5 years in the United States (Ring and Brown 2003). Although indigenous peoples tend to have higher mortality right across the disease spectrum, much of the excess arises from non-communicable chronic diseases. In all four countries cited above cardiovascular and respiratory diseases and

Table 6.7   Millennium development goals: selected health indicators for selected WHO member states, 2000

Member state and population (000)	Children under 5 years of age under-weight for age	One-year-olds immunised against measles	Maternal mortality ratio	HIV prevalence among 15–49-year-olds	Tuberculosis mortality rates	Population with sustainable access to an improved water source	
	%	%	(per 100 000 live births)	%	(per 100 000)	% Urban	Rural
Australia (19,544)	0	93	6	0.1	0	100	100
China (1,302,307)	10	79	56	<0.1	21	93.7	66.1
Cuba (11,271)	3.9	99	33	<0.1	1	99	95
France (59,850)	N/A	84	17	0.3	2	N/A	N/A
Germany (82,414)	N/A	89	9	0.1	1	N/A	N/A
Guatemala (12,036)	24.2	91	240	1.0	13	98	88
India (1,049,549)	46.7	56	540	0.8	41	95	79
Indonesia (217,131)	27.3	76	230	<0.1	67	90	69
Netherlands (16,067)	0.7	96	16	0.2	1	100	100
New Zealand (3,846)	N/A	85	7	0.1	1	100	N/A
Papua New Guinea (5,586)	29.9	58	300	0.3	57	88	32
South Africa (44,759)	9.2	72	230	19.6	46	99	73
Sweden (8,867)	N/A	94	8	<0.1	1	100	100
UK (59,068)	1.3	85	11	0.1	1	100	100
USA (291,038)	1.4	91	14	0.6	0	100	100

Source: Data drawn from *www.who.int/* healthcare info/ World Health Organisation health statistics and health information systems: death and DALY estimates for 2002 by cause for WHO member states.

endocrine illnesses (mainly diabetes) and neoplasm account for most of the excess deaths among indigenous people. These conditions collectively account for 70% or more of excess mortality in indigenous people. This is significant because of the avoidable nature of much chronic disease (Ring and Brown 2003). Indigenous populations generally have a lower life expectancy than non-indigenous populations, a higher incidence of most diseases including diabetes, mental disorders and cancers and experience third world diseases like TB and rheumatic fever in developed countries (Durie 2003a). Although the standards of health of indigenous peoples show differences, similarities exist in worldviews, patterns of disease, health determinants and healthcare strategies (Durie 2003a). It is nevertheless important to recognise that there has been a substantial narrowing of the gap in health between indigenous and non-indigenous people although the evidence suggests that in Australia the gap is widening (Ring and Brown 2003).

How can these patterns of health and illness be explained? How can the relationship between where we live, how long we live for and the quality of our lives be explained? The next section looks at the factors that determine health.

The determinants of health

A number of different perspectives can be employed to explain inequalities in health. Historical and cultural analyses will shed light on the history surrounding the health status of a population or a social group. See, for example, Friedrich Engels on the social and economic conditions of Victorian England and Mason Durie on the experiences of Maori in New Zealand (Engels 1999; Durie 1994, 2003a, 2003b). Political, sociological, biological and genetics explanations will yield different explanations.

Compared to many other countries the UK has a strong tradition of producing robust data over time to describe patterns of inequalities and these data have been compiled in a number of high-profile sources over many decades. However, the evidence in relation to why these patterns exist is less robust and raises political questions about the relative roles and responsibilities of individuals, families, the community and society and the state (Baggott 2000). The authors of the UK Black Report describe four theoretical explanations of the relationship between health and inequality. These are artefact explanations, theories of natural/social selection, materialist/structuralist explanations and cultural/behavioural explanations. They conclude that the most significant causes are those relating to materialist/structuralist explanations and base their recommendations for action on this perspective (Townsend and Davidson 1982). Durie argues that explanations for current indigenous health status can be grouped into four main propositions: genetic vulnerability, socio-economic disadvantage, resource alienation and political oppression. All four propositions can be conceptualised as a causal continuum. Short–distance factors at one end (such as the impact of abnormal cellular processes) and at the other end long–distance factors such as government polices. Midway factors include values and lifestyles (Durie 2003a).

Wilkinson and Marmot (2003) focus upon the social determinants of health that affect populations and distinguish this perspective from the role that individual factors such as genetic susceptibility play in health and illness. The key social factors, a brief summary of the evidence base and the implications of this for public policy, based on Wilkinson and Marmot, is presented in Table 6.8. The research evidence for the summaries of 'what is known' and the 'policy implications' are fully sourced in the original publication, which is available on the European Public Health Alliance (EPHA) website (see useful websites at the end of this chapter). The relative influence of these factors is influenced by economic and political factors:

> Economic growth and improvements in housing brought with them the epidemiological transition from infectious to chronic diseases – including heart disease, stroke and cancer. With it came a nutritional transition when diets, particularly in Western Europe change to over consumption of energy dense fats and sugars producing more obesity. (Wilkinson and Marmot 2003: 26)

Given the evidence for the important role of social factors in determining health, what role should or could formalised healthcare systems play?

The contribution of healthcare to health status: healthcare in perspective

Until the 1970s it was commonly assumed that the improvements in health experienced in many countries during the last century had occurred as a consequence of advances in medical care. Marmot and Wilkinson's work summarises the evidence demonstrating that the health of people, patients and populations is influenced by many factors that exist outside of formalised systems of healthcare (Wilkinson and Marmot 2003). The amount of money spent on healthcare, measured by the proportion of GDP spent on health (see Table 6.9) within a system is not in itself a direct and causal contributor to the health profile of the nation.

During the 1970s there was a fundamental change in western societies' attitudes to medicine and the 'self–evident' efficacy of medicine. The validity of medical knowledge has also been increasingly challenged. These challenges came from a number of sources both within and outside of medicine (Cochrane 1972; Illich 1977a, 1977b; Kennedy 1983, McKeown 1979). However, some recent publications have suggested the need for a reappraisal of the role of medical and heathcare (Bunker 2001 and Nolte and McKee 2004; Craig et al. 2006). As Craig (2006: 1) states: 'The idea that successfully changing society and the environment will

Table 6.8   The social determinants of health

What is known: key points	*Policy implications*
Health inequalities • Poor social and economic circumstances affect health status from birth to old age. • Differences between social and economic groups exist for most disease categories and causes of death. • The effects upon health accumulate during the life cycle.	• Policy should address social and economic circumstances in policy areas such as housing and minimum wages. • Critical transitions in life – for example, starting school and moving from primary to secondary school – can affect health and should be the focus of policy interventions.
Stress • Poor social and psychological circumstances can cause long-term stress. • Anxiety, insecurity, low self-esteem and social isolation affect health status due to the physiological effects of stress on the immune and cardiovascular system.	• As well as managing the biological changes associated with stress attention should be focused 'upstream', i.e. on the causes and not just on the effects. • The quality of the social environment and material security in schools, workplaces and the wider community are important.
Early life • Infant experience is important to later health for biological, social and psychological reasons. • Insecure emotional attachment and poor stimulation can lead to low educational attainment and problem behaviour. • Slow or retarded physical growth in infancy is associated with reduced cardiovascular, respiratory, pancreatic and kidney development and function, which increase the risk of illness in adulthood.	• Improved preventive healthcare before the first pregnancy and for mothers and babies in pre- and postnatal services and through improvements in the educational levels of parents and children. • Policies for improving health in early life should aim to increase the general level of education, provide good nutrition, health education and health and preventive care facilities and adequate social and economic resources before and during pregnancy and in infancy and support parent–child relationships.
Social exclusion • Poverty, relative deprivation and social exclusion have a major impact on health and premature death. • The unemployed, many ethnic minority groups, guest workers, disabled people, refugees and homeless people are at particular risk of both absolute poverty (a lack of the basic material necessities of life) and relative poverty (being much poorer than most people in society).	• All citizens should be protected by minimum incomes guarantees, minimum wages legislation and access to services. • Interventions to reduce poverty and social exclusion at both the individual and the neighbourhood levels. • Legislation can help protect minority vulnerable groups from discrimination and social exclusion. • Public health policies should remove barriers to health and social care, social services and affordable housing. • Labour market, education and family welfare policies should aim to reduce social stratification.

Table 6.8   continued

What is known: key points	*Policy implications*
Work	
• In general having a job is better for health than having no job.	• Improved conditions at work will lead to a healthier workforce, which will lead to greater productivity.
• Stress at work plays an important role in contributing to inequalities in health, sickness absence and premature death.	• Appropriate involvement in decision making is likely to benefit employees at all levels of an organisations.
• Health also suffers if people have little opportunity to use their skills and low decision-making authority.	• Good management involves ensuring appropriate rewards (money, status and self-esteem).
• The psychosocial environment at work is an important determinant of health and contributor to the social gradient in ill health.	• Workplace protection includes legal controls and workplace healthcare.
Unemployment	
• High rates of unemployment cause more illness and premature death. Unemployed people and their families suffer a substantially increased risk of premature death.	• Policy should aim to prevent unemployment and job insecurity; to reduce the hardship suffered by the unemployed and to restore people to secure jobs.
• The health effects of unemployment are linked to psychological and financial consequences.	
• Job insecurity has been shown to increase effects on mental health, self-reported ill health and heart disease.	
Social support	
• Social support provides people with emotional and practical resources.	• Good social relations can reduce the physiological response to stress.
• Supportive relationships may also encourage healthier behaviour patterns.	• Reducing socio-economic inequalities can lead to greater social cohesiveness and better standards of health.
• Social isolation and exclusion are associated with increased rate of premature death and poorer chances of survival after a heart attack.	• Improving the social environment in schools, at work and in the community will help people feel valued and supported.
• The amount of emotional and practical social support people get varies by social and economic status.	• Designing facilities to encourage meeting and social interaction in communities could improve mental health.
• Social cohesion (quality of social relationships, trust and respect in wider society) helps to protect people and their health.	• Practices that treat some groups as socially inferior or less valuable should be avoided, as they are socially divisive.
Addiction	
• Drug use is both a response to social breakdown and an important factor in worsening the resulting inequalities in health.	• Support and treatment of addictions.
	• Address underlying social deprivation.
• Alcohol dependence, illicit drug use and cigarette smoking are all closely associated with social and economic disadvantage.	• Regulate availability of drugs.
	• Health education about less harmful forms of administration.
	• The broad framework of social and economic policy must support effective drug policy.

Table 6.8   continued

What is known: key points	Policy implications
Food • A good diet and adequate food supply are central for promoting health and well-being. • A shortage of food and lack of variety cause malnutrition and deficiency diseases. • Excessive intake of food is also a form of malnutrition – obesity contributes to a number of diseases including cardiovascular disease, diabetes, and cancer. • More deprived people are more likely to be obese. In many countries the poor substitute cheaper processed foods for fresh foods. Dietary goals to prevent chronic diseases emphasise eating more fresh vegetables, fruits and pulses and more minimally processed starchy foods but less animal fat, refined sugars and salt.	• Local, national and international government agencies, non-governmental organisations and the food industry should ensure: • The integration of public health perspectives into the food system to provide affordable and nutritious fresh food, especially for the most vulnerable. • Democratic, transparent decisionmaking and accountability in all food regulation matters. • Support for sustainable agriculture. • A stronger food culture for health, for example, through school education.
Transport • Healthy transport means less driving and more walking and cycling supported by better public transport systems. • Cycling, walking and using public transport provide exercise, reduce fatal accidents, increase social contact and reduce air pollution.	• Improve public transport and change incentives to encourage use of public transport. • Encourage cycling.

Source: Wilkinson and Marmot (2003).

result in improved health is uncontentious. However, it does not follow that healthcare has little role to play.'

Access to appropriate, acceptable and good quality healthcare is an important contributor to health and this is the case across all social and ethnic groups. Even where this is demonstrated, there is not a direct relationship between the availability of effective healthcare and health because of inequalities in access where those in greatest need of healthcare have least access (Tudor-Hart 1971). Wilkinson and Marmot suggest:

> Health policy was once thought to be about little more than the provision and funding of medical care: the social determinants of health were discussed only amongst academics. This is now changing. While medical care can prolong survival and improve prognosis after some serious diseases, more important for the health of the population as a whole are the social and economic conditions that make people ill and in need of medical care in the first place. Nevertheless, universal access to medical care is clearly one of the social determinants of health. (Wilkinson and Marmot 2003: 7)

Table 6.9 Expenditure on health for a selection of WHO member states

Member state and population (000)	Total expenditure on health as a proportion of GDP				
	1997	*1998*	*1999*	*2000*	*2001*
Australia (19,544)	8.5	8.6	8.7	8.9	9.2
China (1,302,307)	4.6	4.8	5.1	5.3	5.5
Cuba (11,271)	6.6	6.6	7.1	7.1	7.2
France (59,850)	9.4	9.3	9.3	9.4	9.6
Germany (82,414)	10.7	10.6	10.7	10.6	10.8
Guatemala (12,036)	3.8	4.4	4.7	4.7	4.8
India (1,049,549)	5.3	5	5.2	5.1	5.1
Indonesia (217,131)	2.4	2.5	2.6	2.7	2.4
Netherlands (16,067)	8.2	8.6	8.7	8.6	8.9
New Zealand (3,846)	7.5	7.9	8	8	8.3
Papua New Guinea (5,586)	3.1	3.8	4.2	4.3	4.4
South Africa (44,759)	9	8.7	8.8	8.7	8.6
Sweden (8,867)	8.2	8.3	8.4	8.4	8.7
UK (59,068)	6.8	6.9	7.2	7.3	7.6
USA (291,038)	13	13	13	13.1	13.9

Many healthcare systems across the world have made fundamental changes to the management and delivery of healthcare in attempts to reduce inequalities in both health status and access to health services. Space prohibits a systematic or comprehensive review here. However, to illustrate a range of strategies in different settings, examples from selected countries in Europe and from countries addressing the health status of indigenous people will be given.

Addressing health inequalities: examples of European experiences

In an analysis of policy developments on health inequalities in different European countries, Mackenbach and Bakker (2003) found that countries are in widely different phases of awareness of and willingness to take action on inequalities in health. Their international comparisons suggest that the UK is ahead of continental Europe in developing and implementing policies to reduce socio-economic inequalities in health and is 'on the brink of entering a stage of comprehensive, coordinated policy'. They identified factors that supported or inhibited action on inequalities, including the availability of descriptive data, the presence or absence of political will and the role of international agencies such as WHO. Innovative approaches were identified in five main areas: policy steering mechanisms, labour market and working conditions, consumption and health-related behaviour, healthcare and territorial approaches:

1 *Policy steering mechanisms* such as quantitative policy targets and health inequalities impact assessment. In the Netherlands, for example, quantitative policy targets were set for the reduction of inequalities in 11 intermediate outcomes including poverty, smoking and working conditions.
2 *Labour market and working conditions* can be addressed universally or in a targeted approach. An example of a universal approach comes from France where occupational health services offer annual check-ups and preventive interventions to all employees. An example of a targeted approach is job rotation among dustmen in the Netherlands.
3 *Consumption and health-related behaviour.* Again universal and targeted approaches are identified. In the UK women on low income are targeted using multi-method interventions to reduce smoking. In Finland a universal approach is adopted by serving low-fat food products through mass catering in schools and workplaces.
4 *Healthcare.* Examples of innovative practices here include working with other agencies. In the UK, for example, there are community strategies led by local government agencies but integrating care across all the local public sector services.
5 *Territorial approaches* include comprehensive strategies for deprived areas such as the health action zones in the UK (Mackenbach and Bakker 2003).

Although there were some similarities, for example, the UK, Netherlands and Sweden have comprehensive strategies to reduce inequalities informed by national advisory committees, their analysis found considerable variations in approaches which they suggest is a symptom of intuitive as opposed to rigorous evidence-based approaches to policymaking. They conclude: 'Further international exchanges of experiences with development, implementation and evaluation of policies and interventions to reduce health inequalities can help to enhance learning speed' (Mackenbach and Bakker 2003: 1409).

Addressing the health status of indigenous peoples

Mason Durie identifies two broad directions for improving health services for indigenous health in New Zealand – increasing the responsiveness of conventional services and establishing dedicated indigenous
programmes. In New Zealand both these approaches are endorsed in
legislation and government health policy. Section 8 of the New Zealand
Public Health and Disability Act (2000) requires health services to
recognise the principles of the Treaty of Waitangi – the 1840 agreement
that saw sovereignty exchanged for Crown protection (Durie 2003b).
The New Zealand strategy is broad in its approach, seeking to influence
macro policies such as labour market policies, public health population
approaches to health and personal health services. In this respect it is
consistent with the Maori holistic approach to health and intersectoral
determinants of health.

Indigenous health services provide a range of healing methods, including conventional professional services and traditional healing. Durie
argues that their most significant contribution is improved access to
health services for indigenous people, enabling earlier intervention, ener-
getic outreach, higher levels of compliance and a greater sense of community participation and ownership. Indigenous services tend to be built
around indigenous philosophies, aspirations, social networks and economic realities (Durie 2003b). For Durie coexistence of conventional
and indigenous healthcare is not problematic:

> While there is some debate about which approach is likely to pro-
> duce the best results, in practice conventional services and indigen-
> ous services can exist comfortably together. More pertinent is the
> type of service that is going to be most beneficial to meet a particu-
> lar need. In general indigenous health services are more convincing
> at the level of primary health care. Higher rates of childhood
> immunisation, for example seem to be possible with services that are
> closely linked to indigenous networks, and early intervention is
> embraced with greater enthusiasm when offered by indigenous pro-
> viders. (Durie 2003b: 409)

The importance of partnership and collaborative working is identified as
a crucial component for success:

> Conventional health services and indigenous services need, however
> to work together within a collaborative framework. Clinical acu-
> men will be sharpened by cultural knowledge and community
> endeavours will be strengthened by access to professional expertise.
> It makes sense to build health networks that encourage synergies
> between agencies, even when philosophies differ. (Durie 2003b:
> 409)

Devadasan et al. (2003) describe an initiative working with tribes in
India where a health system specifically targeted at tribal people had a

remarkable impact on infant and maternal mortality. Over 10 to 15 years immunisation coverage increased from 2% to over 75%. Use of hospital services was three times the national average in a population that initially refused to go to hospital because 'only dead spirits circulate there'. They identified the main features that characterised the success of this initiative:

- It was nested within larger development services, such as agriculture, education and housing.
- It was owned by the people. From the beginning tribal communities participated in planning and implementing the scheme. Most of the staff were from the tribal community.

The health system was developed with the worldview of the tribal community in mind. For example, initially the hospital did not have beds as patients found it more comfortable to sleep on mats on the floor (Devadasan et al. 2003).

The role of healthcare managers

The strategies increasingly being adopted by many countries are broad public policies in recognition that progress in health depends on a wide range of social determinants, in addition to individual susceptibility to specific illnesses. Strategies are therefore broad and the proximity of interventions to specific illness in individuals may not be apparent. Managers and professionals must recognise the importance of partnership working and collaborative working and communicate the relevance of these strategies to health. The emphasis placed on the importance of intersectoral gains and partnership working highlights the need for effective, evidence-based mechanisms for achieving this. The evidence supporting the effectiveness of health service interventions needs to be better understood by managers, healthcare professionals, the public health community and individual users of services. At the same time the relevance of interventions outside the health service such as welfare reforms, agricultural polices and pollution control needs to be understood by the same key stakeholders. Change requires cultural changes within the healthcare workforce and organisation but also a recognition and acceptance of the significance of culture to definitions and experiences of health and illness.

To meet the challenge of implementing broad-based public policies, the development of an appropriate and effective workforce is essential. A number of developments are apparent here ranging from joint appointments between local government and healthcare organisations for the public health workforce in the UK (Fotaki et al. 2004) to New Zealand where the development of the workforce is a common theme in the development of indigenous health. The similarities and contrasts between different countries suggest the value to be had from sharing good practice and developing research through international links.

Conclusion

This chapter has argued that health is much more than the absence of disease by providing evidence in support of the WHO's (1946) definition of health: 'Health is a state of complete physical, mental and social well-being and not merely the absence of disease or infirmity.' The responsibility for health and healthcare extends beyond formalised systems of healthcare. Nevertheless the role of healthcare and healthcare managers is crucial in ensuring access to healthcare interventions that improve the health of their populations alongside wider public policies that address the social determinants of health:

> The evidence that health is determined by social, environmental and economic influences throughout a person's life is not at issue. What is lacking is secure evidence that many broad public health interventions are effective. Priority must be given to addressing this lack of evidence. In the meantime, instead of polarized positions, an appropriate balance needs to be struck between the contrasting strategies of developing health services and intervening outside the health system. (Craig et al. 2006: 1)

Summary box

- Definitions of health and illness are the product of the complex interaction of the individual with cultural, social and political factors within their environment.
- The relative burden of the three major disease categories varies considerably between different countries. Poorer developing countries continue to suffer high death rates from infectious diseases whilst richer countries have experienced the epidemiological transition from infectious diseases to the non-communicable chronic diseases.
- Routine data conceal considerable inequalities between different socio-economic, cultural and ethnic groups within countries.
- The key social factors determining health are inequalities in health, stress, early life, social exclusion, work, unemployment, social support, addiction, food and transport.
- Access to appropriate, acceptable and good quality healthcare is also an important determinant of health.
- The evidence supporting the effect of health services interventions needs to be better understood by managers, healthcare professionals, the public health community and individual users of services.
- Change requires cultural changes not only within the healthcare workforce and organisation but also a recognition and acceptance of the significance of culture to definitions and experiences of health and illness.

Self-test exercises

Describing and explaining inequalities in health

1 Using the data presented in Table 6.2, *describe the relationship* between sex and life expectancy for each country. What are the similarities and differences in this data for the 15 countries listed?

2 Why do women live longer than men? Using Wilkinson and Marmot's list of the ten social determinants of health, develop hypotheses about why women live longer than men.

3 Can (and if so how) the healthcare systems that you use or work in *influence* these facts?

Identifying innovative practice

1 Reflect on the public health policies being developed and implemented in your country. Can you identify innovative approaches in any of the five main areas identified by Mackenbach and Bakker (2003):

- policy steering mechanisms
- labour market and working conditions
- consumption and health-related behaviour
- healthcare
- territorial approaches?

2 Do you think that these policies have been developed through the application of rigorous evidence or are they a symptom of intuitive policymaking?

References

Baggott, R. (2000) *Public Health: Policy and Politics.* Basingstoke: Palgrave Macmillan.

Blaxter, M. (1990) *Health and Lifestyles.* London: Tavistock-Routledge.

Bunker, J.P. (2001) *Medicine Matters After All: Measuring the Benefits of Primary Care, a Healthy Lifestyle and a just Social Environment.* London: Nuffield Trust for Research and Policy Studies in Health Services.

Cochrane, A.L. (1972) *Effectiveness and Efficiency: Random Reflections on Health Services.* London: Nuffield Provincial Hospitals Trust.

Craig, N., Wright, B., Hanlon, P. and Galbraith, S. (2006) Does health care improve health? Editorial. *Journal of Health Services Research*, 11(1): 1–2.

Davey, B., Gray, A. and Seale, C. (eds) (2001) *Health and Disease: A Reader*, 3rd edn. Maidenhead: Open University Press.

Devadasan, N., Menon, S., Menon, N. and Devadasan, R. (2003) Use of health services by indigenous population can be improved. Letters. *British Medical Journal*, 327: 988.

Dubos, R. (1987) *Mirage of Health*. Rutgers: Rutgers University Press.

Dunnell, K. and Cartwright, A. (1972) *Medicine Takers, Prescribers and Hoarders*. London: Routledge and Kegan Paul.

Durie, M. (1994) *Whaiora: Maori health development*. Auckland, Oxford University Press.

Durie, M. (2003a) The health of indigenous peoples. *British Medical Journal*, 326: 510–11.

Durie, M. (2003b) Providing health services to indigenous peoples. *British Medical Journal*, 327: 408–9.

Engels, F. (1999) *The Condition of the Working Class in England*. Oxford: Oxford University Press.

Fotaki, M., Higgins, J. and Mahon, A. (2004) *The Development of the Public Health Role in Primary Care Trusts in the North West*. Manchester: Centre for Public Policy and Management, University of Manchester.

Helman, C. (2001) Feed a cold, starve a fever. In B. Davey, A. Gray, and S. Seale (eds) *Health and Disease: A Reader*, 3rd edn. Maidenhead: Open University Press.

Hughner, R.S. and Kleine, S.S. (2004) Views of health in the lay sector: A compilation and review of how individuals think about health. *Health*, 8(4): 395–422.

Illich, I. (1977a) *Disabling Professions*. London: Boyars.

Illich, I. (1977b) *Limits to Medicine: Medical Nemesis – the Expropriation of Health*. New York: Penguin.

Kennedy, I. (1983) *The Unmasking of Medicine: A Searching Look at Healthcare Today*. St Albans: Granada.

Kleinman, A. (1985) Indigenous systems of healing: Questions for professional, popular and folk care. In J. Salmon (ed.) *Alternative Medicines: Popular and Policy Perspectives*. London: Tavistock.

McDermott, R. et al. (2003) Sustaining better diabetes care in remote indigenous Australian communities. *British Medical Journal*, 327: 428–30.

Mackenbach, J.P. and Bakker, M.J. (2003) Tackling socio-economic inequalities in health: Analysis of European experiences. *The Lancet*, 362: 1409–14.

McKeown, T. (1979) *The Role of Medicine: Dream, Mirage or Nemesis?* Princeton: Princeton University Press.

Nolte, E. and McKee, M. (2004) *Does Healthcare Save Lives? Avoidable Mortality Revisited*. London: Nuffield Trust.

Ring, I. and Brown, N. (2003) The health status of indigenous peoples and others. *British Medical Journal*, 327: 404–5.

Smith, R. (2003) Learning from indigenous people. *British Medical Journal*, 327.

Townsend, P. and Davidson, N. (eds) (1982) *Inequalities in Health: The Black Report*. Harmondsworth: Penguin.

Tudor-Hart, J. (1971) The inverse care law. *The Lancet*, 1: 405–12.

Wadsworth, M., Butterfield, W.J.H. and Blaney, R. (1971) *Health and Sickness: The Choice of Treatment*. London: Tavistock.

Wilkinson, R. and Marmot, M. (eds) (2003) *Social Determinants of Health: The Solid Facts*, 2nd edn. Geneva: World Health Organisation.

World Health Organisation (WHO, 1946) Preamble to the Constitution of the World Health Organisation as adopted by the International Health Conference, New York, 19–22 June 1946; signed on 22 July 1946 by the representatives of 61 States (Official Records of the World Health Organization, 2: 100) and entered into force 7 April 1948.

www.who.int/ healthcare info/World Health Organisation Health statistics and health information systems: death and DALY estimates for 2002 by cause for WHO Member States (accessed 2 February 2006).

Websites and resources

Association of Public Health Observatories (APHO). Facilitates collaborative working of the Public Health Observatories (PHOs) and their equivalents in England, Wales, Scotland and Ireland. It provides a forum for disseminating good practice, sharing methodologies, co-ordinating action and providing a focus for links with national organisations: *www.apho.org.uk*

Department of Health. Provides detailed summaries of policies and good practice in addressing inequalities in health in the English NHS: *www.dh.gov.uk/PolicyAndGuidance/HealthAndSocialCareTopics/HealthInequalities/*

European Public Health Alliance (EPHA). Represents over 100 non-governmental and other not-for-profit organisations working in public health in Europe: *www.epha.org*

Part II
Managing healthcare organisations

7 Managing in primary care
Judith Smith

The defining moment in contemporary history of primary healthcare is generally considered to have been the declaration, at a World Health Organisation conference in 1978, of what primary healthcare should provide to people within communities and nations. This declaration, known as Alma Ata after the name of the town in the Russian Federation where the conference took place, sets out the following statements about the nature of primary healthcare:

> [Primary healthcare] . . . forms an integral part of both the country's health system of which it is the central function and the main focus of the overall social and economic development of the community. (WHO 1978: Section VI)

> Primary health care addresses the main health problems, providing preventive, curative, and rehabilitative services accordingly . . . but will include at least: promotion of proper nutrition and an adequate supply of safe water; basic sanitation; maternal and child care, including family planning; immunization against the major infectious diseases; education concerning basic health problems and the methods of preventing and controlling them; and appropriate treatment of common diseases and injuries. (WHO 1978: Section VII)

These definitions are striking in their holistic assessment of primary healthcare as being what Tarimo (1997) has termed an 'approach to health development', namely all those elements of care and community development that together enable people to lead healthy and meaningful lives. A view of primary healthcare as an approach to health development holds that it is central and foremost within a healthcare system, comprising all those activities and conditions that go towards ensuring the public health. 'Primary' therefore implies that this area of care is fundamental, essential and closest to people's everyday lives and experiences. The Alma Ata declaration goes on to call for countries of the world to address the structural causes of ill health and in this way the WHO declaration defines primary healthcare as a central part of a strategy for social action.

The Alma Ata conception of primary care as an approach to health development is striking in its difference from what is traditionally considered to be 'primary care' within many health systems, and particularly within countries in the more developed world where hospitals and more technical forms of care tend to dominate people's understanding of a health system. In these countries, primary care tends to be viewed as one part of the biomedical spectrum of health services provided to people who are ill, with primary care being the point of 'first contact' with the health system. Thus primary care is often viewed as what Tarimo has termed 'a level of care', in contrast to the broader understanding of primary healthcare as an approach to overall health development.

The work of Barbara Starfield draws together these two main conceptions of primary care, viewing primary care as a level in a healthcare system, but at the same time considering it to be crucial and central to that system and to the health of populations:

> . . . [Primary care is] that level of a health service system that provides entry into the system for all new needs and problems, provides person-focused (not disease-orientated) care over time, provides for all but very uncommon or unusual conditions, and co-ordinates or integrates care provided elsewhere by others. (Starfield 1998: 8–9)

Starfield sets out what she considers to be the four central features of effective primary care:

1 The point of first *contact* for all new needs.
2 Person-focused rather than disease-focused *continuous* care over time.
3 Providing *comprehensive* care for all needs that are common in the population.
4 *Coordinating* care for both those needs and for needs that are sufficiently uncommon to require special services.

These 'four Cs' are held by many commentators to define what is essential about primary care, and Starfield uses these dimensions as a way of assessing the degree of effectiveness of a country's primary care system. Indeed, Starfield's extensive research into the quality and nature of primary care in the international context has revealed a clear link between the strength of a country's primary care system (as measured against the four Cs) and the degree of cost effectiveness of that system, and more importantly, the level of health outcomes achieved for the population (Starfield 1998). Having ranked the primary care systems of twelve industrialised nations, Starfield (1998) noted that 'countries with a better primary care orientation tend to have better rankings on health indicators than countries with a poor primary care orientation' (p. 355).

Managing in primary care

Given the acknowledged importance of having a strong primary healthcare orientation to a health system, it is striking that relatively little has been written about the management (as opposed to the delivery) of primary care, particularly in comparison with the amount of analysis accorded to the management of hospital services. However, the management of primary care has in recent years been given greater prominence in both academic and practitioner communities, as people have increasingly come to view primary care as the main locus for seeking to improve health and control health system costs (e.g. Tarimo 1997; WHO Europe 1998; WHO 2002; Peckham and Exworthy 2003; Shi et al. 2003; Starfield et al. 2005). For example, in 1998, the WHO asserted:

> A more integrated health sector is needed, with a much stronger emphasis on primary care . . . Secondary and tertiary care, which are largely provided in hospital, should be clearly supportive to primary care, concentrating only on those diagnostic and therapeutic functions that cannot be performed well in primary care settings. (WHO Europe 1998, Target 15: 25).

The rationale for placing such a strong emphasis on primary care as the central function within a health system is that primary healthcare can play a particular role in improving people's health, and thus in preventing illness and the need for hospital and other medical care (see Chapter 6). In order to bring about this stronger health improvement element within a health system, it is acknowledged that primary care itself needs to be strengthened and developed, including the provision of a wider range of services in community settings outside hospitals and extending access to primary care for disadvantaged communities (Starfield 1998; Hefford et al. 2005; Starfield et al. 2005). A further role ascribed to primary care in some health systems, and one seen as being a lever to enable health improvement and primary care development, is that of primary care-led commissioning. This function, whereby primary care practitioners and organisations assume a role in the funding, planning and purchasing of healthcare on behalf of populations registered with local general practices, has been used most enthusiastically by state policymakers in England and by managed care insurers in the United States, and also in more limited ways in experiments with primary care budget holding in Sweden and New Zealand. Taken together, the use of primary care as a locus for health improvement, primary care development and service commissioning points to a general policy intention on the part of many governments to bring about a more primary care based health system. Such a system embodies the principles of Alma Ata and more recent interpretations of WHO and other international health policy, namely that health managers should seek to develop strong primary care as a way of bringing about improved public health and community well-being.

Thus we can identify the following four functions for the management of primary care:

- managing for health improvement
- managing for primary care service development
- managing for primary care led commissioning
- managing for a primary care based health system.

These functions reflect an increasing international trend towards viewing primary care as a part of the health system that can be used to manage and influence change in health and health services, one that has been coined 'managed primary care' (Smith and Goodwin 2006). These functions associated with the management of primary care are used here as the basis for exploring what is distinctive and important about managing in primary care.

Managing for health improvement

As noted above, a robust primary care system has been demonstrated as important to the delivery of good and equitable health outcomes (Starfield 1998). Shi et al. (2003) similarly assert that managing and improving primary care is a key strategy for policymakers seeking to reduce health inequalities but lacking the political power or mandate to influence factors outside the health sector. These authors point to evidence that an improvement in people's primary healthcare can, to some extent, act as a counterweight to health-damaging environmental conditions. Thus the point is made that the management and development of primary care is crucial to improving people's health, and in turn to the amelioration of some of the inequalities in health status that exist in most of not all countries. In order to identify the key areas for action by primary care managers seeking to manage for health improvement, Starfield's 'four Cs' provide a useful organising framework. These functions are set out in Box 7.1.

Box 7.1   Starfield's four Cs as an organising framework

1 Point of first contact – system of primary care gatekeeping, a single point of access to most services provided by the health system.
2 Person-focused continuous care over time – registration of patients with a single primary care practitioner or practice.
3 Comprehensive care for all common needs – multidisciplinary primary care and community health services that can assess, diagnose and treat common conditions.
4 Co-ordination of care provided elsewhere – role as the individual's advocate within and guide through the wider health system, including the guardian of overall patient information.

Source: Adapted from Starfield (1998).

Primary care 'gatekeeping' is considered by many researchers and analysts (Fry and Horder 1994; Starfield 1998; Peckham and Exworthy 2003; Wilson et al. 2006) as being crucial to the management of an effective health system, both in relation to cost and clinical effectiveness. What gatekeeping entails is the identification of a single point of access to the health system for most of the health needs that people experience and traditionally this has been a general practice staffed by family doctors and their teams. Within a system of primary care gatekeeping, patients cannot access hospital specialists or associated diagnostic services unless they have first consulted their family doctor. The strength of such a system is seen as being the ability of the family doctor to take a holistic view of a person's care, assuring only appropriate referrals to more specialist services, and thus avoiding unnecessary expensive and possibly invasive tests and care in hospital settings. Gatekeeping is a function typically associated with tax-funded health systems such as those in the UK, New Zealand, Denmark, Italy and Sweden. Critics of gatekeeping assert that it limits patients' rights and choices within a health system. Countries that have a strong libertarian tradition such as France, Israel and the United States typically baulk at the concept of limiting people's choice of point of access to care in this way, although for reasons of medical cost inflation all three of these countries have been experimenting with pilot projects of gatekeeping.

The *registration of patients* with a single practice or practitioner is viewed by public health practitioners and policymakers as being vital in relation to both individual and population health. For individuals, it is considered to enable the development of a long-term and continuous relationship between patient and family doctor (or doctors' practice), meaning that the doctor can have an overview of a person's medical history, firmly located within a knowledge and understanding of their broader social context, including family situation, employment status, housing provision, and education. For populations, a system of registration provides managers in a health system with a register of people that sets out key health data (e.g. age, sex, any chronic ill-health problems, family situation) and thus represents the basis for carrying out population-focused health interventions such as calls for health screening, immunisation campaigns, child health surveillance and health monitoring associated with specific age categories. The importance of a system of registration has been powerfully demonstrated by the recent experience of New Zealand, where the government has explicitly developed a Primary Health Care Strategy (Minister of Health 2001) that seeks, among other things, to develop a system of patient registration, and where, just a few years later, there is evidence that levels of access to care and health promotion services have shown a significant improvement from their previously low base in comparison with other developed countries (Hefford et al. 2005).

The provision of *comprehensive and multidisciplinary primary and community services* is a goal that is clearly set out in Alma Ata as being a key element in enabling effective primary healthcare. This underlines the

WHO vision of primary care as being the centre of a health system, and not the bottom of a pyramid of care as is often implied or asserted in management and clinical circles. The specific nature of comprehensive primary care differs both within and between countries, but typically entails a locally based practice or health centre that offers (or can easily refer to) community-based services such as:

- general practice (family medicine)
- primary care nursing
- public health nursing
- child health surveillance
- chronic disease management
- community mental health
- physiotherapy
- speech and language therapy
- community dietetics
- dentistry
- pharmacy.

Together with the role of gatekeeping and patient registration, comprehensive provision of services in a community setting is seen as a key element in supporting people in maintaining good health and managing much of their ill health and longer term conditions. Despite the common perception among the populations of many countries that a health system is synonymous with hospitals, the majority of people's healthcare takes place within primary care, at least in those countries where there is effective gatekeeping of the wider health system.

The role of *coordinating a person's care* within the health system is perhaps the most problematic function that is ascribed to 'ideal' primary care, given the ever more complex nature of healthcare interventions. For example, many approaches to chronic disease management are founded on the principle of a clinical professional taking responsibility for the coordination of care for an individual, this role encompassing needs assessment, monitoring of health, organisation of care and advocacy for the individual if admitted to hospital care. There is a body of research evidence that points to the difficulties in achieving effective coordination of care for people with complex needs (whether in community or hospital settings), and an analysis of the associated issues is set out in Chapter 17. Nevertheless, analysis of primary healthcare in the international context highlights primary care as the most appropriate location for the coordination of care for individuals, especially when combined with effective gatekeeping and patient registration (Starfield 1998).

When managing for health improvement, policymakers and managers face a dilemma in relation to how far they focus on the concerns and priorities of individual patients or citizens, and how far they address the health needs of the wider population. For example, a system of primary care gatekeeping enables cost-effective use of a nation's health resources, but compromises an individual's ability to choose their care provider. Similarly, the development of a system of individual care managers for people with long-term conditions may enable personal choice in care management, but could lead to fragmentation of overall care, unless there is careful integration of the activity of care managers within an overall local health plan. This patient/population tension is a further manifestation of Tarimo's two alternative approaches to understanding primary healthcare – as a level in the health system (that provides care to patients) or as an approach to health development (that seeks to improve public health). Others see this tension as an expression of the fact that two medical disciplines, general practice and public health, seek to own and manage what is typically understood as primary care. On the one hand, general practice traditionally sees its role as providing medical care for individual patients, whereas public health seeks to improve the health of whole populations.

One management and organisational solution to this patient/population tension in recent years has been the development of 'primary care organisations'; bodies that are set up to manage and develop primary care services in order to both improve population health and enable effective and high quality general practice provision (Ham 1996; Malcolm et al. 1999; Mays et al. 2001; Dowling and Glendinning 2003; Smith and Goodwin 2006). Primary care organisations are a specific manifestation of the move towards more managed primary care in a number of health systems, and represent a managerial solution to the dilemma of how to draw together often diverse and autonomous general practices and other community services into a coherent local plan for improving health. Further analysis of the role of primary care organisations is set out below.

Managing for primary care service development

The management of primary care service delivery and development continues to be, in many health systems, the most pressing and time-consuming challenge for primary care managers. This typically takes the form of planning, funding and managing two main areas of service delivery: general practice (family medicine) and associated services such as practice nursing and chronic disease care; and community health services including public health nursing, child health surveillance, continuing care of older people and health promotion. The relative importance of these two areas of primary care service provision varies between countries. For example, in Australia, general medical practice continues to represent the primary form of care provision outside of hospitals, albeit that there are moves towards greater use of community health teams incorporating nursing, physiotherapy and other allied health professions. In the UK, although general medical practice continues to feature in most people's mind as the first point of entry to the health system, in reality more and more primary care services are delivered directly by community nurses, public health nurses, community pharmacists and social care staff, even if these services are nominally or actually managed by a general practice.

At the other end of the spectrum, in some developing countries such as Tanzania community health workers or nurses form the backbone of the primary care system, acting as public health and health promotion advisers to local communities, signposting people towards medical and nursing services as and when they need them. In the context of the Alma Ata definition of primary healthcare, it can be argued that a community health approach to the provision of primary care, and based on strong public health nursing, is more appropriate to developing overall community health than a system based on medical practice. However, general medical practice has dominated the provision of primary care in many industrialised countries and the challenge for managers is how they can make a system of general practice work in such a way that it achieves wider public and community health goals.

General medical practice is often organised on the basis of independent self-employed doctors working in small groups (or singly), and contracting with local health authorities to provide services to a registered local population. This system operates in the UK, Netherlands, Denmark and Canada. In other countries, doctors similarly work in independent practices but levy fees directly from patients who can in some cases seek reimbursement of fees from their state or private health insurance. General practitioners levy fees from patients in countries such as New Zealand, France and the USA. The practice-based system of primary care is not confined to general medical practice, but is also commonly found in community dentistry, optometry and pharmacy.

A system of independent practice in primary care poses a range of challenges to those seeking to manage primary care service delivery and development. There is a fundamental decision for a health system to make in respect of how it will structure its relationship with general practice and thus seek to bring about change with that part of the health sector. Options available for managing the relationship between the health system and general practice include the following:

- Managing through *a system of contracts* between the health system and individual general practices or practitioners, thus using financial incentives and/or quality indicators as a way of bringing about desired changes to services (e.g. UK, Danish and Australian general practice).
- Letting a *market* develop whereby fee-paying patients (or their insurers) choose their practice or practitioner, and services are developed in response to patient (or insurer) demand, and prices regulated largely by the market (e.g. traditional New Zealand general practice, French general practice, US family medicine).
- Providing centrally run (by the state or by insurance organisations) *primary care centres* with salaried doctors and associated staff, with standards and services defined by the state or insurer (e.g. Swedish health centres, US managed care organisations, Netherlands sickness fund health centres).
- Developing *primary care organisations* as intermediary bodies that seek to influence primary care provision using options such as letting contracts with providers of services; making specific payments to practices

or others develop or extend services; establishing specialised services; shifting resource from other parts of the health system in order to facilitate service development in primary care (e.g. English primary care trusts, New Zealand primary health organisations, Australian divisions of general practice, Welsh local health boards).

• Establishing other non-governmental organisational forms such as *community or social enterprises* as a vehicle for developing and providing care in innovative ways that are appropriate to specific population groups, in particular those traditionally excluded from general practice (e.g. New Zealand by Maori for Maori, or Pasifika healthcare organisations; community health enterprise organisations in the UK; US care organisations for people with long-term conditions).

The choice as to how to structure the relationship between the health system and primary care providers is likely to involve multiple and 'blended' solutions as a means of influencing the behaviour of practitioners (Gosden et al. 2001). In health systems that are increasingly complex, and with more and more patients living to an older age and with long-term conditions, managers need to find solutions that not only assure the development of primary care services for different groups of the population, but also ensure the achievement of wider health system goals. In addition to the structuring of the relationship with primary care as set out above, they may also seek to use other tools in developing primary care services including: the establishment of new community health centres that provide a wide range of health and social care for local communities; walk-in assessment centres for emergency primary care; telephone or internet based advice services; and out-of-hours care centres that involve paramedic, nursing, general practice and perhaps hospital emergency room practitioners.

What is clear is that health systems are increasingly seeking to coordinate and manage a diverse range of providers of primary care, trying at once to develop and improve primary care services whilst improving the public health. This poses specific management challenges, including assuring the quality of services provided to patients and the public, delivering value for money for taxpayers and insurers, enabling continuity and coordination of care for individuals and their carers, and finding ways of developing a workforce for current and future community health services. These management challenges are now finding their way into the health strategies of many countries, with primary care being seen as a key element in wider health plans. Examples of countries that are taking a more primary health care focused approach to strategy development include New Zealand with its Primary Health Care Strategy, Wales and Northern Ireland with their clearly public-health oriented plans for national health, and Australia with its investment in developing primary care organisations. At an international level, the WHO continues to press for a stronger primary healthcare orientation to health systems, and for the development of primary care to be seen as the heart and not periphery of a healthy care system.

Managing for primary care led commissioning

Primary care led commissioning (or purchasing as it is often known) is a key management function at the disposal of primary care managers and has been defined as follows:

> Commissioning led by primary health care clinicians, particularly GPs, using their accumulated knowledge of their patients' needs and of the performance of services, together with their experience as agents for their patients and control over resources, to direct the health needs assessment, service specification and quality standard setting stages in the commissioning process in order to improve the quality and efficiency of health services used by their patients. (Smith et al. 2004: 5)

In other words, it concerns the use of primary care practices or organisations for the planning and funding (or purchasing through the placing of contracts) of health services for a defined population (e.g. a practice or locality population). Primary care led commissioning typically takes the form of a total or partial delegated budget that is managed by GPs, nurses and primary care managers, with the intention of using this resource as a means of buying services that will support the achievement of local (and often national) primary care development and health improvement goals. In this way, it offers a further tool for primary care managers seeking to both develop primary care and improve health. Its particular potential is considered to be the ability for primary care budget holders to redesign health services in such a way that they are refocused on community and primary care, with less of a reliance on hospital care.

Primary care led commissioning is an area of primary care management that is regarded as a key feature of some health systems, whilst being eschewed or not even considered in others. The English NHS is the system that has most consistently held faith with primary care led commissioning, seeking to use primary care practices and organisations as the main location for the planning and purchasing of health services. Other countries that continue to pursue or have experimented with primary care purchasing or budget holding include New Zealand (independent practitioner associations and community-governed organisations); Australia (divisions of general practice); United States (independent practice associations, health maintenance organisations); Sweden and Estonia (GP budget holding); Scotland, Wales and Northern Ireland (GP fundholding in the 1990s).

There is a significant base of research evidence concerning the management challenge primary care led commissioning, particularly in relation to the process of implementing and developing such approaches. An analysis of this evidence base points to the following factors known to facilitate effective primary care led commissioning, as set out in Box 7.2.

Where some or all of the above conditions are met, research evidence suggests that a health system is likely to experience: demonstrable improvements in the delivery of primary and intermediate care services;

> **Box 7.2 Factors facilitating effective primary care led commissioning**
>
> - Stability in the organisation of healthcare, especially the structure of commissioning bodies.
> - Sufficient time to enable clinicians to become engaged, and strategies for commissioning to be developed and implemented.
> - Policy that supports offering patients and commissioners a choice of providers.
> - Policy that enables resources to be shifted between providers and services.
> - A local service configuration that enables commissioners to choose between providers.
> - A local primary care system that is sufficiently developed to provide additional services.
> - Incentives that engage general practitioners and practices in seeking to develop new forms of care across the primary–secondary care interface.
> - Effective management and information support for practice-based commissioners.
> - Appropriate regulation to minimise conflicts of interest arising from general practitioners being both commissioners and providers.
>
> *Source:* Smith et al. (2005: 1398).

some marginal changes to the quality and responsiveness of secondary care; greater engagement of doctors, nurses and other professionals in the planning and funding of care; and a stronger overall primary care orientation in the health system (Smith et al. 2004). There will, however, remain some apparently intractable problems for managers of primary care including: trying to make a significant or strategic impact on the delivery of secondary and tertiary (i.e. hospital) services; shifting resource from hospital to community settings; and reshaping the pattern of delivery of emergency and unscheduled care (Smith et al. 2004). These challenges (as witnessed in Chapter 12) are not unique to primary care led approaches to commissioning, and are faced by planners and funders of care in almost all health systems. They are, however, significant for managers of primary care who, in their attempts to improve the quality and range of primary care services as part of an overall attempt to develop the public health, might consider primary care led commissioning as a tool in their armoury. What is clear is that primary care led commissioning has real and evidence-based potential as a means of developing primary care (and thus, over time, in enabling improvements to health as envisaged by Starfield and others), but that it remains to be proven as to whether it can play a significant role in more widescale redesign of health services across health systems.

Managing for a primary care based health system: what are the main challenges?

In line with WHO policy, many countries seek to develop less of a sickness and more of a health focused system, based on strong primary healthcare. In so doing, they espouse the research of Starfield, Shi and others that advocates strong primary care as a vital prerequisite for improved health outcomes that are achieved in a manner that is cost effective for overall health systems. Whilst the WHO's assertion of primary care as the centre of a health system, with secondary care playing an important (but essentially secondary in both senses of the word) role, can seem somewhat idealistic, there is international evidence of countries seeking to redress the balance of health funding, activity and management effort away from hospital care in favour of primary care. For example, the New Zealand Ministry of Health is embarked on the implementation of an ambitious primary healthcare strategy that is the main focus of current financial investment in health in that country and that has the aims set out in Box 7.3.

Box 7.3   Aims of primary healthcare strategy, New Zealand

- To work with local communities and enrolled populations.
- To identify and remove health inequalities.
- To offer access to comprehensive services to improve, maintain and restore people's health.
- To co-ordinate care across service areas.
- To develop the primary healthcare workforce.
- Continuously to improve quality using good information.

Source: Minister of Health (2001: vii).

Similarly, the Welsh Assembly has specified the strengthening and development of family health services as a key health priority, including improvements to community health services and the extension of availability of free eye care and prescriptions along with other public health measures (Welsh Assembly Government 2005). The policy being pursued in Wales is strikingly more primary care focused than that of its neighbour England where improvements in access to secondary care services have been the main focus of policy and management attention in recent years (DH 2000). These examples indicate the possibility of countries adopting a specific policy focus on primary healthcare (in its widest Alma Ata sense) as the guiding framework for health policy. As can be seen in both cases, the management response to such a policy direction requires a range of tools and approaches including: the use of health improvement goals and activities that aim to reduce health inequalities; the development of policies directed at improving primary care services (use of incentives for practices and practitioners, establishing contracts for services, establishment of new forms of service); and a commitment to shift resource from elsewhere in the system to support improvements to primary care. Primary care led commissioning is not being used to any significant extent in New Zealand and Wales, but research evidence would suggest that it has the potential to further incentivise improvements to and extensions in the range of services provided outside of hospitals, as is believed by English policymakers who are introducing a policy of 'practice-based commissioning' (DH 2004) as a way of engaging GPs in wider health system goals and in the hope that this will result in improved management of the demand for secondary care services (Smith et al. 2005).

The major challenges faced by those seeking to manage primary care are therefore those related to the two dimensions of primary care that were considered at the start of this chapter – namely trying to improve the relative strength and power of primary care within the health system and thus realise its potential as an approach to health development (Tarimo 1997). Primary care, although being targeted as an area for specific policy and management attention in many health systems, typically remains the poor relation in respect of attracting significant investment, particularly in comparison with the power of large hospitals that attract political and public visibility and support. There are many reasons for this disparity, including the somewhat diffuse and networked nature of primary care providers in comparison with the institutional power and status of hospitals. Likewise, GPs have traditionally been perceived to wield less power within health systems compared with hospital specialists, mainly on account of their commonly held status as self-employed business people working in small groups or as individuals, whilst specialists operate in larger clinical teams. There are, however, significant potential health and cost effectiveness gains to be made if health systems can become more primary care focused. This is even more the case in the context of rising incidence of chronic disease in developed countries, and infectious diseases such as HIV/AIDS and malaria in developing countries (see Chapter 6), for these public health trends are particularly amenable to primary healthcare solutions. However, if the potential of primary care based approaches to health policy and management are to be realised by those with the power to influence resource allocation and future policy development, managers need to have in place robust measures that can demonstrate the degree to which more managed primary care can deliver improvements to both primary care itself and to the wider public health (Box 7.4).

Conclusion

For managers in primary care, as has been demonstrated, the main challenges relate to how they can act in order to improve health, develop primary and community care, enable primary care led commissioning,

---

Box 7.4   The main challenges for managing in primary care

* Putting in place an effective system of primary care gatekeeping.
* Ensuring the registration of the public for primary care and public health purposes.
* Developing primary care provision that is comprehensive and multidisciplinary in nature.
* Having a clear primary care based co-ordination function for individual patients being cared for elsewhere in the health and social care system.
* Developing an appropriate balance between the provision of family medicine (general practice) and community health services.
* Working out the appropriate blend of approaches and techniques for managing the relationship between general practice and the wider health system.
* Determining the degree to which primary care led commissioning or budget holding is relevant to the wider achievement of primary care and public health goals.
* Working to ensure that system-wide strategy is primary care focused.
* Seeking to strengthen the overall position and power of primary care within the health system.
* Having measures in place that can demonstrate progress towards the achievement of primary care and public health goals.

---

and thus have a more clearly primary care based health system. In so doing, they need to find ways of meeting the main challenges of managing in primary care.

Summary box

* Primary healthcare is concerned with enabling and improving healthy communities and societies.
* In many countries, however, primary healthcare has been seen as synonymous with first contact care in the healthcare system and with general practice in particular.
* Primary healthcare is fundamental to both healthcare and health improvement, and the existence of a strong primary care orientation in a health system has been shown to improve health outcomes and cost effectiveness.
* The management of primary care is increasingly receiving policy and research attention, in particular with reference to improving health, developing primary care services and as a basis for commissioning services elsewhere in the health system.
* In managing primary care for health improvement, key functions include the development of effective gatekeeping, patient registration and care coordination.
* In managing primary care for the development of primary and community services, there is a balance to be struck between the emphasis on family medicine and community health services.

- The management of the relationship between a health system and family medicine is crucial for primary care managers and can be achieved through various means including the use of contracts, financial incentives, and the development of primary care organisations.
- Primary care led commissioning is a management function used by some primary care managers as a means of developing primary care and increasing overall primary care influence within a health system.
- Ultimately, the main challenge for the management of primary care is to increase its influence in a health system in relation to the power and resources of hospital services.
- If this shift in influence can be achieved, primary healthcare can become a route to improving health and developing stronger and more sustainable communities.

Self-test exercises

1 Make an assessment of your own country's health system in relation to its degree of primary care orientation according to Starfield's 'four Cs'. In so doing, assess on a scale of 1–10 (where 1 = not at all, and 10 = completely) your health system's

- degree of gatekeeping in primary care
- extent of primary care and public health registration
- provision of comprehensive primary care and community health services
- ability to provide primary care focused coordination of care for individuals.

2 Make the same assessment for the health system of another country with which you are familiar through personal experience or your studies. How do the two countries' health systems compare in respect of primary care orientation?

3 Find out how these same two countries compare in relation to health outcomes data and cost effectiveness of the overall health system. Is there any relationship between what you have observed in relation to primary care orientation and system health and cost outcomes?

References and further reading

Department of Health (DH, 2000) *The NHS Plan. A Plan for Investment, A Plan for Reform*. London: The Stationery Office.

Department of Health (DH, 2004) *Practice Based Commissioning: Promoting Clinical Engagement*. London: Department of Health.

Dowling, B. and Glendinning, C. (eds) (2003) *The New Primary Care, Modern, Dependable, Successful*. Maidenhead: Open University Press.

Fry, J. and Horder, J. (1994) *Primary Health Care in an International Context.* London: Nuffield Provincial Hospitals Trust.

Gosden, T., Forland, F., Kristiansen, I., Sutton, M., Leese, B., Giuffrida, A., Sergison, M. and Pedersen, L. (2001) Impact of payment method on behaviour of primary care physicians: A systematic review. *Journal of Health Services Research and Policy*, 6(1): 44–55.

Ham, C. (1996) Population centred and patient focused purchasing: The UK experience. *Milbank Quarterly*, 74(2): 191–214.

Hefford, M., Crampton, P. and Macinko, J. (2005) Reducing health disparities through primary care reform: The New Zealand experiment. *Health Policy*, 72: 9–23.

Malcolm, L., Wright, L. and Barnett, P. (1999) *The Development of Primary Care Organizations in New Zealand: A Review Undertaken for Treasury and the Ministry of Health.* Lyttelton: Aotearoa Health.

Mays, N., Wyke, S., Malbon, G. and Goodwin, N. (eds) (2001) *The Purchasing of Health Care by Primary Care Organisations. An Evaluation and Guide to Future Policy.* Buckingham: Open University Press.

Minister of Health (2001) *The New Zealand Primary Health Care Strategy.* Wellington: Ministry of Health. *http://www.moh.govt.nz/*

Peckham, S. and Exworthy, M. (2003) *Primary Care in the UK – Policy, Organisation and Management.* Basingstoke: Palgrave Macmillan.

Shi, L., Macinko, J., Starfield, B., Wulu, J., Regan, J. and Politzer, R. (2003) The relationship between primary care, income inequality and mortality in US states, 1980–1995. *Journal of the American Board of Family Practice*, 16(5): 412–22.

Smith, J.A. and Goodwin, N. (2006) *Towards Managed Primary Care: The Role and Experience of Primary Care Organizations.* Aldershot: Ashgate.

Smith, J.A., Mays, N., Dixon, J., Goodwin, N., Lewis, R., McLelland, S., McLeod, H. and Wyke, S. (2004) *A Review of the Effectiveness of Primary Care-Led Commissioning and its Place in the NHS.* London: Health Foundation.

Smith, J.A., Dixon, J., Mays, N., Goodwin, N., Lewis, R., McClelland, S., McLeod, H. and Wyke, S. (2005) Practice-based commissioning: Applying the evidence. *British Medical Journal*, 331: 1397–9.

Starfield, B. (1998) *Primary Care: Balancing Health Needs, Services and Technology.* Oxford: Oxford University Press

Starfield, B., Shi, L. and Macinko, J. (2005) Contribution of primary care to health systems and health. *Milbank Quarterly*, 83: 457–502.

Tarimo, E. (1997) *Primary Health Care Concepts and Challenges in a Changing World – Alma-Ata Revisited.* Geneva: World Health Organisation.

Welsh Assembly Government (2005) *Designed for Life: Creating World Class Health and Social Care for Wales in the 21st Century.* Cardiff: Welsh Assembly Government.

Wilson, T., Roland, M. and Ham, C. (2006) The contribution of general practice and the general practitioner to NHS patients. *Journal of the Royal Society of Medicine*, 99: 24–8.

World Health Organisation (WHO, 1978) *Declaration of Alma Ata.* Geneva: WHO.

World Health Organisation (WHO, 2002) *Innovative Care for Chronic Conditions: Building Blocks for Action.* Geneva: WHO.

World Health Organisation Regional Office for Europe (1998) *Health 21 – An Introduction to the Health for All Policy Framework for the WHO European Region.* Copenhagen: WHO.

Websites and resources

World Health Organization. *www.who.int/about/en*
World Health Organization European Regional Office. *www.euro.who.int/.*
Australian Primary Health Care Research Institute. *www.anu.edu.au/aphcri*
New Zealand Ministry of Health (see primary health care and PHOs pages). *www.moh.govt.nz*
Canadian Health Services Research Foundation (see primary healthcare policy pages). *www.chsrf.ca*
World Association of Family Doctors. *www.globalfamilydoctor.com/*
National Primary Care Research and Development Centre, Manchester. *www.npcrdc.man.ac.uk/*
King's Fund (see primary care policy pages). *www.kingsfund.org.uk*
Health Services Management Centre, Birmingham (see primary care pages). *www.bham.ac.uk/hsmc*

8 Managing in acute care

Dave Evans

Introduction

Managing in acute care can be complex and challenging. Perhaps the biggest test facing policymakers, clinicians and managers in modern acute care is to focus on providing just that part of the healthcare process which genuinely constitutes acute care, and to do so in an integrated way that connects effectively with primary care services and is focused on the needs of the individual patient.

This chapter first outlines the development of acute care, the issues and challenges of managing acute care provision and current developments within the acute care sector and the impact these will have for patients. It then reviews the development of acute care in three countries with very different systems for financing and providing healthcare: the United States, with its highly diverse and market-based healthcare system in which many innovations in acute care have been pioneered; the United Kingdom, with its state-financed and provided National Health Service in which acute services are rapidly changing; and the Czech Republic, which has transitioned from a state-run healthcare system to one based on the European model of social insurance, but still has a largely traditional acute care sector. The chapter concludes by exploring how the future development of acute care will shape healthcare systems and provision for patients.

Acute care services – the traditional approach, new forms and alternative models

Acute care usually means treatment for a short-term or episodic illness or health problem which a patient may often receive in hospital. Acute care embraces both emergency and elective or planned treatment for health problems that may arise through accident or trauma, or through the occurrence of disease. The defining characteristic of acute care has often been the place of delivery – in an acute hospital, with all the diagnostic facilities, inpatient accommodation and therapeutic paraphernalia that might be needed available in one place. But much of what such hospitals do is not necessarily acute care and much acute care can be delivered outside the hospital setting.

According to the World Health Organisation (WHO 2000), the conventional model of acute care based in hospitals has been in existence for a little over a century. Prior to this life expectancy was shorter, the curative capacity of medicine was more limited, and in a low technology society the majority of people would never have visited a hospital. As modern medicine developed during the twentieth century the hospital increasingly became the setting for the delivery of a growing proportion of healthcare services. Some services (for example, maternity care) moved into hospitals even though birth had been widely regarded as a normal process and had previously had been carried out at home with care provided by midwives. It could be argued that from a sociological perspective the rise of the secondary care sector, and of medically dominated hospitals especially, came about as a result of the increased organisation and political power and influence of the medical profession. It was certainly not the result of a deliberate process of strategic planning of the development of services provided in individual acute hospitals.

In most countries, the acute care sector now accounts for a majority of overall healthcare spending – for example, in the UK hospitals consume 55% of the NHS budget (DH 2005) – although most patients are cared for by primary care services and do not need or use hospital services. The cost pressures on acute care, through technological, demographic and other changes, are considerable, and the financial problems of many national healthcare systems are often rooted in the performance of the acute care sector.

Traditionally, the secondary care sector – hospitals – has been the foundation of acute care delivery, with hospitals serving local populations with a wide range of emergency and elective care across most medical and surgical specialities, on both an inpatient and outpatient basis. In the UK this model has its roots in the Dawson Report (1920) and it is a model used in most developed countries. The package of facilities at an acute hospital has included a wide range of diagnostic services, including radiology and pathology services, together with a range of interventional facilities including operating rooms, intervention/treatment rooms and associated inpatient beds being used for investigations. In effect the hospital-based acute care model has therefore been a mixture of acute care, routine investigations and chronic disease management

In the UK, since Enoch Powell's Hospital Plan of the early 1960s, the secondary care sector has been based around the concept of the district general hospital (DGH) – a hospital serving a local population of around 250,000 people, though in fact for reasons of geography and history the population actually served has ranged from 150,000 to 500,000 (West 1998). Whilst the DGH may not be a model that has been universally adopted, in most countries acute care is also provided in hospitals that serve the needs of a geographic local population. The typical hospital facility in most health systems provides a wide range of medical services including:

- emergency department
- general medicine
- care of older people (geriatric medicine)
- obstetrics
- gynaecology
- paediatrics
- general surgery
- critical care (including intensive care)
- trauma and orthopaedics.

These services are, of course, interdependent in many ways, with the ability of a DGH to maintain its emergency department, for example, dependent on the availability of services like general surgery, paediatrics and trauma and orthopaedics. This means that the withdrawal of one or two services in any DGH may threaten a cumulative disintegration of other services on which they were codependent. In addition, the secondary care sector has also provided many specialist services in areas like cancer care and cardiology. Some specialist services (such as neurosurgery, organ transplantation, specialist paediatric services, and so on) are often delivered through tertiary hospitals on a subregional, regional or even national basis. As the growing subspecialisation of medicine has created more and more specialties, each with distinctive staffing, skill and expertise requirements, the ability of DGHs to provide a full range of services has come under considerable pressure and the 'critical mass' of staff, beds, facilities and specialties deemed necessary for a DGH has expanded. In many areas, reconfigurations of acute care services and hospital mergers have been driven by these pressures to sustain the viability of acute care.

It can be argued that much of what has been seen as acute care, or more accurately much of what has traditionally been delivered by the secondary care sector, is not necessarily acute care and could be more appropriately delivered in other sectors, particularly in primary care, closer to the communities they serve (Black 2006). Additionally, it can be argued that by structuring the healthcare system into primary, secondary and tertiary care (as described in Chapter 3), policymakers, clinicians and managers have created artificial organisational and financial barriers that by their nature obstruct cross-sector and joint sector working, reduce the ability of the healthcare system to deliver seamless care for patients, make it more difficult for patients and the public to navigate and understand, and make it more difficult to innovate in the way acute services are delivered.

There has been a fundamental shift in many countries' economies over the past decade from central state control to more market based mechanisms, with a concomitant reduction in state intervention and control. That trend – evident in a wide range of public services – has resulted in the introduction and development of markets in healthcare in many countries. In place of direct state ownership of healthcare provision, and to sustain government's capacity to set health policy and to influence and shape the healthcare system, many countries have increasingly introduced regulatory and governance frameworks in their emerging healthcare markets. These changes present some new challenges for acute services operating in a competitive market regardless of how that market is configured and regulated. The market may be in commissioning (for example, the European social insurance model in the Netherlands, Germany and Switzerland) or in healthcare provision (for example, the UK NHS) or in both (as in the USA).

In recent years a number of developments have resulted in changes and challenges to the traditional secondary care hospital model, including:

- an increasing range and number of procedures being carried out on an ambulatory or daycase basis, and so no longer requiring the use of inpatient beds
- reductions in length of stay across all specialities in acute hospitals, meaning both that fewer inpatient beds are required and that the overall acuity of the inpatient mix has become more complex as convalescing patients are discharged earlier and earlier
- separation of emergency and elective care delivery so that elective services are not disrupted by emergency needs and can be run more efficiently
- increasing focus of commissioners (and users) on quality outcomes as information about the quality of care provided by hospitals has become more widely available
- a recognition that much of the demand for healthcare is predictable and that flow and process analysis tools used widely in other industries can be brought to bear in understanding patient flow in acute care and redesigning care processes
- a move away from the remuneration of acute care providers on a block or cost and volume contract basis, in which their funding is inflexible but secure, to payment systems based on actual levels of delivered activity, which give great incentives to increase activity and productivity and are both more flexible and less secure
- a rise in consumerism on the part of the public and patients, resulting in pressures on acute care providers to be more responsive to patient expectations about the way care is delivered
- developments in care models that do not require acute care beds or require fewer such beds, including intermediate care, rehabilitation services, chronic disease management, etc.
- recognition that care packages should be designed across the whole of the health system, not just around the acute care episode, resulting in the development of integrated delivery systems and disease management in some markets
- shortages of staff and skills in some professional groups, particularly doctors and nurses, which have resulted in changes to the way such

professionals are used in acute care and pressures to find new ways of working which make optimal use of scarce skilled staff
- an increasing regulatory framework focusing on clinical quality, in which acute care providers are held much more to account for the quality of care they deliver
- the move away from a health delivery system based on planning and assessed need to one that is more driven by markets, competition, and consumer demand.

The impact of these changes can be clearly seen in trends in the acute care sector over the last decade. For example, there have been marked increases in day case rates for elective care, reductions in numbers of acute beds, and a drop in the average length of stay in almost every OCED country. While acute care facilities and usage still vary very widely between countries, the trend almost everywhere is the same. For the OECD countries there has been an average reduction in length of stay of 2.1 days in the period 1992 to 2001 (see Figure 8.1) and a similar reduction in bed numbers (see Figure 8.2).

Acute care in the USA: pioneering change

The USA spends more per capita and as a proportion of GDP than any other OECD country on healthcare. This is despite a significant proportion of the population (around 17%) having no health insurance and so having at best very limited access to healthcare. The continually rising costs of healthcare in the USA over the last two decades have been one of the most important drivers of change in acute care provision – the most expensive part of the US healthcare system. Many of the acute care innovations now being adopted by healthcare systems in other OECD countries originated in the USA, and were a fruit of its constant search for ways to control healthcare costs.

The development of separate elective and emergency care facilities started in the USA in the early 1970s with the creation of the first Surgicentre to deliver routine elective care outside the traditional hospital. The underlying principle was that by separating elective care out of the acute hospital there would be increased efficiency. Over time this has coincided with the gradual increase in the number and range of procedures that can safely be carried out on a daycase basis due to changes in anaesthetics and the development of laparoscopic surgical techniques. There has been a significant growth in Surgicentres in the USA over the past 30 years and they now account for over 8 million operations a year, with over 4000 Surgicentres across the USA (FASA 2005). Surgicentres can be either single speciality or multi-speciality and are attractive to doctors and insurers. Doctors like them (and many are part or wholly owned by doctors), as they enable them to plan their workload and operate unencumbered by the potential delays in surgery due to

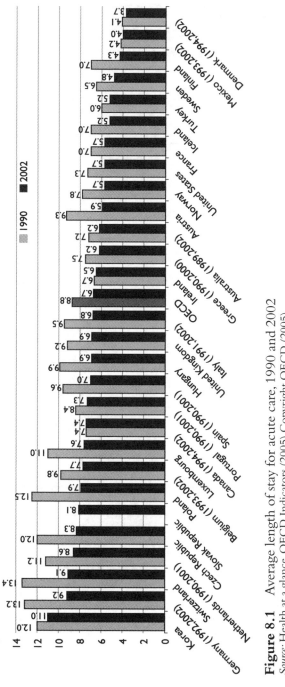

Figure 8.1 Average length of stay for acute care, 1990 and 2002
Source: Health at a glance, OECD Indicators (2005) Copyright OECD (2005).

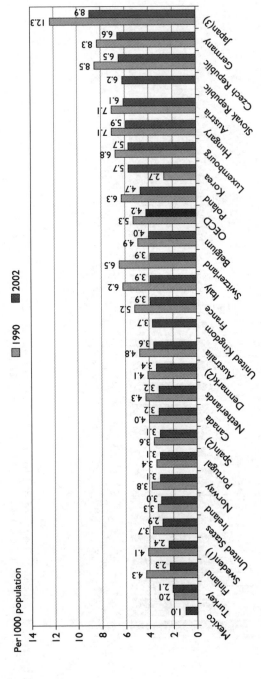

Figure 8.2 Acute care hospital beds per 1000 population, 1990 and 2002
Source: Health at a glance OECD Indicators (2005) Copyright OECD (2005).

emergencies. Insurance companies have favoured this approach as it means that high degrees of throughput and efficiency can be achieved and thus from a cost perspective care is cheaper than in a conventional acute hospital. According to FASA (2005) the average cost of an operation in a Surgicentre is 47% less than the cost at a traditional hospital. This is also an attractive option for self-paying patients.

Another development pioneered in the USA has been the creation of integrated care delivery systems across primary and secondary care, through managed care models used by health maintenance organisations (HMOs). The fundamental aims of these systems include reducing, as far as possible, admission to hospital. This can take a number of forms, including patient education and homecare programmes, particularly in relation to management of chronic disease. Increasingly these integrated systems are enabling greater numbers of patients to be treated away from the conventional hospital, which is more convenient for patients and reduces infrastructure costs over the long term in acute care facilities.

Kaiser Permanente is a not-for-profit health maintenance organisation based in California (but operating in a number of states). It is a very large organisation with over 8 million members (the majority of them in California) and both commissions and provides care (albeit as separate arms of the business) and directly employs all of the medical staff in Kaiser facilities. Both in terms of size and function therefore, Kaiser, it has been suggested, is not dissimilar to the NHS (Feachem et al. 2002). When direct comparisons are made, particularly in relation to acute care costs, performance and bed utilisation, Kaiser appears to perform significantly better than the NHS. Feachem et al. (2002) have argued that when a number of adjustments are made for different demographics, socio-economic factors, etc. there is little difference in costs (on a per capita basis) between the two systems. They found, however, that there were significant differences in a number of other areas, including length of stay within the acute hospital environment. Ham et al. (2003) have demonstrated that the NHS uses a significantly greater number of bed days than Kaiser, particularly for patients in the over-65 age group. Dixon et al. (2004) believe that in general terms there are lessons for the UK in how HMOs like Kaiser Permanente in the USA manage care and use a range of operational techniques to minimise hospital admissions. They also suggest that in HMOs clinicians are more involved managerially and that there is greater coherence between managers and clinicians in the way the organisation is run. In addition, there are often strong financial incentives to provide care in accordance with agreed guidelines or pathways. Whilst there has been some small-scale experimentation with fee for service models in the UK, it would appear from the US and elsewhere that giving clinicians financial incentives, either through ownership or other methods, helps to secure clinical engagement and change. The integrated delivery model that Kaiser Permanente and other HMOs use offers a number of advantages, both for patients and commissioners of services. With a shift in service away from the acute sector there has also been a shift in the provision of diagnostic services, particularly radiological investigations. Patients who are seen in a primary care setting will receive the majority of their diagnostic investigations outside an acute hospital, either in a primary care clinic setting or a freestanding imaging centre which offers a range of radiological investigations including magnetic resonance imaging, with some larger centres now offering PET scans. With increasing use of technology it is no longer necessary for radiologists to be on site to interpret images as this can be carried out at distance by telecommunication links. Similarly, if as a result of investigations patients require hospitalisation, the care they receive is very focused, ensuring that there are no delays in discharge to an alternative care setting as soon as practicable.

Acute care in the UK: the politics of change

The first point to note in reviewing acute care provision in the UK is that since the introduction of devolved administrations in Scotland, Wales and Northern Ireland, each of the four countries now essentially operate as four separate National Health Services, with different priorities and policies set by politicians and policymakers. Whilst this may mean that the approaches adopted may be different in each country, nevertheless the fundamental challenges are the same. There has been a year-on-year increase in numbers of emergency admissions – in England and Wales there has been a 10% increase in the two-year period 2002–3 to 2004–5 alone. In England, the traditional approach to rising numbers of emergency admissions (and in particular when a peak or surge of such admissions occurs) has been to cancel routine elective surgery, with emergency admissions taking priority when beds are short. This inevitably has led to delays in treatment for patients waiting for elective surgery and has impacted on waiting times for treatment. Increasingly, such delays for elective acute care have been seen as politically unacceptable.

As a result, policymakers in England (and to a lesser extent in Scotland) have started to separate significant elements of routine elective care into separate facilities, which are protected from emergency admissions. In England, this has taken the form of the Treatment Centre programme, the main driver of which initially was to create additional elective capacity in the NHS to cut waiting times for routine surgical procedures. This was usually for the procedures that traditionally had the longest waiting times and were most at risk of cancellation due to a lack of beds resulting from high numbers of emergency admissions. Borrowing heavily on the US Surgicentre model (although there are also influences from the central European polyclinic model), it was anticipated that the creation of a network of freestanding Treatment Centres would both help to reduce waiting times and encourage NHS acute care providers to learn to alter their processes for care delivery and to adopt the US ambulatory model, in which care is closely managed and changes in anaesthesia and pain management in particular enable a wide range of surgery to be carried out on a daycase basis. Subsequently, there has been a significant expansion of the Treatment Centre programme with significant investment in building and running treatment centres by the private sector in England. Ostensibly the rationale for this was expansion of elective capacity, of which there was a clear shortfall (NHS Plan 2000), but it has also served a wider policy purpose for the Labour government of creating plurality and contestability in acute services and opening up the NHS to a new market in elective care. Indeed, the government has made it clear that at least 15% of elective activity will be delivered by non-traditional providers in future.

However, the Treatment Centre programme is not the only element of reconfiguration that has been taking place in England. In the UK generally the debate on reconfiguring services has been advanced by the medical profession in the shape of the Royal College of Physicians, the Royal College of Surgeons and the British Medical Association which argued in 1998 that 'comprehensive medical and surgical care of the highest quality requires the concentration of resources and skills into larger organisational units' (BMA et al. 1998). Black (2002) states that the Department of Health estimated that three-quarters of English hospitals are involved in some form of debate regarding the reconfiguration of services. Proposals by both Royal Colleges have indicated that the population size served by DGHs would need to be in the region of 500,000 – or twice the typical population served by a DGH only a decade or so ago. That poses a significant challenge to the way that acute services are organised in the UK, particularly in those parts of the four countries with large rural populations, and creates some challenging equity of access dilemmas for healthcare managers and policy makers.

It is clear that any wholesale change resulting in the closure (perceived or otherwise) of local acute hospitals is deeply unattractive to local populations and therefore politicians. The events in the West Midlands town of Kidderminster are a potent reminder of what can happen when proposed alterations to acute services are forced on a community (Raftery and Harris 2005). In Kidderminster, as part of a countywide restructuring, it was proposed that the accident and emergency department and inpatient medical and surgical beds would be moved to two other hospitals approximately 20 miles away. This was greeted with such concern and hostility by the local population that, following various stages of protest, a political party, Health Concern, was formed with the single campaign issue of saving the Kidderminster hospital. A Health Concern candidate was elected as MP in 2001, unseating a Labour government minister and the party also won the local council elections and took control of the local authority. In response to this and some other contentious reconfiguration debates in other parts of England, the Department of Health re-examined the whole issue of acute care reconfiguration, looking at examples from other areas of the UK and overseas of how services have been reconfigured as well as how technological changes, for example, telemedicine could be used. This work formed the basis of a Department of Health report *Keeping the NHS Local* (DH 2003) which highlighted some of the projects being supported by the Department of Health to enable services to be delivered in smaller local hospitals.

There are a number of approaches being taken to ensure that there continues to be local delivery of acute services, which at the same time begin to reshape and redefine healthcare delivery for patients. In the UK this has taken the form of the development of managed clinical networks. These are multidisciplinary clinical teams working to predefined clinical pathways (either speciality or disease specific) that map the total patient journey through the healthcare system. In so doing they identify what should be happening to patients in terms of care management at any given moment and also involving patients and their carers in both care delivery as well as involvement in the decision-making process. There are similarities therefore with the integrated delivery systems in the USA. Managed clinical networks were first established in Scotland in the late 1990s as one of the outputs of an acute services review (Scottish Office 1998). The aim is to enable patients to be seen locally wherever and whenever possible, in part through investment in IT and technology in areas such as telemedicine either in terms of remote consultation with other members of the clinical team or in the transmission of information for interpretation at a specialist centre. There is clear evidence to support the use of telemedicine for clinical care, with benefits including reduced length of stay and improved data analysis (Rendina et al. 1998; Loane et al. 2000). The Scottish Acute Services review (Scottish Office 1998) identified a number of advantages of the model including:

- optimal use of resources
- improved equity of access
- reduction in waiting times for diagnosis or treatment
- improved quality of patient care
- improved multidisciplinary team working
- improved communications
- lead clinician taking responsibility for care delivery.

The concept of the managed clinical network has also been introduced into other parts of the UK, most notably in England with the establishment of a series of geographically based cancer networks which have focused on specific cancer types, bringing together the whole of the multidisciplinary team involved in the patient's care. The National Audit Office (2005) has concluded that the development of the cancer networks has made improvements in the delivery of cancer services. An example of how a regional clinical network can operate across the total health spectrum is outlined in Table 8.1.

Finally, there is a growing recognition that the largely hospital-based provision of diagnostic services in English acute care can both delay access to acute care services and impose costs on patients and on primary care services. Around half of the hospital-based diagnostic services activity in areas like radiology and pathology laboratories is actually provided to primary care providers and their patients. The rationale for siting such services in hospitals has been that doing so makes best use of their capital

Table 8.1 Integrated regional vascular service (IRVS)

Service level	Service offered	Development needs
Living at home, not using GP services	Advice	Community pharmacists trained and able to give advice
Local GP surgery	GP consultation, screening for vascular conditions (e.g. aneurysm), onward referral	Joint protocols for managing vascular disease, defined referral criteria agreed with network consultant(s)
Specialist GP surgery	GP specialist undertake some forms of circulatory testing, nurse-led clinics held by visiting vascular specialist nurse or leg ulcer nurse	Training in equipment use, agreed referral criteria, vascular nurse experts, expertise from vascular centre (e.g. technical developments) links to specialist pharmacists
Community hospital	Outreach clinics, local rehabilitation following surgery, community leg ulcer clinic	Minimal equipment needs, links to rehabilitation services with support from Allied Health Professionals (AHPs) and limb-fitting services
Local acute hospital	Day case and inpatient operating (up to intermediate level), emergency receiving operates across area in conjunction with other DGH(s), limited imaging/vascular laboratory service (perhaps on outreach basis)	Agreed operating procedures, managed emergency rotas (running with consultants from network hospitals), consultant with major interest in vascular surgery, general nursing staff (core with specialist vascular interest and skills)
Ambulatory care/ treatment centre	Day case varicose vein surgery	Efficient day case service
Specialist centre in integrated regional vascular service (IRVS)	Major surgery, invasive vascular radiology requiring specialist radiological interest and equipment, centre for limb fitting services and beginning rehabilitation in ward prior to discharge to local area	Specialist vascular physicians, surgeons and radiologists, wards staffed by nurses with specialist interest, vascular laboratory staffed by specialist technicians, rehabilitation skills (nursing and AHPs), good communication networks with transfer of patients to local services for continuation of care.

Source: Joint Working Party (1998). Acute Service Review. (Reproduced under the terms of the click use Licence)

assets (laboratory equipment, MRI scanners and so on), and achieves economies of scale, but technological changes mean that it may now be both more economic and more appropriate to locate many diagnostic services in primary care settings. For example, significant investments are now being made in the provision of routine radiology in primary care organisations in areas such as ultrasound and plain film X-ray facilities, which will result in large numbers of patients having investigations carried out away from the hospital setting. This has the dual benefits of cutting down on unnecessary visits by patients and reducing expenditure.

In addition there has been widespread concern from politicians and the public over waiting times for high end diagnostics such as MRI scans, and in response it is clear that the current Treatment Centre programme will be expanded into diagnostics, with the creation of freestanding diagnostics centres operated on similar principles.

Acute care in the Czech Republic: the need for change

Healthcare provision in the Czech Republic has seen a significant increase in public spending since the end of the communist era, with a rise in the share of GDP spent on healthcare from 5% in 1989 to 7.4% in 2003. At the same time, there has been a shift away from a state-controlled healthcare system towards one based more on a European model of social insurance. In comparison with many western European countries or the USA, the Czech healthcare system has a much higher level of acute care provision based in hospitals and makes more use of those acute care services. It is clear from OECD figures that the Czech Republic has more acute beds than almost any other country in the European Union, with a lower bed occupancy rate than the UK and a longer length of stay. Currently there are approximately 200 hospitals in the Czech Republic serving a population of 10.3 million. Although outpatient and primary care services have been largely privatised, most hospital services are still owned and operated by the government or municipalities. Despite the general overprovision of hospital services, those services are not evenly distributed and there are inequities in acute care delivery with wide regional variations in both the distribution of diagnostic equipment and in the quality of care delivered.

Arguing for radical reform of the Czech healthcare system, Hrobon et al. (2005) suggest that its current problems result partially from having too many hospitals, a lack of integration between hospitals, outpatients and primary care services, and a poorly defined health planning and regulatory framework. They note that many of the changes to acute care seen in other countries and described earlier in this chapter have yet to be taken up in the Czech Republic, and argue that there are substantial opportunities for reconfiguration. This is also borne out by the European Observatory on Health Care Systems (2005) report on the Czech Republic, which highlights the cautious and incremental approach taken so far to acute care reform, and the high level of acute care provision, though it notes there is some growth in homecare and day surgery provision as alternatives to hospital-based acute care. It seems likely that there will need to be a substantial shift in acute care delivery in the Czech Republic towards a more modern integrated model of care. Hrobon et al. (2005) believe that such changes are likely to be driven by the introduction of market-based healthcare reforms with increased competition both in health insurance and in healthcare provision.

Conclusion

In many countries, the acute care sector is changing. The circumstances which led to the rise of the large acute hospital over several decades, with hundreds (or even thousands) of acute care beds and a concentration of diagnostic and therapeutic activity all delivered from a single site, and patients coming to the hospital for a wide range of acute, specialist and diagnostic services, have changed. The totemic significance of hospitals to their communities should not be underestimated, but the rationale for their existence in their current form has been gradually undermined. In their place, commentators like Black (2006) set out a vision of a much smaller, more focused and more specialised acute care sector, better integrated into stronger and better resourced primary care services.

In the future, significant areas of what has traditionally been seen as acute care will be delivered outside the setting of a hospital, with benefits for patients (in being more patient centred and convenient) as well as for health systems (in being more cost effective and efficient at a time of increasing cost pressures). These include outpatient consultations, monitoring, routine investigations and elective surgery, rehabilitation and chronic disease management, as part of the managed care process. These changes will be accelerated by the move to market-based healthcare systems in many countries, and they pose important challenges for acute care clinicians and managers. They need to find new ways to deliver sustainable acute services that are locally based, and which are not reliant on the traditional organisational architecture of the acute hospital.

Summary box

- Acute care usually means treatment for a short-term or episodic illness or health problem which a patient may often receive in hospital. Acute care embraces both emergency and elective or planned treatment for health problems which may arise through accident or trauma, or through the occurrence of disease.
- The defining characteristic of acute care has often been the place of delivery – in an acute hospital. But much of what such hospitals do is not necessarily acute care – and much acute care can be delivered outside the hospital setting.
- The twentieth century saw the progressive expansion and development of the hospital sector, and a focus on providing acute care from large hospital sites with a concentration of facilities and expertise.
- A range of technological, financial and social pressures are driving radical changes in the nature of acute care provision, towards a model which is less hospital based and better integrated into primary care services. Important developments include the provision of freestanding treatment centres for elective surgery; diagnostics centres based in the community; and clinical networks aimed at managing whole patient pathways and keeping patient admissions to hospital to a minimum.

> • In the future, significant areas of what has traditionally been seen as acute care will be delivered outside the setting of a hospital, with benefits for patients (in being more patient centred and convenient) as well as for health systems (in being more cost effective and efficient at a time of increasing cost pressures). These include outpatient consultations, monitoring, routine investigations and elective surgery, rehabilitation and chronic disease management as part of the managed care process.

Self-test exercises

1 Choose a disease or patient group or a major service area with which you are familiar (such as diabetes, childbirth, stroke, cardiac disease, obesity or dermatology) and map out typical current provision using the levels of service framework in Figure 8.1. Now identify areas in which future changes to service provision are likely and consider their impact on acute services provision.

2 Identify an example of changes or reconfiguration in acute care with which you are familiar. Consider what were the drivers for change – professional, technical and economic. How was the case for change made by local healthcare organisations and others and how was it received by the community being served? How were community concerns about the changes addressed and reconciled with the drivers for change?

References and further reading

Black, A. (2002) Reconfiguring health systems. *British Medical Journal*, 325(7375): 1290–93.

Black, A. (2006) *The Future of Acute Care*. London: NHS Confederation.

Department of Health (DH, 2000) *The NHS Plan: A Plan for Investment, A Plan for Reform*. London: Department of Health (available from http://www.dh.gov.uk).

Department of Health (DH, 2003) *Keeping the NHS Local – A New Direction of Travel* London: Department of Health. Available at *http://www.dh.gov.uk*

Department of Health (DH, 2005) *Departmental Report (Summary Report) The Health and Personal Social Services Programmes*. London: Department of Health. Available at *http://www.dh.gov.uk*

Dixon, J., Lewis, R., Rosen, R., Finlayson, F. and Gray, D. (2004) Can the NHS learn from US managed care organisations? *British Medical Journal*, 328(7433): 223–5.

European Observatory on Health Care Systems (2000) *Health Care Systems in Transition Czech Republic*. Brussels: European Observatory on Health Care Systems.

FASA (2005) *The History of ASCs.* Alexandria, VA: FASA (available from http://www.fasa.org).

Feachem, R.G.A., Sekhri, N.K. and White, K.L. (2002) Getting more for their dollar: A comparison of the NHS with California's Kaiser Permanente. *British Medical Journal*, 324(7330): 135–43.

Ham, C., York, N., Sutch, S. and Shaw, R. (2003) Hospital bed utilisation in the NHS, Kaiser Permanente, and the US Medicare programme: analysis of routine data. *British Medical Journal*, 327(7426): 1257.

Hrobon, P., Machachek, T. and Julinek, T. (2005) *Health Care Reform for the Czech Republic in the 21st Century Europe*. Prague: Health Reform.cz. Available at *http://www.healthreform.cz*

Joint Working Party of British Medical Association, Royal College of Physicians of London, Royal College of Surgeons of England (1998) *Provision of Acute General Hospital Services*. London: Royal College of Surgeons.

Kennedy, I. (2001) *Learning from Bristol – The Report of the Public Inquiry into Children's Heart Surgery at the Bristol Royal Infirmary 1984–1995*. Bristol: Bristol Royal Infirmary Inquiry. Available at *http://www.bristol-inquiry.org.uk*

Loane, M., Bloomer, S., Corbett, R., Eedy, D., Hicks, N., Lotery, H., Mathews, C., Paisley, J., Steele, K. and Wootten, R. (2000) A randomized controlled trial to assess the clinical effectiveness of both realtime and store-and-forward teledermatology compared with conventional care. *Journal of Telemedicine and Telecare*, 6: S1–S3.

Lord Dawson of Penn (1920) *Interim Report on the Future Provisions of Medical and Allied Services*. United Kingdom Ministry of Health. Consultative Council on Medical and Allied Services. London: HMSO.

National Audit Office (2005) *The NHS Cancer Plan: A Progress Report*. London: The Stationery Office.

OECD (2005). *Health at a Glance. OECD Indicators 2005*. Paris: OECD Publications.

Raftery, J.P. and Harris, M. (2005) *Kidderminster Health: Monitoring and Evaluating the Reconfiguration of the NHS in Worcestershire*. Birmingham: HSMC, University of Birmingham.

Rendina, M.C., Downs, S.M., Carasco, N., Loonsk, J. and Bose, C.L. (1998) Effects of telemedicine on health outcomes in 87 infants requiring neonatal intensive care. *Telemedicine Journal*, 4(4): 345–51.

Scottish Office Department of Health (1998) *Acute Services Review Report*. Edinburgh: Scottish Office. Available at *http://www.scotland.gov.uk/library/documents5/acute-00.htm*

West, P. (1998) *Future Hospital Services in the NHS: One Size Fits All?* London: Nuffield Trust.

World Health Organisation (WHO, 2000). *The World Heath Report, Health Systems: Improving Performance*. Geneva: World Health Organisation. Available at *http://www.who.int*

Websites and resources

Nation's Healthcare. Independent UK treatment centre operator – wide variety of information for patients: *www.nationshealthcare.co.uk*

Kaiser Permanente. HMO in the US. Site provides information about the company and also a wide variety of information for patients: *www.kaiserpermanente.org*

Federated Ambulatory Surgery Association. Provides a variety of information on ambulatory surgery. One of the main accreditation bodies for Surgicentres and publishes data on outcomes from its members: *www.fasa.org*

European Observatory on Health Systems and Policies. Details of acute care provision in HiT reports on individual countries: *http://www.euro. who.int/observatory*

Department of Health. Policies, guidance and supporting information on acute care services and reconfiguration: *http://www.dh.gov.uk/PolicyAndGuidance/OrganisationPolicy/SecondaryCare/ConfiguringHospitals/fs/en*

Scottish Office. Resources on acute services: *http://www.healthmanagement online. co.uk/toolkit/toolkit.asp?p=*da

9 Managing in mental health

Steve Onyett and Helen Lester

Introduction

Managing in mental health is a complex task, carried out at times in a climate of uncertainty. Mental health managers are moving from an environment focused on secondary care services with limited partnership working towards a future focused on integrated working practices across multiple care sectors. What is also increasingly clear from both a policy and practice perspective is that the task of working to achieve better outcomes for service users goes beyond 'care' to include a range of activities encompassing mental health promotion, social inclusion and the promotion of self-management. It also increasingly requires managers to have in mind more than just service structures, as we might tradition-ally understand them, and include the wider range of social supports available to all citizens.

This chapter will outline some of the key challenges that currently face those managing mental health services, focus on specific issues in man-aging new mental health teams, describe strategies for engaging key stakeholders across the wider system and suggest ways to address some of these challenges through effective leadership and management.

Defining mental health

The World Health Organisation (WHO) describes mental health as 'a state of well-being in which the individual realises his or her abilities, can cope with the normal stresses of life, can work productively and fruitfully, and is able to make a contribution to his or her community' (WHO 2001). This definition introduces the theme of building on strengths and stresses the role of the individual as a contributor to the life of their local communities. It also underlines the aspiration that each individual should be socially included and able to participate effectively in community life. Mental 'ill health' includes mental health problems and strain, impaired functioning associated with distress, symptoms and diagnosable mental disorders such as schizophrenia and depression.

Mental health problems are increasingly common (see Table 9.1). The WHO has projected that depression will soon become the second greatest disease burden facing developed economies (WHO 2003). The health ministers of all 52 countries in the European Region have recently signed up to a declaration embodying 12 action points in the pursuit of the promotion of mental well-being, reduction of stigma and discrimination, prevention of mental ill health and suicide, access to good primary healthcare and incorporation of mental health as a vital part of public health policy (WHO Europe 2005). The latter has been reflected in the United Kingdom (UK) public health policy agenda (DH 2004a) which advocates equality between mental health and physical health, recognising that mental well-being is 'fundamental to the quality of life and productivity of individuals, families, communities and nations, enabling people to experience life as meaningful and to be creative and active citizens' (WHO Europe 2005).

The challenge of delivery: fiscal issues

In spite of the recognition that the consequences of mental ill health account for at least a third of all healthcare costs, many countries in the European Region spend less than 3% of their health budgets on mental healthcare (WHO 2003). In England, mental health remains one of the top three health priorities along with heart disease and cancer (DH 2000), yet according to estimates prepared by the Department of Health for the Wanless Review of health spending (Wanless 2002), expenditure on adult mental health services will need to double in real terms over the next ten years to meet the identified needs. There has been a reported increase in National Health Service (NHS) and local authority combined expenditure on mental health of over 19% in the period 1999–2000 to

Table 9.1   Prevalence of mental disorders in men and women (rates per 1000)

	Men	*Women*	*Total*
All neurosis	135	194	164
Mixed anxiety and depression	68	108	88
Generalised anxiety	43	46	44
Depression	23	28	26
Phobias	13	22	18
Obsessive-compulsive disorder	9	13	11
Panic	7	7	7
Personality disorder	54	34	44
Probable psychosis	6	5	5

Source: Singleton et al. (2001)

2002–03 (Appleby 2004). However, the trend in expenditure is towards spending on mental health falling increasingly behind total NHS expenditure. The NHS financial climate is additionally complicated by current concerns over debts of at least £200 million, with estimates that the 'real' figure may be closer to £800 million. A similar pattern is seen in the United States (US) where statistics from the Surgeon General Report (1999) suggest that the US spends about $170 billion, that is 8% of its total healthcare expenditure on mental healthcare. This, however, represents a slower rate of growth in spending compared to expenditure on the rest of healthcare.

Insufficient funding is compounded by difficulty tracking mental health resources, a growing distance between strategic planning, the operational processes of managing financial resources and of agreeing and monitoring service level agreements (SCMH 2003). Complex resource allocation decision-making structures, inadequate financial data and the poor status of mental health services in comparison to acute trust needs also contribute to the complexity (Mahoney et al. 2004). However, even reports highlighting the financial difficulties concede that more could be done by provider trusts to improve the efficiency of existing expenditure and to accelerate the transfer of resources to new services (SCMH 2003).

The challenge of delivery: the policy context

The NHS in England is currently subject to a policy waterfall, both within and beyond the arena of mental health services. Many of the policy imperatives encourage a more integrated approach to delivering services, often within a primary care context. This direction of travel can also be found in some small-scale programmes in the US and Canada (Kate et al. 1997; Druss et al. 2001). It is, however, difficult to implement and manage new working practices within a system that is in a constant state of change. As Means et al. (2003: 214) have suggested, there is 'the impression of a modernisation muddle in which managers and field level staff are struggling to keep pace with the demand for policy change and the ever increasing flood of directives, guidelines and indicators'.

More positively, the policy context for mental health service development and delivery has perhaps never been better aligned with user and carer aspirations. Policy initiatives and the supporting performance management frameworks continue to stress the importance of mental health promotion, social inclusion and choice. Overcoming stigma and discrimination, race equality, problems associated with dual diagnosis and with people who have both a learning disability and mental health problems, access to psychological therapies, prison mental health, early intervention and user and carer participation are also issues that currently command attention in policy circles. These issues need to be addressed across the whole age range and underpinned by effective joint working between agencies across transitions.

The challenge of delivery: the rhetoric/reality gap

Whilst it is important to recognise the complexities of the policy environment for mental health service development, the day-to-day reality for many managers and service providers continues to be one of massive underprovision (WHO 2003; Layard 2004), discrimination (DH 2005b) and failure to meet basic standards for those who manage to get services. The Commission for Healthcare Audit and Inspection (2005) survey of 26,555 users found that less than half of those responding felt that they definitely had enough say in decisions about their care and treatment. The proportions of people who would have liked help with aspects of their care but did not receive any were 50% with respect to accommodation needs, 52% for help with finding work, 73% for help with getting benefits and 57% for information about local support groups. Since this was based upon a response rate of 41%, we can only speculate what those who did not reply might have felt about their care. Stakeholder consultations by the Healthcare Commission and Commission for Social Care Inspection also highlighted the need to empower service users and carers to get involved both in their own care and the strategic delivery of mental health services. This picture is reflected, to some extent, in a recent national survey in the US to determine the extent of consumer empowerment in the public mental health system. The survey found that although the concept gained considerable momentum in the late 1990s, it was by no means universal across states (Geller et al. 1998).

The immediate management challenges

Mahoney et al. (2004) described the most frequently cited challenges for mental health communities in one English region over the previous five to eight years as follows:

- Underdeveloped community and primary care services and the need to shift away from an over-reliance on inpatient services.
- Determining the correct number of inpatient beds. Formulaic approaches to determining bed numbers fail to take account of the potential for new ways of working to decrease pressure on beds. The introduction, for example, of the gatekeeping of beds by adequately resourced crisis resolution teams offering home treatment provides a viable alternative to more inpatient stays. Early indications from a national survey of crisis resolution teams suggest that disputes with local consultant psychiatrists remain one of the most significant obstacles to effective implementation of these new ways of working.
- Poor social care resources. This was framed as a problem both in terms of a lack of access to resources (e.g. to a range of appropriate

accommodation to reduce occupied bed days) and difficulty in keeping a social care perspective privileging outcomes concerned with recovery, social inclusion and quality of life on the agenda.

- Too much money going out of area because of weaknesses in local provision which further compounded the lack of local investment.
- A tendency to prioritise resources initially for new developments due to the pressure to implement targets within the National Service Framework for Mental Health (DH 1999) while existing core services remain inappropriate or poorly developed.
- The constant neglect of hard-to-reach or marginalised groups such as black and minority ethnic communities, travelling and homeless people, people diagnosed with personality disorder and other people with complex and multiple needs. Serving the prison population through mainstream mental health services and now primary care trusts (PCTs) provides a further challenge in this area.
- Inequities in investment between areas, stemming from problems achieving informed commissioning. Good commissioning strategies are underpinned by effective needs assessment, good information and benchmarking, strong public health support, commissioning expertise and effective leadership and management, not all of which are readily available (see chapter 12 for further discussion).
- The need to promote a 'whole person' perspective that tackles social exclusion and overcomes discrimination.

Many of these issues are encapsulated by the challenges of managing new mental health teams in a way that makes sense to team members, service users and their supports.

Managing new mental health teams

In the UK, since the early 1980s, multidisciplinary community mental health teams (CMHTs) have been the main vehicle for delivering coordinated comprehensive community-based mental health services. More recently, the notion of generic CMHTs responsible for all aspects of care for people with mental health problems has been reassessed. CMHTs now provide the core around which newer functionalised teams, for example, early intervention, assertive outreach and home treatment teams, have been developed. Policy guidance is not prescriptive about the relationships between CMHTs and the newer functionalised teams, although it suggests that 'mutually agreed and documented responsibilities, liaison procedures and in particular transfer procedures need to be in place when crisis resolution, home treatment teams, assert-ive outreach teams and early intervention teams are being established' (DH 2002: 17). However, in practice there is evidence of difficulties as teams compete for funding within a finite budget allocation and of functionalised teams perceived as 'elites' compared to generic teams (Lester and Glasby 2006). Mental health managers need to be aware of the potential for mistrust and misunderstanding, working with new and established teams to create clear channels of communication and an appreciation of respective strengths and weaknesses.

The concept of what it means to be part of a 'team' is of itself contentious. Nine out of ten people in the last NHS Staff Survey (Dawson et al. 2005) reported that they worked in teams. However, this collapsed to only 43% when a definition of effective team working was supplied that included clear objectives, close working with other team members to achieve these objectives, regular meetings to discuss effectiveness and no more than 15 members. The situation is further complicated in mental health in that practitioners and team developers have to consider what makes a team effective and also how their team complies with a range of organisational features for the new team configurations required by the Department of Health.

Since 1999, there have been annual autumn reviews of the extent to which new team configurations comply with the Mental Health Policy Implementation Guides. Latterly, there has been a noticeable maturing of the debate, with greater flexibility allowed to respond to local circumstances provided that the proposed model meets the functions specified in the relevant guidance. Variations also need to be supported by local implementation teams (particularly users and carers) and not simply proposed because they are cheaper (NIMHE 2003). The means by which these issues of team organisation are resolved are central to both local management concerns, and in particular the balance of provision across both different types of teams and between community and inpatient provision. Resolving these issues locally requires a shared understanding across agencies about the strengths and weaknesses of the current system of care and the needs of the client group.

Unfortunately, such collaborative and informed governance processes are still not universal. Mahoney et al.'s (2004) commentary gives a flavour of the lack of consensus about ways forward. Feelings about the merits of the requirements of the post-NSF world vary hugely even among clinicians, and there is often an absence of consensus about team structures and functions. A generic problem appears to have been a paucity of good information to drive local development, not least in the area of how services are experienced by service users and carers.

As mental health managers, the application of improvement methods that can then inform more systematic evaluation of demand and capacity in different parts of the local system are critical tools to help unlock some of these issues. Process mapping, as a means of effectively incorporating a user view of the current situation and involving them from the outset in thinking about improvement, seems to be the most evidence based of the improvement methodologies (McNulty and Ferlie 2002; McLeod 2005). Within the mental health field, the Creating Capable Teams Toolkit has been designed to help teams integrate the new roles of the consultant psychiatrist with other mental health professionals. It is being piloted by the Sainsbury Centre for Mental Health (SCMH) and NIMHE and should be widely available by the end of 2006.

Engaging senior stakeholders across the wider system

Reinertsen et al. (2004: 3) suggest: 'The most common reason for failure of large systems to change is the failure of the senior leadership team to function as an effective team with the right balance of skills, healthy relationships, and deep personal commitment to the achievement of the goals.' In the new commissioning environment heralded by *Commissioning a Patient-Led NHS* (DH 2005a), the task of creating this effective team may increasingly fall to commissioners concerned with creating a more pluralistic range of providers, with a stronger role for the voluntary and independent sector. It suggested, for example, that greater coordination is expected between primary care trusts and local authority social service boundaries, with a greater emphasis on contestability in healthcare provision in primary as well as secondary care. This followed in the wake of the formal national Compact to govern relations between the voluntary and community sector (VCS) and the state (1998) and the first Strategic Agreement between the Department of Health, the NHS and the VCS which proposed making the VCS part of mainstream health service provision (DH 2004b).

Mental health managers will have to consider what type of cross-community leadership team they will need to achieve choice, social inclusion and race equality for users and their supports. Processes will be needed that achieve the required integration of vision and activity both horizontally across organisations and vertically across hierarchical strata. There is useful guidance available on how to use joint mechanisms for coordinated planning across localities in pursuit of performance management targets, for example, local strategic planning mechanisms and the use of local area agreements. However, clarifying shared objectives, prioritising actions and finding a shared language for collaboration remains a significant challenge (see also Cameron et al. 2003; NIMHE 2005). The following case study illustrates some of these issues.

Case study 1: mental health provision in North Tyneside

Papworth and Crosland (2005) describe the implementation of a large whole systems intervention across organisations concerned with mental health provision in North Tyneside. It consisted of a large whole systems event (Weisbord and Janoff 1995) and subsequent phased service mapping and project work running over three years. The main reported benefit of the intervention was that it was seen as providing a catalyst for deeper systemic change through challenging existing values and assumptions about mental health services. Its primary care orientation also raised the profile of mental health beyond the usual boundaries of specialist services. As one interviewee described: 'It [the project] has actually made people sit up and say "how can we do this better?" and "what can we do?" It has got the whole system seriously looking now at how they can contribute to a more co-ordinated approach' (p. 525). However, the authors also highlighted the following problems in achieving concrete actions as a result of the approach:

- Creating a widely shared understanding of what a whole systems approach really means can be difficult.
- The process can become identified with a particular agenda to the extent that certain stakeholder groups may become alienated from the process.
- Stakeholders can be suspicious of the motives of the approach, believing there to be 'hidden agendas'.
- Action plans can be difficult to achieve as the planning was often devolved back to existing task groups rather than creating new structures to undertake novel initiatives.
- Developing an appropriately inclusive approach can be challenging. One key organisation, for example, was excluded because it had not contributed to the funding of the intervention.
- There may be difficulty in engaging the people who should be involved in implementation (in this case the therapists).
- Employing an internal facilitator meant that this individual was often seen as taking responsibility for actions where an external facilitator may have been better placed to ensure wider ownership of agreed action plans.
- The long timescale meant that organisations changed over the period of the programme and became more engaged with external demands rather than the aims of the intervention.

Overall, the evaluation concluded that there is merit in short-term, large whole-systems events to orientate people towards shared objectives, articulate values and challenge assumptions about the nature of mental health services and the roles of the respective stakeholders. However, this case study suggests that a more embedded approach is needed to sustain action over the longer term.

Embedding change in the system

Bolden's (2004: 23) review of the impact of leadership concluded: 'At an organisational level, management and leadership appear to have an effect on a range of outcomes, but only as part of a more general set of [human resource management] practices. It is the leader's influence on employee motivation and commitment that appears to have the greatest impact, rather than any specific characteristic or behaviour of the leader per se.' This chimes with research on leadership that highlights the much greater concern that staff have with their immediate managers rather than leaders at the top of their organisations (Shamir 1995; Alimo-Metcalfe and Alban-Metcalfe 2004). Leadership is an enabler of optimal staff performance, building from the best values they bring to their work, and shaped by the needs of the prevailing circumstances. West and Markiewicz (2004) described the challenge of improving the morale and effectiveness of the workforce as helping staff achieve clarity about what they should be doing and creating environments in which they felt valued, supported and respected. As a values-based framework, the mental health field benefits from having a formulation of 'Ten Essential Shared Capabilities' developed through focus groups with service users, carers, managers, academics and practitioners (Hope 2004; see Table 9.2) The shared capabilities can also form the basis of a framework for appraisal and personal development plans for both professional and non-professionally affiliated mental health staff. Some of these leadership issues are illustrated in the overleaf case study.

Table 9.2   The ten essential shared capabilities for mental health practice

1 **Working in partnership**. Developing and maintaining constructive working relationships with service users, carers, families, colleagues, lay people and wider community networks. Working positively with any tensions created by conflicts of interest or aspiration that may arise between the partners in care.

2 **Respecting diversity**. Working in partnership with service users, carers, families and colleagues to provide care and interventions that not only make a positive difference but also do so in ways that respect and value diversity including age, race, culture, disability, gender, spirituality and sexuality.

3 **Practising ethically**. Recognising the rights and aspirations of service users and their families, acknowledging power differentials and minimising them whenever possible. Providing treatment and care that is accountable to service users and carers within the boundaries prescribed by national (professional), legal and local codes of ethical practice.

4 **Challenging inequality**. Addressing the causes and consequences of stigma, discrimination, social inequality and exclusion on service users, carers and mental health services. Creating, developing or maintaining valued social roles for people in the communities they come from.

5 **Promoting recovery**. Working in partnership to provide care and treatment that enables service users and carers to tackle mental health problems with hope and optimism and to work towards a valued lifestyle within and beyond the limits of any mental health problem.

6 **Identifying people's needs and strengths**. Working in partnership to gather information to agree health and social care needs in the context of the preferred lifestyle and aspirations of service users, their families, carers and friends.

7 **Providing service user centred care**. Negotiating achievable and meaningful goals, primarily from the perspective of service users and their families. Influencing and seeking the means to achieve these goals and clarifying the responsibilities of the people who will provide any help that is needed, including systematically evaluating outcomes and achievements.

8 **Making a difference**. Facilitating access to and delivering the best quality, evidence-based, values-based health and social care interventions to meet the needs and aspirations of service users and their families and carers.

9 **Promoting safety and positive risk taking**. Empowering the person to decide the level of risk they are prepared to take with their health and safety. This includes working with the tension between promoting safety and positive risk taking, including assessing and dealing with possible risks for service users, carers, family members, and the wider public.

10 **Personal development and learning**. Keeping up to date with changes in practice and participating in lifelong learning, personal and professional development for oneself and colleagues through supervision, appraisal and reflective practice.

Source: Department of Health (2004).

Case study 2: Worcester Mental Health Partnership

The Worcester Mental Health Partnership Trust achieved the worst possible NHS performance star rating in 2004. A critical report from the Commission for Healthcare Improvement suggested it needed to improve its governance structures, risk management and clinical audit mechanisms (Box 9.1). In its journey from the worst to the best performance rating, some key lessons were learned (see Forrest 2005 for a fuller account).

Box 9.1   Leadership issues

- An initial focus on getting the right people into the right jobs with attention to basic good human resource practice was key.
- Recognition, particularly by the chair and non-executive directors of the board, that a schism existed between the trust board and the staff, was instrumental in turning the trust around. There was a need to promote ownership of organisational performance, so the chair and chief executive devoted considerable attention to 'earthing' themselves in the grassroots of the organisation by getting out to places where care was delivered.
- The team realised they needed high calibre leadership throughout the organisation, including new board membership and middle management changes.
- New ways of working were encouraged, for example, by giving permission for the consultant to not see every user.
- A 15-member project board was established to develop a detailed service development plan. This included clear protocols, each with an identified director responsible for implementation, a service lead, the desired outcome and a target date for completion.
- A forum was created where new ways of working could be discussed.
- A positive culture of risk taking, with risk management an integral part of the organisation's service development plan, was created.
- The Care Programme Approach was remodelled to reflect new ways of working.
- Strong medical leadership was achieved with generic leadership skills developed in the medical workforce.

Source: Forrest (2005)

Conclusion

There is a series of future challenges for individuals managing in mental health. The increasing presentation and recognition of mental health problems means there are considerable pressures to increase the current mental health workforce (Appleby 2004; Layard 2004). The demands of the new policy agenda and the aspirations of users and their supports require that managers in mental health create new partnerships and work within the new mechanisms for planning and delivery. Strong leadership will be needed to establish and manage mental health teams within this challenging environment.

In essence, mental health managers will need to be able to help professionals from different backgrounds communicate effectively both within and between teams. Leadership and improvement work will need to be better integrated and conducted in contexts where there is effective vertical (across hierarchies) and horizontal (across teams, organisations, sectors) integration. At local levels, different leaders and management initiatives will need to be better coordinated to achieve a multiplier effect. Leadership development itself needs to be well led to avoid perpetuating the 'silo mentality' that characterises much health and social care (Edmonstone and Western 2002). Whilst the new commissioning environment provides an opportunity to achieve many of these aspirations, leaders will need to work cooperatively to develop new governance arrangements that increase the role of users and their supports in commissioner-led, continuous quality improvement. Perhaps, above all, managers of mental health services will need to model values concerned with recovery, choice, equality and social inclusion.

Summary box

- Mental health managers are working in an environment of policy change and fiscal constraints.
- Good management is ultimately demonstrated through improvement in provision for services users and their supports.
- Engaging the hearts and minds of the right breadth of stakeholders is a longstanding challenge. Working appreciatively and respectfully at the level of people's own beliefs about the current situation and their aspirations may offer a way forward.
- Management and leadership are enacted through relationships and for much of health and social care this means relationships within teams. Good team design and support is therefore critical.
- Managers of mental health services need to model values concerned with recovery, choice, equality and social inclusion.

Self-test exercises

1 As manager of an early intervention team, the health purchasing/ insurance organisation informs you that the funding stream for next year is less than predicted and you need to think how to best reshape your service. What issues does this raise in terms of service delivery, team morale, future service development and relationships between your team and other mental health teams in your locality? What tools could you use to help you in your decision making process?

2 In your capacity as a mental health manager, describe how you could use the Ten Essential Shared Capabilities for Mental Health Practice (see table 9.2) to help you reflect on team development, recruitment policies and procedures, your organisation's annual appraisal processes and outcomes for people who use services.

3 As a senior manager in a mental health provider organisation you receive a letter from a local service users' group asking for greater involvement in decisions about the development of community mental health services in your locality. Think about how you would respond to this request, who you might involve, how you might manage opposition from other stakeholders to this request and strategies you would need to put in place to ensure the process was positive and productive.

References and further reading

Alimo-Metcalfe, B. and Alban-Metcalfe, J. (2004) Leadership in public sector organisations. In J. Storey (ed.) *Leadership in Organisations: Current Issues and Key Trends*. Abingdon: Routledge.

Appleby, L. (2004) *The National Service Framework for Mental Health – Five Years On*. London: Department of Health.

Bolden, R. (2004) *What is Leadership?* Leadership South West Research Report. South West Development Agency. www.leadershipsouthwest.com

Cameron, M., Edmans, T., Greatley, A. and Morris, D. (2003) *Community Renewal And Mental Health: Strengthening the Links*. London: King's Fund.

Commission for Healthcare Audit and Inspection (2005) *Survey of Users 2005. Mental Health Services*. London: Healthcare Commission.

Dawson, J., West, M. and Beinart, S. (2005) *NHS National Staff Survey 2004. Summary of Key Findings*. London: Commission for Healthcare Audit and Inspection.

Department of Health (DH, 1999) *National Service Framework for Mental Health: Modern Standards and Service Models*. London: Department of Health.

Department of Health (DH, 2000) *The NHS Plan*. London: Department of Health.

Department of Health (DH, 2002) *Mental Health Policy Implementation Guidance: Community Mental Health Teams*. London: Department of Health.

Department of Health (DH, 2004) *The Ten Essential Shared Capabilities: A Framework for the whole of the Mental Health Workforce*. Department of Health, London.

Department of Health (DH, 2004a) *Choosing Health: Making Healthy Choices Easier*. London: The Stationery Office.

Department of Health (DH, 2004b) *Making Partnership Work for Patients, Carers and Service Users. A Strategic Agreement between the Department of Health, the NHS and the Voluntary and Community Sector*. London: Department of Health.

Department of Health (DH, 2005a) *Commissioning a Patient-Led NHS*. London: Department of Health.

Department of Health (DH, 2005b) *Delivering Race Equality in Mental Health*

Care: An Action Plan for Reform Inside and Outside Services and the Government's Response to the Independent Inquiry into the Death of David Bennett. London: Department of Health.

Druss, B., Rohrbaugh, R., Levinson, C. and Rosenheck, R. (2001) Integrated medical care for patients with serious psychiatric illness. A randomised trial. *Archives of General Psychiatry,* 58: 861–8.

Edmonstone, J. and Western, J. (2002) Leadership development in healthcare – what do we know? *Journal of Management in Medicine,* 16(1): 343–7.

Forrest, E. (2005) Stars in their eyes. *Health Service Journal,* 20 October: 22–4.

Geller, J.L., Brown, J.M., Fisher, W.H., Grudzinskas, A.J. and Manning, T.D (1998) A national survey of 'consumer empowerment' at the state level. *Psychiatric Services,* 49: 498–503.

Healthcare Commission and Commission for Social Care Inspection (2005) *Partnership Review of Community Mental Health and Social Care Services for Adults aged between 18 and 65. Report on Consultation and Engagement Events.* London: Healthcare Commission.

Hope, R. (2004) *The Ten Essential Shared Capabilities. A Framework for the Whole of the Mental Health Workforce.* London: NIMHE.

Kate, N., Craven, M., Crustolo, A.M., Nikolaou, L. and Allen, C. (1997) Integrating mental health services within primary care. A Canadian programme. *General Hospital Psychiatry,* 19: 324–32.

Layard, R. (2004) *Mental Health: Britain's Biggest Social Problem?* Paper prepared for No. 10 Downing Street Strategy Unit. *www.strategy.gov.uk/downloads/files/mh_layard.pdf*

Lester, H.E. and Glasby, J. (2006) *Mental Health Policy and Practice.* Basingstoke: Palgrave Macmillan.

McLeod, H. (2005) A review of the evidence on organisational development in healthcare. In E. Peck (ed.) *Organisational Development in Healthcare.* Oxford: Radcliffe.

McNulty, T. and Ferlie, E. (2002) *Re-engineering Healthcare: The Complexities of Organisational Transformation.* Oxford: Oxford University Press.

Mahoney, C., Nixon, D. and Aubery, R. (2004) *Strengthening the Capacity and Capability of Mental Health Commissioning Systems in Cheshire and Merseyside to Deliver the Modernisation Programme.* North West Development Centre, Hyde: NIMHE.

Means, R., Richards, S. and Smith, R. (2003) *Community Care: Policy and Practice,* 3rd edn. Basingstoke: Palgrave Macmillan.

NIMHE (2003) *Counting Community Teams: Issues In Fidelity And Flexibility.* London: NIMHE.

NIMHE (2005) *Making it Possible: Improving Mental Health and Wellbeing in England.* London: NIMHE.

Papworth, M. A. and Crosland, A. (2005) Health service use of whole system interventions. *Journal of Management Development,* 24(6): 519–29.

Reinertsen, J.R., Pugh, M., Bisognano, M., Pearce, J. and Beasley, C. (2004) *What Will It Take to Move the Big Dots?* Briefing Paper. Institute of Healthcare Improvement. *www.ihi.org*

SCMH (2003) *Money for Mental Health; A Review of Public Spending on Mental Health Care.* London: Sainsbury Centre for Mental Health.

Shamir, B. (1995) Social distance and charisma: Theoretical notes and an exploratory study. *Leadership Quarterly,* 6: 19–47.

Singleton, N., Bumpstead, R., O'Brien, M., Lee, A. and Meltzer, H. (2001)

Psychiatric Morbidity Among Adults Living in Private Households, 2000. London: The Stationery Office.

US Department of Health and Human Services (1999) *Mental Health: A Report of the Surgeon General–Executive Summary*. Rockville, MD: National Institutes of Health, National Institute of Mental Health.

Wanless, D. (2002) *Securing Our Future Health: Taking a Long-Term View*. London: HM Treasury.

Weisbord, M.A. and Janoff, S. (1995) *Future Search*. San Francisco: Berrett-Koehler.

West, M. A. and Markiewicz, L. (2004) *Building Team-based Working*. Oxford: Blackwell.

WHO (2001) *Strengthening Mental Health Promotion*. Fact sheet no. 220. Geneva: World Health Organisation.

WHO (2003) *Mental Health in the WHO*. European Region Fact sheet EURO/03/03. Geneva: World Health Organisation.

WHO Europe (2005) *Mental Health Declaration for Europe*. Copenhagen: World Health Organisation.

Websites and resources

Auseinet. Australian network for promotion, prevention and early intervention for mental health, and suicide prevention (Auseinet): *www.auseinet.com/*

Canadian Mental Health Association. Nationwide charitable organisation that promotes the mental health of the whole population and supports a recovery focus within mental health services: *www.cmha.ca/bins/index.asp*

Care Services Improvement Partnership. Launched in 2005 and aims to support positive changes in services and in the well-being of people with mental health problems, learning disabilities, people with physical disabilities, older people with health and social care needs, children and families with health and social care needs and people with health and social care needs within the criminal justice system: *www.csip.org.uk*

Health management online. Scottish-based generic health management website with a good library and a range of updated policy documents and useful links: *www.healthmanagementonline.co.uk/index.asp*

Improvement leader's guides. Provide practical advice on key improvement tools that will enhance local decision making such as process mapping, involving users and carers effectively, and mapping demand and capacity: *www.wise.nhs.uk*

International Initiative for Mental Health Leadership. Joint endeavour of the UK National Institute for Mental Health in England, US Substance Abuse and Mental Health Service Administration (*www.samhsa.gov/*) and the Mental Health Director of the Ministry of Health New Zealand (*www.moh.govt.nz/mentalhealth.*). It is intended to facilitate the sharing of best practices and to provide needed support and collaboration for leaders of mental health services to develop robust managerial and operational practices: www.iimhl.com

NHS-based Health Management Specialist Library. Aims is to provide timely and efficient access to high quality information resources for health managers, clinical managers and leaders and those involved in commissioning health services: *http://libraries.nelh.nhs.uk/healthManagement*

NHS Networks. Means of promoting and connecting the many networks which exist throughout the NHS and encouraging the formation of new ones: www.networks.nhs.uk

Sainsbury Centre for Mental Health. Works to improve the quality of life for people with mental health problems, carries out research, analysis, training and development to improve practice and influence policy in public services; ranges from national research into the key issues in mental health to local development projects that tackle some of the most difficult issues services face: www.scmh.org.uk

US National Institiute of Mental Health. Lead Federal agency for research on mental health problems, including basic science and clinical studies and a programme to educate the public about mental health issues: www.nimh.nih.gov/

10 Service and capital development

Andrew Hine

Introduction

This chapter looks at how to develop a business case for a new healthcare service or capital development. It considers first the broader environment facing healthcare providers, taking into account expected patient demand, competition and available resources. It then moves on to examine a seven-step approach to developing a business plan for capital investment, including the use of sophisticated evaluation and financial modelling techniques to help make more objective choices. The various sources of funding for capital development are discussed, with an emphasis upon the use of private finance initiatives (PFIs) and other new schemes.

The increasing focus in some health systems on the creation of a market for customers in public healthcare fundamentally alters the way that planners assess the viability of a new service. In the past, funding would often have been in the form of guaranteed block payments whereas now the income in most cases has to be earned on an ongoing basis. As with any private business, revenues are not guaranteed, with customers (patients) having the choice to go elsewhere for their treatment. This introduces a much greater level of uncertainty and risk, with planners having to be more rigorous in drawing up a business case, taking into account the expected level of demand for the service, the alternatives available to patients, the options for delivering the service and the expected lifespan of the service. Ultimately, any new service would only be developed if projected income could cover its costs. Moving towards such a market-based approach requires a big change in mindset for planners, and not all will find it easy to adapt to this new commercial reality. Building up a comprehensive business case brings a new level of rigour to the planning process with the use of modelling techniques and sensitivity analysis, all designed to minimise the risk of launching a service. One important development is the need to engage stakeholders such as clinicians, service managers, commissioners and patients at an early stage to get buy-in.

An example of a more rigorous private sector approach to healthcare capital development is that of the private finance initiative (PFI) in the NHS. Within PFI, the onus on meeting deadlines and budgets is placed firmly in the hands of the private sector, with penalties applied to those failing to meet targets. The consortia backing these schemes are in turn attracted by predictable revenue streams as the payment terms tend to be 25 to 30 years. With customer choice becoming more widespread and the emergence of private sector providers of core services, public–private partnerships have become a permanent feature of healthcare provision in the UK and many other health systems.

Section 1: Developing a business plan

Planning new medical services in the acute or primary care sector needs to follow a similar approach to new product development in a commercial organisation, taking into account patient demand and competition for services, and effective use of resources. Rather than putting forward a single proposal, planners must evaluate a number of options in a rigorous fashion and we set out here a process for such an appraisal.

Assessing demand – is there a need for the new service among the catchment population?

The first step is to research the level of need for the proposed service, taking into account age profiles, income levels, ethnicity and access to transport. The planner should also consider epidemiological needs within the local health economy, major health issues facing the population, mortality rates, hospitalisation rates by key disease areas and the health profile of the population by disease area. For those elective services where the patient can choose his or her provider, this research should also extend to surrounding localities. At the end of this process, the planner should have a good idea of the number and type of potential patients per year.

Competitive analysis – what level of competition will you face in providing the service?

In an open market, where the patient can choose from a number of providers, it is important for a provider to be able to assess how competitive their new proposed offering will be. This entails an analysis of the strengths and weaknesses of existing providers, and the threats and opportunities in the overall market place. Michael Porter's model of the competitive environment (2004) represents an effective analytical tool in this context. Two key questions for a provider to ask are:

- If there are no existing competitors, how easily could a new provider emerge?
- Are there barriers to entry such as high capacity costs, scarce resources and lack of access to appropriate technology?

These factors can clearly affect the attractiveness to a provider of entering a particular market for a service.

Political, social and technological forces

The competitive environment within which a healthcare provider is located could also be affected by changes in the political, social and technological landscape, all of which have an impact on the potential success of the new service.

Political factors

Despite the move towards a more open market in healthcare services in some countries, healthcare markets are usually still tightly regulated and controlled through government policy. Any service provision developments must therefore take into account foreseeable changes in policy and attempt to mitigate such risks.

Social factors

Demand for particular services could be adversely affected by broader societal trends such as an improved health consciousness and a move towards more localised provision of healthcare.

Technological factors

Are there new technologies – such as superior equipment – in the pipeline that could supersede the proposed service and reduce future demand?

Service design options – how can the service best be delivered?

An acute hospital provider has a number of options available when designing a new service and needs to weigh up the pros and cons of various delivery models including:

- service redesign
- refurbishing existing capacity
- privately financed, self-financed or publicly financed new build (depending on the national policy context)
- buying capacity in other facilities and providing the service from these sites
- contracting with another public or private sector provider (outsourcing)

- redesigning existing services to accommodate the new service
- some blend of the above.

Resources

The planner needs to consider where the services would be based and whether any additional technical capacity is needed. Human resource requirements such as availability of consultants, GPs, nurses and allied health professionals must also be assessed, including any relevant training needs.

Guidelines

At the very least, any proposition must meet appropriate national guidelines, for example, in the English NHS this would include those outlined in national service frameworks (NSFs) and in National Institute for Health and Clinical Excellence (NICE) policies (DH 1998). If any of the options do not meet these basic standards they should be eliminated from further consideration.

Risks

When presenting the various options, it is important to use a series of standardised headings, highlighting the differences between the options. In particular there should be a clear indication of how the patient pathway is affected; that is, how the patient would move through the system from first contact with the service through to discharge. For each option there is also a need to assess the level of risk; for example, is there sufficient workforce capacity available to deliver the new service? What are the clinical risks within an option? What are the financial risks? What are the political, social and technology risks?

Engaging stakeholders

Given that the success of any service will ultimately be determined by its acceptability to users and those who deliver the service, it is vital to get the views of key stakeholders such as clinicians, service managers, commissioners and patients. This helps with testing of the attractiveness of a new idea as well as gaining valuable buy-in from those likely to use the new service.

Evaluation criteria – narrowing down the options

Faced with multiple options about how to develop a service, the planner needs to have a robust way of reducing these to a more manageable number. A formal evaluation should take into account criteria such as financing, income, clinical viability, human resource implications and access to services and organisational capacity. By giving each of these a weighting, the various options can be ranked according to their overall attractiveness. If this process is carried out at the option development stage, any low-scoring service concepts can be eliminated early on and planners may decide upon some absolute thresholds that all options have to meet in order to be viable.

Costing options – will projected revenue cover your cost base?

At the service design stage it is reasonable to include cost and income assumptions at a general rather than a detailed level. The following stage of development, the outline business case (OBC), will go into more depth and this is explored in the next section of this chapter. The objective at this point is to get a sufficiently broad view of the costs and revenues to be able to draw up a shortlist of two to three preferred alternatives.

In estimating costs, planners should call on experts with experience within their own organisation as well as with relevant service providers. When making income projections, the cost of service delivery needs to be compared with any current national schedule of tariffs for that particular service. To provide an accurate reflection of costs for the service, the cost models should incorporate human resources costs for service delivery, including all medical professional staff, management costs, cost of supplies and infrastructure maintenance costs. These overall costs should be matched against anticipated activity to calculate the cost per full consultant episode (or whatever the standard unit of activity used for health services) that can then be compared to the tariff. By carrying out a sensitivity analysis, the planner can assess how increases or decreases in activity would affect the tariff and therefore the overall income of the healthcare providers.

Partnering in service development and delivery – adding a new dimension to service delivery

Of the various options available to develop better services, the area that is significantly underexploited in some health systems is the use of partnerships. In the English NHS, the creation of a more plural market in healthcare provision has expanded the number of choices available to commissioners and patients and this trend seems set to continue. At the primary care level there has been an international move towards greater integration of social and primary care for older people's services and long-term condition management (see Chapter 7). However, for acute service planners and commissioners there is an opportunity to make radical alterations to service delivery through the development of partnerships with the private and voluntary sectors. Within this new environment, hospital providers can explore partnering with GPs, independent sector providers and technology companies to deliver innovative models of care and this offers the organisation the potential of gaining a true competitive advantage.

Section 2: Developing a business case for capital investment

Many new services require significant investment in buildings and equipment. An outline business case (OBC) brings a high degree of analytical rigour to the selection and evaluation of different capital options. This will ensure that any decision is cost effective and in line with the provider's and commissioner's broader strategic objectives. The process inevitably combines quantitative analysis with professional judgement and the general principles outlined earlier in this chapter can be applied in a seven-step framework that represents commercial best practice for developing a business case, involving the carrying out of a full cost–benefit analysis and the use of financial modelling techniques. The NHS *Capital Investment Manual* recommends using three phases for planning a capital project (DH 1994), as set out in Figure 10.1. Although the overall degree of analysis carried out should reflect the size and complexity of the project, all investments should, however, receive a rigorous and systematic appraisal.

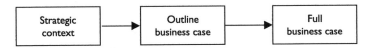

Figure 10.1   Three phases of planning a capital project

Setting the strategic context – making sure the service is consistent with the broader strategy of the organisation

In the course of its strategic planning process, a provider will develop service proposals that require capital investment. Any new service should therefore be sustainable and fit clearly into the wider vision. Setting the strategic context will normally include an initial appraisal of the various delivery options and in all cases an assessment of the potential funds that could be raised, to ensure that the project is at the very least affordable. This will prevent time and money being spent on business cases that could never come to fruition. The strategic plan should take into consideration the broader objectives of the organisation and the competitive environment including:

- commissioner requirements and the service delivery objectives of the provider
- forecast changes in service demand
- prospective changes in care models and methods of service delivery
- the financial position of the organisation
- the estate, its condition and contribution to achieving the business objectives of the organisation
- the local/regional healthcare market and likely future developments.

The strategic context will also outline the framework within which investment decisions are to be evaluated. The overall seven-step framework for developing a business case is set out in Figure 10.2.

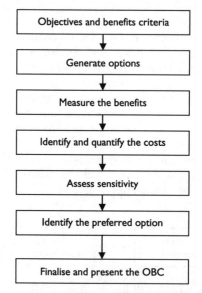

Figure 10.2   Seven-stage framework for developing a business case

Stage 1: Objectives and benefits criteria – setting clear goals for the project

Having identified a need for a new service, a set of clear achievable objectives must be agreed and these will be the foundation for the business case. Any options that are developed should meet these key objectives as well as providing clinical and economic benefits such as:

- improved service access
- improved clinical standards
- earlier interventions
- improved cost efficiency.

Such benefits criteria must be clearly defined for each option and will be a benchmark for judging the overall attractiveness of the investment.

Stage 2: Generating options – seeking creative solutions

By encouraging free and open thinking from a wide range of stake-holders, planners will give themselves the best chance of drawing up a strong list of options. Contributions should be sought from service users (patients), service professionals and external advisers, whilst brainstorming sessions could be used to generate a range of ideas. It may also be helpful to look at how other healthcare organisations approach similar challenges. However, the process must be rigorous and objective in developing a number of options, avoiding the situation where a preferred option is steamrollered through without duly considering alternatives. A shortlist would typically include four to six options including a 'do-nothing' scenario.

Stage 3: Measuring the benefits – enabling meaningful comparisons of options

To carry out a full economic analysis, there is a need to measure the extent to which each investment option meets the agreed benefit criteria. In some cases it may also be possible to place a cost on each benefit to allow a true cost–benefit analysis. Likewise, there will be a need to assess the level and type of benefit. For this, a ranking matrix should be used as follows:

1 Agreeing a weighting for each benefit criterion according to its level of importance.
2 Scoring each option against each benefit criterion using an agreed ranking scale (e.g. 1 = least satisfactory, 5 = most satisfactory).
3 Calculating a weighted benefit score for each option by combining the individual scores and the weightings attached to each benefit criterion.

The ranking process is inevitably to some extent subjective and it is therefore helpful to include as wide a range of stakeholders as possible to even out any bias. In addition to healthcare managers, both health professionals and service users (patients) should be involved.

Stage 4: Calculating the costs – creating a flexible model

There are two types of cost associated with each option:

• financial costs: capital and revenue
• economic costs: the opportunity costs of using resources already owned and the additional costs that would be borne by others.

Different projects have different lifespans, so the net present value (NPV) should be calculated for each option to allow a fair comparison, using an agreed discount rate. Whilst the cost estimates should be as accurate as possible, one should avoid spending an excessive amount of time pulling together highly detailed numbers. Ideally, one should put together a fairly sophisticated financial model that will assess the impact of changes to specifications for each option. This will let planners refine the design of each option and will be useful for the sensitivity analysis.

Stage 5: Assessing sensitivity

Any assumptions about costs and benefits for each option are subject to changes in the environment. These changes can alter the assessment and ranking positions and therefore the model needs to be flexible enough to cope, allowing a sensitivity analysis to be carried out on the following:

- the weighting applied to each of the benefits criteria
- the scores attributed to each option against each benefit criterion
- the resource assumptions (e.g. buildings specification, staffing levels) of each option.

By testing the sensitivity of various types of changes one can identify those variables that have the greatest impact upon the overall scores. The probability of such changes should be taken into consideration when carrying out the assessment and rankings.

Stage 6: Identifying the preferred option – towards objective decision making

All the information should now be brought together in one table incorporating the weighted benefits scores and the estimated total costs for each option. These may show that one option clearly outperforms the rest, but equally the results may be inconclusive, as illustrated in Table 10.1.

Table 10.1   Weighted benefits scores and estimated costs

	Option 2	Option 3
Scenario 1		
Weighted benefits score	13.7	14.6
Total costs (NPV)	£2.4 m	£2.3 m
Scenario 2		
Weighted benefits score	13.7	14.6
Total costs (NPV)	£2.4 m	£2.4 m
Scenario 3		
Weighted benefits score	13.7	14.6
Total costs (NPV)	£2.4 m	£2.56 m
Scenario 4		
Weighted benefits score	13.7	14.6
Total costs (NPV)	£2.4 m	£2.7 m

In scenario 1 in Table 10.1, the decision is straightforward with option 2 having both the highest weighted benefits score and lowest cost and the same is true of scenario 2, where option 2 has equal costs to option 1 but a higher benefits score. Scenario 3 is more difficult to interpret. Option 2 has a higher weighted benefits score and total costs which are both marginally higher than for option. With scenario 4, the benefits score of option 2 is still a little higher but its total costs are 12.5% higher and may lead you to favour option 1. These examples show up the limitations of this approach, and where there is no clear winner a degree of subjective judgement will have to be employed. These tables do not take into account the sensitivity of the various options to changes, which could affect the rankings – and the cost estimates – still further.

Stage 7: Developing and presenting the outline business case (OBC) – letting key decision makers reach an informed judgement

The OBC must be presented in a report that summarises the results of the strategic review and the investment appraisal. This document must be concise and easy to digest, with consistency between the qualitative and quantitative findings. The level of detail for cost and benefits assessments should be tailored to meet the particular requirements of the decision makers and be proportionate to the nature and scale of the proposed project.

Full business case (FBC) – developing a project blueprint

This includes the findings of the outline business case plus plans for managing and monitoring the project, post-project evaluation and guidance on how to manage any risks that might impact its success. However, the FBC will vary according to the type of financing adopted. If private funding is the chosen route within the NHS, then the planners will have to go through the various stages of the Private Finance Initiative (NHS Executive 1999) procedures before completing the full case. This is in contrast to more conventional capital finance appraisal, and the NHS *Capital Investment Manual* (DH 1994) has a separate section offering guidance for PFI projects.

The physical design of the proposed building is an important consideration when presenting the FBC, as this has significant implications for both the delivery of services and the overall project costs. Those involved in design should seek advice and help from health professionals delivering the services and service users (patients), and also refer to government guidelines and general best practice. Where possible it will be beneficial if they could incorporate innovative features into the design.

Section 3: Capital schemes – from option appraisal to commissioning

Public sector capital projects have traditionally been considered by poli-cymakers to be relatively poorly managed, often coming in late and over budget. The move towards public–private partnerships in the NHS was designed to introduce greater efficiency into the process. The health service has been in the vanguard of the private finance initiative in public sector in England, with both the infrastructure and the associated services being funded privately and paid for over time by the NHS. This concept is now also being applied in other countries in Europe, notably Portugal, Spain, France and more recently Greece. PFI schemes are based around long-term partnerships between the public and private sectors, and in the case of the NHS it is the health service that continues to be responsible for the provision of clinical care to patients. The private sector partner will generally take the form of a consortium made up of a construction company, a facilities management company and a financier providing equity and will typically assume responsibility for the management of facilities and support services within the new hospital, as part of the overall PFI contract.

The PFI in the NHS – progress to date

At the time of writing there have been around 680 completed PFI deals worth some £40 billion across all sectors in the UK. In the acute hospital sector alone there are over £5 billion of schemes that have reached financial close and over £2 billion across 24 schemes are operational. A further £6 billion is currently at the procurement stage, including the scheme at Barts and the London NHS Trust, which has a total capital value well in excess of £1 billion. A further £4 billion of schemes were approved in July 2004 and have yet to start procurement, although in early 2006 there were signs that the government was starting to challenge the financial framework of some PFI schemes (O'Dowd 2006).

A recent survey into the effectiveness of PFI has been carried out by KPMG in cooperation with the Business Services Association. This con-cluded that PFI contracts are operationally effective and that their com-pliance with service level agreements is high, with 98% of respondents reporting that they were meeting their service level agreements. This supported the overwhelmingly positive views that respondents held about the performance of their projects.

However, there has been considerable criticism and questioning of PFI policy in the academic literature (Pollock et al. 1997; Gaffney et al. 1999; Pollock et al. 1999, 2002), with much of this focused on assertions that PFI ultimately costs more than public financing (due to the require-ment to make a return for private sector investors) and hence incurs a long-term debt to be serviced by taxpayers and NHS funders over the long-term. Indeed, Allyson Pollock, the best-known critic of PFI, has asserted that PFI more than doubles the cost of capital as a percentage of NHS trusts' operating income (Pollock et al. 2002). Others such as Sussex (2001) have developed a critique of PFI that asserts that whilst there are acknowledged potential benefits from the policy (e.g. lower construction costs, quicker delivery of projects and better maintained hospitals) there are also some clear (and increasingly recognised) limitations in relation to higher costs of borrowing and how far risk is really transferred to the PFI provider.

Guidance for PFI projects

Developing a common approach

The Capital Prioritisation Advisory Group (CPAG) was established in the NHS in 1997 to advise ministers on how to prioritise capital schemes on the basis of health needs. The CPAG also assesses whether individual schemes are affordable and has ultimate responsibility for deciding whether projects go ahead or not. In 1999 the NHS Executive (as it then was) published the guidance document: *Public Private Partnerships in the National Health Service: The Private Finance Initiative* (1999) which provides practical advice to NHS bodies considering a PFI scheme. Part 2 of the Guidance set outs the PFI procurement process. This was followed by the publication of the NHS Standard Form Project Agreement and Schedules.

In the NHS, many PFI schemes have been completed since the publication of guidance in the 1990s. The Private Finance Unit (PFU) has published a substantial body of standard documents including procurement documentation, output specifications and good practice guides. A strategic outline case (SOC) is required for all capital schemes with an expected value of £25 million or more with strategic health authorities approving all trust and primary care trust schemes up to £25 million. The Department of Health's delegated limit for PFI and IT schemes is £100 million and HM Treasury approval is required for all cases over £100 million.

The procurement process – achieving a competitive and comprehensive bid

Within a PFI process such as that in the NHS, after a scheme has been initially prioritised at a national level, an outline business case will be developed and carefully assessed. The Department of Health then requires a draft 'Invitation to Negotiate' as well as outline planning consent before procurement can start, with projects typically being advertised in the *European Journal*. The tender proposal request should have clear objectives and guidelines to ensure that all bids can be compared on an equal basis. Having made a choice, a preferred bidder letter should be produced, for this is now a mandatory Private Finance Unit requirement in the NHS and confirms the status of the preferred partner, the principal contract terms, the timetable to close and most significantly the (unitary) payment for the entire tenure of the contract term. The bidders' financiers are also required to confirm their support and agreement by countersigning the letter.

Local Improvement Finance Trusts (LIFT) – helping fund smaller developments

Capital schemes are needed for small as well as large-scale capital developments and a solution adopted by the English NHS in 2001 has been the development of a PFI hybrid. This alternative funding route – Local Improvement Finance Trust (LIFT) – was so named as it was designed to provide a 'lift' to primary and community care in areas of high health need. Traditional PFI for single one-off acute hospital developments has not been considered appropriate when building a number of relatively small, new, community-based healthcare facilities. Although LIFT is broadly similar to PFI and subject to the same European Union procurement process, it has two main differences. First, the public sector entities (Partnerships for Health, a joint venture entity between the Department of Health and Partnerships UK, and the local primary care trusts) have a 40% stake in 'Liftco' (the principal LIFT entity). Second, each scheme anticipates a number of smaller developments over time as part of the local Strategic Service Development Plan. Forty-two LIFT projects were announced in the first three waves of schemes and at the time of writing 41 of these have reached financial close and a number have signed second and third tranche schemes in their areas. The initiative has been recognised by the National Audit Office as being effective, providing good value for money and offering 'an attractive way of securing improvements in primary and social care' (National Audit Office 2005).

Why choose a PFI?

Although NHS trusts are required to consider the PFI option when making a capital investment decision, there are still a large number of conventional schemes funded purely by public money, although these tend to be smaller in scale. As NHS foundation trusts get more freedom over borrowing limits (Walshe 2003), a wider range of funding schemes emerge. However, the accounting treatment of capital schemes in the NHS continues to favour PFI, for some people assert that traditional funding offers poor value for money (a claim challenged by the work of Pollock and others), and crucially PFI expenses add to the nation's public sector borrowing figure, meaning that the cost of the asset is capitalised and charged against a trust's external financing limits.

The way in which capital schemes are accounted will affect the level of risk and therefore their overall attractiveness and the main risk indicators commonly applied are:

- design risk
- performance risk
- pricing risk
- demand risk
- operating cost risk
- residual value risk.

There is extensive guidance on this aspect that is available on Department of Health and Treasury websites. A summary of the main alleged benefits and challenges (risks) of a PFI approach to capital development to be considered by healthcare providers when reviewing the potential options open to them is as follows.

Principal benefits of PFI

- Brings private sector skills and expertise.
- Brings private sector finance and capital.
- Delivers budgetary certainty.
- Delivers quality of service over life of contract.
- Organisations only pay when service is delivered.
- Transactions can be accounted off the balance sheet.

Principal challenges or risks

- Market appetite and capacity may not be sufficient.
- PFI or public–private partnership procurement can be a lengthy and costly process.
- Relatively inflexible contracts and structures over the long term.
- Private sector cost of finance is relatively higher than its public sector equivalent.
- There is no absolute transfer of risk from the health system to the private provider.

Financing: a review of the options available

The type of finance package chosen for a healthcare capital development will affect the level of risk for the funding. Larger PFI schemes are generally funded by either bank financing, bonds or (in the case of larger projects) a combination of both, with the European Investment Bank also providing backing that usually comes with a bank guarantee. Some projects have been funded by the private sector without any need for third party finance and refinancing is often also considered once the new facilities have been completed and there is no further construction risk.

This allows a PFI consortium to lower the cost of capital and therefore reduce the revenue payments charged to the healthcare organisation.

Whatever type of funding is used, equity will also be required from the project sponsors or third party specialist equity providers. This is the most expensive type of funding as it carries the highest risk should any problems arise. Bank financing consists of debt that is issued by commercial banks. This usually comprises the bulk of the funding requirement and is the first form of funding to be repaid during the contract period. NHS trusts and their commissioners (funders) are not prepared to accept the risk of variable payments and therefore have to make fixed, index-linked payments agreed in the long-term contract.

Conclusion

This chapter has demonstrated that healthcare capital developments, being concerned with high-value and complex schemes, require the same rigour and detail of planning and analysis as parallel developments in other sectors. Whatever the overall funding of a healthcare system, the processes by which capital schemes are proposed, planned, evaluated and funded need to be stringent and in accordance with best business practice. Schemes also need to be able to demonstrate value for money, whether the funder is the taxpayer, a health insurer, or individuals paying for their care. In many countries, public–private partnerships are being used as a way of managing the investment and risk associated with capital development. Whilst such an approach has some clear benefits in terms of responsiveness, it also brings potential problems in relation to the cost of borrowing and the extent of transfer of risk. What is clear is that capital development requires significant management expertise and acumen, and as healthcare provision continues to develop (see Chapter 4), so the need for flexible and responsive approaches to developing new buildings, equipment and services will be heightened.

Summary box

1 Private finance is now an accepted way of funding health service projects in many health systems.
2 Any new service must show that it satisfies latent demand in the market and is consistent with the broader strategy of the acute trust.
3 The development of a business case should adopt the same approach as that used in a commercial organisation.
4 A range of options for delivering the service should be developed and rigorously assessed using objective criteria.
5 Financial modelling and cost–benefit analysis will help in selecting an option that is affordable and meets the needs of patients and other stakeholders.

6 A private sector partner will generally be a consortium made up of a construction company, a facilities management company and a financier.
7 With PFI, the risk of late completion and overspend is firmly in the hands of the private sector.
8 However, PFI also entails significant risks to the health system, particularly in relation to the long-term nature of the financial commitment in a context where service provision is changing rapidly.
9 The procurement process for capital development should be transparent and competitive.
10 New types of PFI solutions are being developed to help fund smaller healthcare facilities and offer significant potential as patterns of care shift towards more community-based models.

Self-test exercises

1 What do you consider to be the biggest factors influencing the success or failure of a new service? How can you counter these risks when developing a service development proposal?
2 In your experience, are business cases developed in a thorough and objective manner, taking into account a range of options? If not, then how could you implement a more professional approach?
3 How could you get a clear enough understanding of costs to build a NPV and sensitivity analysis?
4 What are the pros and cons of a PFI approach as opposed to more traditional capital funding methods?

References and further reading

Department of Health (DH, 1994) *Capital Investment Manual*. London: Department of Health.
Department of Health (DH, 1998) *A First Class Service*. London: Department of Health.
Gaffney, D., Pollock, A.M., Price, D. and Shaoul, J. (1999) The private finance initiative: NHS capital expenditure and the private finance initiative – expansion or contraction? *British Medical Journal*, 319: 48–51.
National Audit Office (2005) *Innovation in the NHS: Local Improvement Finance Trusts*. London: The Stationery Office.
NHS Executive (1999) *Public Private Partnerships in the National Health Service – The Private Finance Initiative*. London, NHS Executive.
O'Dowd, A. (2006) Three hospital PFI schemes are delayed while government looks at their cost. *British Medical Journal*, 332: 196.
Pollock, A.M., Dunnigan, M., Gaffney, D., Macfarlane, A. and Majeed, F.A. (1997) What happens when the private sector plans hospital services for the NHS: Three case studies under the private finance initiative. *British Medical Journal*, 314: 1266.

Pollock, A.M., Dunnigan, M., Gaffney, D., Price, D. and Shaoul, J. (1999) The private finance initiative: Planning the 'new' NHS: downsizing for the 21st century. *British Medical Journal*, 319: 179–84.

Pollock, A.M., Shaoul, J. and Vickers, N. (2002) Private finance and 'value for money' in NHS hospitals: A policy in search of a rationale? *British Medical Journal*, 324: 1205–9.

Porter, M. E. (2004) *Competitive Strategy: Techniques for Analyzing Industries and Competitors*. New York: Free Press.

Sussex, J. (2001) *The Economics of the Private Finance Initiative in the NHS*. London: Office of Health Economics.

Walshe, K. (2003) Foundation trusts: A new direction for NHS reform? *Journal of the Royal Society of Medicine*, 96: 106–10.

Websites and resources

Department of Health. Public–private partnerships site (England): *http:// www.dh.gov.uk/ProcurementAndProposals/PublicPrivatePartnership/fs/en*

HM Treasury Private Finance Initiative. Key documents: *http://www.hm-treasury.gov.uk. /documents/public_private_partnerships/key_documents/ ppp_guidance_index.cfm*

National Audit Office. PFI and PPP recommendations: *http://www.nao.org.uk/ recommendation/*

Office of Health Economics. Independent research and advisory service that has published reports on capital development and PFI: *http://www.ohe.org/*

Partnerships UK. A joint venture that links public and private sector interests in relation to public–private partnerships: *http://www.partnershipsuk.org.uk*

Scottish Executive. Financial Partnerships Unit: *http://www.scotland.gov.uk/ topics/government/finance/18232/12255*

World Bank. Infrastructure development resources and reports, including links to 'private participation' resources: *http://web.worldbank.org/WBSITE/ EXTERNAL/EXTABOUTUS/ORGANIZATION/EXTINFNET-WORK/0,,menuPK:489896~pagePK:64158571~piPK:64158630~ theSitePK:489890,00.html*

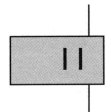

11 Healthcare system strategy and planning

Neil Goodwin

Introduction

This chapter explores health service planning and strategy in the context
of future healthcare policy and organisation. The term 'strategy' is from
the Greek *strategos*, which means 'general'. In the Greek city-states, the
military general was responsible for formulating and implementing a plan
for bringing the legislature's policy decisions to fruition. The terms
'strategy' and 'planning' are often used interchangeably, and grand plans
can be viewed as strategies and vice versa. But the terms 'policy',
'strategy' and 'resources' have quite different meanings. Policy is the goals
and objectives of a government, or of an organisation or of services
provided by an organisation. Strategy and plans determine how those
goals and objectives are to be implemented using resources such as
capital, revenue, leadership capacity, organisational structures and the
workforce. Resources are sometimes confused with tactics but both are
related to how strategy is achieved. Tactics refers to the 'know-how' of
implementation, meaning the decisions and actions needed for successful implementation; whereas resources are the strategy's 'with-what' of
implementation (Davies 2000).

Strategies and plans can be formulated at different levels – government,
interorganisational partnership or network, organisation, service and
department. Organisations will often refer to their 'corporate strategy'
meaning strategy that is used to achieve corporate-level policy goals and
objectives. Although, at a simple level, strategy is a design or plan for how
policy is to be achieved, 'almost no consensus exists about what corporate
strategy is, much less how a company should formulate it' (Porter 1987).
It is therefore not surprising that the concept of strategy can be viewed in
a number of different ways. Having said that strategy and planning are
interchangeable terms, defining strategy solely as a plan is rarely sufficient
because the implementation of strategy is equally important as its content. In that sense, strategy becomes a pattern in a stream of actions,
meaning strategy is consistency of behaviour by the organisation and its
leaders. Strategy can also be a position, specifically a means of locating an

organisation or service in its environment or context. Strategy may also be a ploy, meaning a specific manoeuvre intended to outwit another organisation such as a competitor. Finally, strategy is also a perspective. If strategic position looks outwards, seeking to locate the organisation or service in the external environment, then strategic perspective looks internally. In that context, strategy becomes the ingrained way of perceiving the world.

What is most important to remember about strategy and planning is that healthcare organisations and the services they provide do not stand still. In common with other public service organisations and those in the commercial and charitable sectors, organisations providing healthcare are dynamic entities constantly evolving because their external world is constantly changing and developing. Consequentially, strategies rarely get finished and fully implemented before an organisation's external operating context forces further change if the organisation or service is to survive. For these reasons understanding the policy context and the current and future operating environments of healthcare provision is crucial to strategic planning success.

The healthcare context: change and reform

Along with technological or clinical developments in patient treatment, the economic and operating contexts for governments and healthcare organisations will drive the development of their strategies and plans. The major challenges facing hospitals and other providers of healthcare across the world stem from international macro-economic and demographic health changes. For example, countries across Europe are facing a set of four pressures that will challenge not only the European Union and national politicians but also the local leaders of healthcare organisations and clinical professionals across every country (Goodwin 2005, see Box 11.1). Healthcare in the United States is not immune from these pressures and challenges. The US system, which is subject to more competition

---

Box 11.1   The pressures facing healthcare today

- The drive for greater efficiency, productivity and cost control.
- The growing demand for healthcare as a result of ageing populations and improvements in medical technology and pharmaceuticals.
- The need to devise effective and sustainable responses to increasing consumer demands for greater patient choice, better and faster access to services and the growing number of patients' rights movements.
- The need to manage long-term or chronic diseases such as diabetes, heart disease and obesity, precipitated by increasing longevity, lifestyle and environmental changes.

than virtually anywhere else in the world, has registered unsatisfactory cost and quality performance over many years (Porter and Teisberg 2004).

The pressures facing healthcare systems today apply whether organisations are in competition with each other within a regulated market or quasi-market system or are hierarchically directly managed by national or regional government. Also, although improving efficiency in the healthcare sector is a requirement for national governments, it is also relevant to the wider economic performance of developed countries and to commercial organisations because of their business interest in having a healthy, productive and cost-efficient workforce; for example General Motors spends over $2 billion per year on healthcare (Wigdahl and Tomqvist 2004).

In the late 1980s many European governments began to re-examine the structure of governance in their healthcare systems (Saltman and Figueras 1997; WHO 1996). In particular, the role of the state as being the central player in healthcare is being reassessed and national policy-makers of many countries have felt compelled by a combination of economic, social, demographic, managerial, technical and ideological forces to review existing authority relationships and structures. Europe seems to have experienced widespread disillusionment with large, centralised and bureaucratic institutions and in almost every country, whether economically developed or not, the same drawbacks of centralised systems are being identified: low levels of efficiency, slow pace of change and innovation, and the lack of essential environmental and socio-economic changes to improve population health. The result is that some state functions have been devolved to regional and municipal authorities. At the same time as accelerating the decentralisation of administrative responsibility, most countries are in the process of establishing or strengthening national bodies separate from government to oversee or regulate professional training, quality assurance and the economic performance of healthcare organisations.

Many governments are responding to increasing consumer demand by pursuing national strategies to reduce access times for diagnostic testing and patient treatment, and demanding that providers of healthcare services offer high-quality services in line with international standards. Also, governments are struggling to respond to the lack of incentives for patients, healthcare providers and commissioners of services (the payers) to restrain what they see as excessive utilisation of healthcare services, particularly hospitals. As a consequence, the structural reform themes that now link countries across Europe are decentralisation and devolution of power. Decentralisation and devolvement of authority place greater pressure on the managerial and clinical leaders of healthcare organisations to develop effective and sustainable strategies and implementation plans to respond to the changing context and operating pressures by, among other things:

- stimulating improvements in service delivery by motivating clinical professionals

- securing the better use of resources according to needs
- reducing inequalities in health
- involving citizens in decisions about priorities and the future structure and accessibility of local healthcare services.

It is not surprising that there has been a global epidemic of healthcare reform because of the increasing general discontent with current methods of financing and delivering healthcare. Since the 1980s the organisation of healthcare across large parts of Europe has undergone major change from a professionally driven service to a managerially driven one. Initially, reforms were underpinned by a quasi-market approach, especially in the Netherlands, UK and Scandinavia, but during the 1990s this was succeeded by the new public management approach. This saw governments applying private sector management practices to public sector organisations through the development of quasi-markets, and the introduction of competition and performance management. Some critics, however, have argued that this has resulted in a proliferation of managers and eroded the so-called public service ethos (Dawson and Dargie 2002), whilst in the US competition is seen to be the root of the problem with healthcare performance (Porter and Teisberg 2004).

The UK NHS provides a prime example of repeated structural reform: in the words of the official historian of the UK's health service, 'the time intervals between episodes of major structural reform have progressively diminished to the point that the NHS risks becoming caught up in a vortex of permanent upheaval' (Webster 1998). Competitive market elements and the separation of functions between providers and purchasers of healthcare were formally introduced into the health systems of the UK in the late 1980s. The aim was to enhance the responsiveness of health services by bringing them closer to users' needs and wants, and also to increase efficiency (Glennerster and Le Grand 1995).

The structure of health services across the UK's four countries typifies the different structural approaches to healthcare provision to meet the above pressures and challenges. In common with developments in Spain, health is now a devolved responsibility across the UK with degrees of local autonomy and growing divergence a core feature of health policy. However, the overriding aim of each of the UK's four countries is to create a health service that delivers equitable access to care for patients according to their clinical needs, without regard for their ability to pay and as efficiently as possible. The Welsh Assembly restructured the NHS in Wales in 2003 to strengthen accountability and create a stronger democratic approach. Local health boards commission services and manage and plan primary care provision, whilst public health, tertiary care and ambulance services are now strategically planned, managed and delivered on a national basis.

In Northern Ireland health and social services are integrated and delivered jointly under a single governmental Northern Ireland structure, although it has recently been decided to restructure health and social services to improve service delivery (Secretary of State 2005). A new statutory strategic health and social services authority, to replace four existing organisations, will be established with responsibility for ensuring strong, systemwide performance management and the effective allocation of resources. Hospital and community-based services, currently delivered through 18 provider trusts, will in future be delivered by five organisations. Finally, to bring decision making closer to communities there will be seven local commissioning groups, each coterminous with local (municipal) government.

The NHS in Scotland has undergone a series of structural changes since 1997, each bringing it nearer to the removal of the UK internal market of the 1990s: closer partnership working and, uniquely in the UK, the establishment of an integrated, whole-system approach encompasses both planning and delivery (Scottish Office 1997). This signalled a new relationship between health boards and NHS trusts, resulting in NHS trusts being dissolved as separate statutory organisations to become operating divisions of their local health board (Scottish Executive 2000). Scotland has also introduced community health partnerships, which are new organisations intended to deliver services in partnership with local (municipal) government, the voluntary sector and other agencies. They will seek to bridge the divide between primary and secondary care and between health and social care, replacing service delivery mechanisms that currently are not naturally integrated (Scottish Executive 2003). Further, the role and number of managed clinical networks will be expanded to strengthen clinical leadership and to bridge the boundaries between primary, secondary and social care.

In England, unprecedented extra funding for the NHS (Wanless 2002), additional central targets and a national framework of regulation, principally to improve quality, have brought about significant improvements in recent years. However, the English NHS is being restructured again in 2006 following the last restructuring in 2002 (DH 2005). There is now a belief that further more fundamental changes are needed, including more powerful incentives to drive performance. Hence the introduction of market-style mechanisms, the plan to move away from state monopolies delivering local services to a diverse range of providers including the private sector, and the aim of devolving power and decision making to a local level by creating foundation trusts, which are non-NHS bodies accountable to their local citizens rather than hierarchically to national government.

Although governments see structural change as a solution to many of the ills facing their country's health service, it is by no means certain that such reforms deliver the intended results. For example, ten years after decentralising its health service, the impact on the organisational and managerial modernisation of the Spanish system is not evident (Saltman and Figueras 1997) Equally importantly, attempts by governments to introduce diversity and plurality of provision by separating out elective surgery from general healthcare raise a number of important questions about future policy, strategy development and planning for healthcare organisations. For example, will the majority of services be subject to contestability and market-based competition or is the intention for markets to be developed in some sectors, such as elective care, whilst collaborative planning is the norm in others, for example, in the provision of emergency care or very specialist services?

The healthcare context and strategic responses

The contextual challenges facing health and healthcare are so complex that they defy simple solutions. Understanding the nature of the healthcare environment, the relationship of the organisation to its environment, and the often conflicting interests of internal functional departments and services requires a broad conceptual paradigm. Many of the strategic planning and management methods adopted by healthcare organisations, both public and private, were developed in the business sector. In many respects, healthcare has become a complex business using many of the same processes and much of the same language as the most sophisticated business corporations.

Across much of Europe a consumerist emphasis on competition and choice lies at the centre of national government policy and healthcare strategy. Having stimulated a consumerist approach to healthcare, governments are now likely to be powerless to remove the notion of choice from the public policy debate (Oliver 2005). This can only raise the expectations of citizens on health systems already under considerable pressure. It is possible that government strategies such as choice and competition may well improve some aspects of healthcare by driving out poor professionalism and service delivery. However, choice is likely to be more appropriate in some segments of healthcare, such as elective surgery and diagnostic services, than in other segments, for example, emergency care. Unfortunately, offering greater choice may also often undermine other core goals assuming that primary care practitioners and their patients embrace the choices that are offered to them. For example, it is possible that choice will raise expectations and meeting expectations is costly but the intention of governments is clear: they want to make healthcare more accessible, more efficient and more responsive. The aim is to create services that meet the rising expectations of patients and public, and yet remain affordable within the constraints of government or insurance funded systems. The only way that these laudable aims can be met without significantly increasing costs is to restructure healthcare provision, which requires the formulation of more imaginative strategies and implementation plans that are acceptable to citizens, politicians and healthcare professionals.

Within healthcare, strategy development and service planning is currently undertaken at a number of levels. Although policy is a legislative function and strategy is an executive function, many governments develop strategies for implementing their own policies, often linking future resource availability for health and healthcare to priorities for action. For example, in England, the government has introduced national service frameworks (NSFs), which are long-term national strategies for improving specific areas of care such as heart disease, cancer, child health, mental health and long-term conditions. The NSFs address whole systems of care and set measurable goals within set time frames. Specifically NSFs:

- set national standards and identify key interventions for a defined service or care group
- put in place strategies and plans to support implementation
- establish ways to secure progress within an agreed time scale
- form one of a range of measures to raise quality and decrease variations in service.

Each NSF is developed with the assistance of an external reference group of stakeholders, which brings together healthcare professionals, service users and carers, managers and non-healthcare agencies. The government is responsible, through national clinical directors appointed by them, for managing the development of NSFs and performance managing their implementation across the NHS.

Regional strategic planning is also common for health, healthcare and related services such as social care. For example, by collaborating with other government agencies and socio-economic regeneration businesses, healthcare organisations can play an important role in the regeneration of cities, towns and regions. The strategic planning of specialist healthcare services tends to be undertaken on a regional basis because fewer people consume these services and so larger populations are often required for cost-effective planning and service provision. Examples include cardiac, cancer, vascular, neuroscience and renal services. Finally, local planning will be undertaken for smaller populations to ensure efficient access to those healthcare services consumed by the majority of the population – primary and secondary care.

Undertaking strategic planning

Formulating strategy means defining the key issues needed to be addressed to enable progress to be made in meeting future vision for an organisation or service, whether at government, regional or local level. Vision is a conceptual precursor to the creation of corporate policy, whereas in contrast, mission statements are derived from corporate policy (Davies 2000). Vision is a positive image of what an organisation or service could become and the path towards that aim. Bennis and Nanus (1985) concluded from interviews with 90 top directors that the process of creating a vision – envisioning – requires translating into realities by communicating that vision to others to gain their support. Consequently, vision is the basis for empowering others.

Because implementation of strategy will often involve change, leadership is essential. Vision is the focal point for transformational change because it provides the leader and followers with a map for where the organisation or service is going as well as providing identity, meaning and motivation (Goodwin 2005). Vision has to evolve within the context of the organisation or service and one of the most important leadership roles is to make the vision meaningful through language, actions and stories. When it is communicated clearly, vision seems simple. Consider Henry Ford's *I will build a motor car for the great multitude*; Federal Express founder Fred Smith's *To deliver all packages within 24 hours*; or more simply, Walt Disney's *To make people happy*. As these examples show, vision needs to be bold and ambitious; otherwise it will be seen as merely another organisational objective or aim.

Other aspects of envisioning that are relevant at different levels of an organisation, or across inter-organisational networks, include the formu- lation of strategies based on a SWOT analysis – strengths, weaknesses, opportunities and threats – of the organisation or service, its resources and the interests of its stakeholders, which in the case of healthcare would be government representatives, insurers, patients and local citizens. For example, Gillies (2003) concluded in his SWOT analysis of the English NHS that the fundamental weakness at the time it was undertaken was access to care (see Box 11.2).

In market-based sectors, which increasingly include healthcare with its underlying policy emphasis on consumerism and competition, the aim of

---

Box 11.2   SWOT analysis of the UK NHS

Strengths

- Cost effectiveness
- Patient registration system with GPs
- Health promotion

Weaknesses

- Access to care
- Lack of integrated care

Opportunities

- Build upon experience to date in electronic health records in primary care
- Basic IT infrastructure established through NHSnet
- Interprofessional working

Threats

- Cost control within a global economic downturn
- Staff retention and recruitment
- Organisational change
- Litigation as a pressure to defensive behaviour
- Inappropriate targets driving primary care

Source: Gillies (2003: 72)

strategic planning is to master a market environment by understanding and anticipating the actions of other economic agents, especially competitors. However, strategic development and management should not be regarded as a technique that will provide a quick fix for an organisation that has fundamental management, leadership or service delivery problems (Swayne et al. 2006). Quick fixes for organisations are rare and successful strategic management often takes years to become part of the values and culture of an organisation. Practically every long-lived and highly successful company attributes the primary source of its business success to its culture (Youngblood 2000).

If strategic development is regarded as a technique or gimmick then it is doomed to failure. For organisations operating in markets or quasi-markets, competitive-based strategy will focus on the development of competitive advantage, meaning something an organisation can do that rivals cannot match. It is important to note that competitive advantages are related to characteristics of the external environment in which an organisation operates, primarily its competitors, and not to its internal practices. This means, for example, that although ongoing operating pressures will force healthcare organisations continually to look for economic efficiencies, these are not a competitive advantage because they can be and usually are adopted by other organisations. Most competitive advantage is generated by three factors – customer or consumer captivity, proprietary technology and economies of scale (Porter 1980).

The practical purpose of strategy is to provide a plan that employs multiple inputs, options and outputs to achieve an organisation's policy goals and objectives. Those responsible for leading the formulation of a strategic plan must be able to formulate and evaluate appropriate organisational or service responses and arrange for implementation in detailed operational plans (Wortman 1982). They will be more effective in undertaking this if they are proficient in gathering ideas and information, thinking logically and learning from past strategic and planning mistakes. As people are promoted through their organisations or service, their personal skills in terms of strategic thinking and planning will have to shift from dealing with concrete matters with short-term consequences and for which all the parameters are known to more abstract issues with greater amounts of uncertainty (Jacobs and Jaques 1987).

There are numerous texts available for helping healthcare professionals and managers to undertake competitive strategic analysis. It is not the intention of this chapter to review these texts, however, in 1980 Michael Porter's seminal work, *Competitive Strategy: Techniques for Analysing Industries and Competitors*, was published. This offered a rich framework for understanding the underlying forces of competition in industries, the important differences among industries, how industries evolved and how organisations can find a unique competitive position. Given the direction of current health policy with its increasing emphasis on competition and consumer choice, understanding competitive strategy and planning has never been so important for healthcare leaders. Porter's work, which brought structure to the concept of competitive strategic advantage through defining it in terms of cost and differentiation, precipitated an industry of publications on strategic and competitor analysis and also led to competitive strategy becoming an academic field in its own right. Consequently, managers looking for concrete ways to tackle strategic planning's difficult questions will find Porter's frameworks to be of enormous benefit.

Although the operating context for healthcare gives the impression of a convergence of global consumer demand, understanding and analysing context remains important in strategic development thinking. The ability to understand and distil context into local meaning is an often underrated leadership skill. Separate local environments are still characterised, in both obvious and subtle ways, by different tastes, different business practices and ways of working, and different cultural norms. The more local an organisation's strategies are, the better the implementation tends to be because local ownership of strategies and plans will be greater. Localism facilitates decentralisation and since the days of Alfred Sloan decentralised management has consistently served as a superior structure for concentrating management attention (Greenwald and Kahn 2005). The consequence of this is that if governments are driven to develop market-based approaches for certain services, for example, diagnostics, primary care and elective secondary care, then although they can stimulate market entry by new providers, the successful development of regional markets for healthcare provision should be a local rather than national strategic activity. What is appropriate and works in one region may be neither appropriate nor workable in another because the local contexts and ways of working are likely to be different.

The formulation of strategic plans by organisation or service leaders is typically a group process involving a number of key participants working together. Although strategic planning, particularly SWOT analysis, provides the structure for thinking about strategic issues, effective strategic planning also requires the exchange of ideas, sharing perspectives, developing new insights, critical analysis, and give and take discussion. Strategic momentum is also important because this is the day-to-day activity of managing the strategy to achieve the strategic goals of the organisation or service. Given the increasing complexity of healthcare context, managers responsible for strategy and planning may find general systems theory or a systems approach to be a useful perspective for organising strategic thinking. Attwood et al. (2003) argue twofold: first, that governments the world over are desperate to find more effective ways of delivering better services and new forms of governance that are responsive to user, citizen and community needs; second, that economic forces and globalisation have pushed these previously domestic matters into a wider international context. Government priorities worldwide are now focusing on stabilising national economies and improving public services such as health and healthcare provision. This underscores the importance for healthcare leaders, from government level downwards, to develop effective and sustainable policies, strategies and implementation plans to respond to these pressures and the resultant changes to health services that will follow.

A system is a set of interrelated elements connected to each other, directly or indirectly. In healthcare, there are many such interconnections across primary, secondary and specialist services as well as with social care. Systems thinking brings a way of understanding complexity. Specifically, a systems approach:

- aids in identifying and understanding the big picture
- facilitates the identification of major components of future change
- helps identify important relationships and provides proper perspective
- avoids excessive attention to a single component part
- allows for a broad scope solution
- fosters integration between components and people
- provides a basis for redesign.

As the term implies, the use of the systems approach requires strategic leaders to define the organisation or service in broad terms and to identify the important variables and interrelationships that will affect decisions (Swayne et al. 2006). By so doing, leaders and followers are able to see the big picture in proper perspective. The potential for using systems thinking in strategic development and planning is exemplified by considering the strategic future of hospitals. Today, many hospitals face an uncertain future because of advances in healthcare technology enabling more hospital-based services to be provided outside in community settings; changes in the workforce, especially a reduction in the hours worked by doctors in training; evidence that if some services are better concentrated in fewer centres they are able to achieve superior outcomes; and as referred to above, government policies designed to increase patient choice and stimulate greater efficiency in the use of resources (Ham 2005). Many countries, particularly across Europe, are responding to these pressures by strengthening the primary care based gatekeeping role for access to secondary care, including those not traditionally known for controlling access to hospital physicians such as France, Germany and Poland. In England the introduction of practice-based commissioning is intended to create stronger incentives for primary care physicians to manage demand for care by offering patients alternatives to hospital, resulting in commissioners being able to use the savings to develop the services they see as priorities.

Ham (2005) has identified at least three possible strategic futures for general hospitals, each of which would also emerge by undertaking a SWOT analysis of the average general hospital's organisational strengths, weaknesses, opportunities and threats. The first strategy is to compete aggressively to maintain and if possible increase market share. The second, is to reduce or cease some activities and focus on improving productivity in areas where they have competitive advantage; in other words, cutting costs by concentrating on providing services for which hospital performance enables them to attract patients and income. In this scenario, hospitals might find advantage in horizontal integration, including partnership with other provider organisations and collaboration with specialist centres to enable patients to access care at different hospital locations. Third, diversify into other services, for example sub-acute and primary care. However, experience from the United States would not be a good indicator for strategic success elsewhere. Hospitals and physician groups decided to broaden their services by merging with or acquiring other institutions, which resulted in some 700 hospital mergers between 1996 and 2000 but with few economic and service quality benefits (Porter and Teisberg 2004). Further, in cases where US hospitals pursued vertical integration, they found it difficult to bring together the different cultures of hospital medicine and primary care (Ham 2005).

Undertaking SWOT analyses of individual clinical services would produce more refined results and probably a wider range of strategic options for consideration than those identified above for whole hospital organisations. This is important because it is the level of individual patient care services that should drive the development of strategies and service improvement plans. The more experienced physicians and teams have in treating patients with a particular disease, the more likely they are to create better quality outcomes of care and ultimately generate improved cost effectiveness of service delivery and treatment. However, It would be virtually impossible to explore each strategic option effectively for every service without taking a holistic, system-wide view in conjunction with staff, patients, citizens and other stakeholders.

Finally, there are pitfalls with strategic planning flowing from developing strategies and the associated implementation plans (see Box 11.3). The two interrelated themes running through the list of pitfalls are process and people. It should be remembered when developing inter-departmental and inter-organisational working, which is an essential precursor to formulating strategies and plans, that it is actually individual people who do business with other people, not the corporate management of services or organisations. Consequentially, the development of sustainable interpersonal relationships is crucial to collaborative success. This is important if citizens and stakeholders are to participate effectively in the development of an exciting and stimulating vision. Process and effective people engagement are also important for the leadership and performance management of implementation plans.

Regulation and strategic planning

Most organisations cannot be left to themselves to deliver effective and excellent services. Healthcare organisations, their leaders and staff know they are subject to a range of influences that may act against the objectives desired by themselves, other organisations and patients. For example, a common complaint is that healthcare services are insufficiently responsive to patients or that productivity could be higher. Perhaps it is not surprising that, for example in the UK the last 25 years have seen the

---

Box 11.3 The pitfalls of strategy and planning

Developing strategic plans

- The vision is insufficiently inspirational, challenging, passionate and motivating.
- The vision is not understood by staff and stakeholders, often because they have been insufficiently engaged in its formulation.
- The strategy has been poorly formulated in terms of implementation steps, performance milestones, resource requirements and supporting structure.
- The strategy is not written down and therefore not understood by staff and stakeholders.
- The strategy does not reflect the culture of the organisation or service.
- Too many organisational or service opportunities are identified resulting in no clear strategy emerging that will act as a decision filter for determining future priorities.

Implementation

- Leadership and managerial accountabilities and workforce resources have not been properly determined resulting in poor implementation and the possibility of senior staff turnover.
- Poor quality leadership results in differing levels of support during implementation and consequentially there is limited implementation.
- Performance management arrangements are poor or non-existent, resulting in an inability to understand and account for progress.
- Insufficient delegation of power and authority for implementation resulting in decisions frequently having to be referred upwards.
- No managerial processes have been identified for responding to unforeseen events resulting in the potential for the strategy to be irrevocably 'blown off course'.

---

governmental pendulum swing back and forth from command and control approaches to decentralised market-type changes (Hunter 2005). In market-based systems regulation is one of the range of policy tools to ensure that the core objectives of health and social care systems are met. In their efforts to improve quality, safety and efficiency, many European countries, in reforming their healthcare systems, have introduced regulatory reform either through recentralising or devolving regulatory powers. There are numerous definitions of regulation including the sustained and focused attempt to alter the behaviour of others according to defined standards or purposes with the intention of producing a broadly identified outcome or outcomes which may involved mechanisms of standard setting, information gathering and behaviour modification (Black 2002).

In many countries there has been an increase in the number of regulatory bodies and activities at state and local level in healthcare with the twofold aim of creating a system that provides incentives to innovate and improve quality and efficiency; and providing information to patients and their carers to facilitate choice. To achieve these aims necessitates balancing safety, equity and innovation.

In market-based industries, regulation often takes the form of protecting the consumer from abuse. In public services there can be some blurring of the boundary between internal and external regulation: the state is largely responsible for improving performance and value for money (through internal regulation or performance management), but external regulation (via independent regulators) is concerned with some activities that could be thought of as internal regulation – for example, the UK's Healthcare Commission is required by statute also to improve the performance and value for money of health services.

Regulation is about licensing and accreditation. It is not about a new way of managing the performance of provider organisations although independent regulators often have significant space to define their activities that may result in them straying into internal regulatory areas such as performance management (Dixon 2005). However, a significant challenge for governments is to determine the type and extent of regulation and performance management that will be needed in the development of market-based systems of competition and consumer choice. Specifically how should a market or quasi-market system be regulated and what are the implications for strategic development and planning? Some commentators argue that inequalities are likely to increase as a consequence of the introduction of a market-based approach (Fotaki and Boyd 2005); and that quality and efficiency may well not improve because market mechanisms introduced into public services, particularly health, rely on oversimplified assumptions. Further, there is evidence that services in the UK have already been deregulated to some extent and made less universal as a result of unrelated and gradually implemented policies rather than strategic planning (Higgins 2004).

Although the role of external regulators is generally not to formulate strategy, their activities will directly influence the strategic planning activities of healthcare organisations in two ways. The first way is as a result of the day-to-day activities of regulation. The publication of regulatory reports on intra-organisational issues and inter-organisational comparisons, such as financial management or performance against quality standards, should precipitate local strategic thinking not only to respond to any immediate adverse performance or failure but also to plan for the longer term sustainability. The second way external regulators will have an impact is via their relationship with national government. The potential temptation for governments is to use concerns arising from regulation reports to formulate or demand greater healthcare strategic activity, which is likely to widen the scope of regulatory inspection and thereby increase the burden of regulation. The result would be increasingly centralised strategic and performance management by another name with consequential little development of strategic planning and implementation skills by local healthcare organisations.

Conclusion

Strategic planning has to be driven by its purpose, which is to achieve the successful implementation of policy – whether that of governments, insurance funds or healthcare organisations and services – but two cautions are needed. The first caution is that where there is no linkage between policy and strategy then strategy becomes a means without an end, or is relegated to merely achieving an operational end and not that of an exciting and visionary design or plan for achieving policy objectives. The second caution is that top-down strategies, grand plans and major change initiatives are rarely successful. Despite the persistent mantra of learning from best practice, much local innovation is rarely widely shared and frequently gets lost in its dissemination.

Healthcare internationally is undergoing far-reaching and potentially radical reform. The pressures continue to grow for new forms and standards of delivery and for local joining up and reconnecting of services to users, citizens and communities. These activities are likely to be undertaken against a backdrop of increasing regulation and new relationships formed between healthcare organisations, regulators, citizens and government. The result will be the consequential need for the development and implementation of effective local strategic plans, the success of which will be judged by the development of new, more accessible configurations of healthcare services; the defining of new roles for the hospital of the future; and the devising of new forms of partnership and local and neighbourhood governance. The personal and organisational challenges facing healthcare leaders to meet these changing and challenging requirements by more effective and sustainable strategic development, implementation and leadership are considerable and should not be underestimated.

Summary box

- Policy defines goals and objectives whilst strategy and plans determine how goals and objectives are to be implemented using available resources.
- Strategy can be formulated at different levels – government, organisation, service and department – and understanding the policy and current and future operating contexts of healthcare is crucial to successful strategic development.
- Formulating strategy means defining the key issues to be addressed to enable progress to be made in meeting future vision and because implementation of strategy often involves change, leadership is essential.
- The aim of strategic planning in a market environment is to understand and anticipate the actions of economic agents, especially competitors. Strategic development is best undertaken using SWOT analysis – strengths, weaknesses, opportunities and threats – of an organisation or service.

- Competitive advantages are related to characteristics of the external environment in which an organisation operates, primarily its competitors, and not to its internal practices. Most competitive advantage is generated by three factors – customer captivity, proprietary technology and economies of scale.
- As people are promoted their personal skills in terms of strategic thinking and planning will have to shift from dealing with concrete matters with short-term consequences to more abstract issues with greater amounts of uncertainty.
- The formulation of strategic plans is typically a group process involving a number of key participants working together and given the increasing complexity of healthcare context, general systems theory offers a useful perspective for organising strategic thinking.
- The pitfalls of strategic planning focus on the process of developing strategic plans and engaging people. Remember, it is people who do business with other people.
- By the publication of reports on intra-organisational and inter-organisational performance, the actions of external regulators directly influence the strategic planning activities of governments and healthcare organisations.
- The personal and organisational challenges facing healthcare leaders to develop more effective and sustainable strategic development, implementation and leadership are considerable.

Self-test exercises

1 Identify the national and local contextual policy, strategic and operational pressures for change facing your organisation, service or network. Make sure you understand the impact that each of the pressures will have, identify which of them will have more impact than others and the timescale when the impact will be felt.

2 Undertake a SWOT analysis for your organisation, service or network. What are the main messages? Identify the competitive advantages when compared to competitor organisations or services. How sustainable do you think the competitive advantages are in terms of timescale and the extent to which competitors can replicate them? Identify the necessary changes to increase sustainability and then formulate implementation strategies and plans for change.

3 What are the main components of the system within which your organisation or service sits? Identify the leaders across the system, the key intra- and inter-organisational/service relationships, the extent of their inter-dependency and the influence they have on the ongoing success of your organisation or service.

4 Reflect on your experience of leading or participating in implementing strategy. Consider what went well and what did not go well in terms of participation, process and decision making. List the learning points from your experience, particularly what you would do differently next time and how.

5 In the light of your career experience to date, coupled with your

understanding of the contextual policy, strategic and operating pressures facing your organisation and system, reflect on your personal development needs for leading or participating in future strategy development and planning. List your main development needs and prepare a personal development plan clearly showing how these needs will be met and within what timescale.

References and further reading

Attwood, M., Pedlar, M., Pritchard, S. and Wilkinson, D. (2003) *Leading Change: A Guide to Whole Systems Working.* Bristol: The Policy Press.

Bennis, W.G. and Nanus, B. (1985) *Leaders: The Strategies for Taking Charge.* New York: Harper and Row.

Black, J. (2002) *Critical Reflections on Regulation.* Discussion paper. Centre for the Analysis of Risk and Regulation. London: London School of Economics.

Davies, W. (2000) Understanding strategy. *Strategy and Leadership,* May: 25–30.

Dawson, S. and Dargie, C. (2002) New public management: A discussion with special reference to the UK. In K. McLaughlin, S.P. Osborne and E. Ferlie (eds) *New Public Management. Current Trends and Future Prospects.* London: Routledge.

Department of Health (DH, 2005) *Commissioning a Patient Led NHS.* London: The Stationery Office.

Dixon, J. (2005) *Regulating Healthcare: The Way Forward.* London: King's Fund.

Fotaki, M. and Boyd, A. (2005) From plan to market: A comparison of health and old age care policies in the UK and Sweden. *Public Money and Management,* 25(4): 237–43.

Gillies, A. (2003) *What Makes a Good Healthcare System? Comparisons, Values, Drivers.* Oxford: Radcliffe.

Glennerster, H. and Le Grand, J. (1995) The development of quasi-markets in welfare provision in the United Kingdom. *International Journal of Health Services, 203–18.*

Goodwin, N. (2005) *Leadership in Healthcare: A European Perspective.* Abingdon: Routledge.

Greenwald, B. and Kahn, J. (2005) All strategy is local. *Harvard Business Review,* September: 94–104.

Ham, C. (2005) Does the district general hospital have a future? *British Medical Journal,* 331: 1331–3.

Higgins, J. (2004). Incrementalism in UK policy-making: Privatisation in healthcare. In H. Maarse (ed.) *Privatisation in European Healthcare. The Comparative Analysis of Eight Countries.* Rotterdam: Elsevier.

Hunter, D.J. (2005) The National Health Service 1980–2005. Editorial. *Public Money and Management* 25(4): 209–12.

Jacobs, T.O. and Jaques, E. (1987) Leadership in complex systems. In J. Zeidner (ed.) *Human Productivity Enhancement.* New York: Praeger.

Oliver, A. (2005) The English National Health Service: 1979–2005. *Health Economics,* 14: S75–S99.

Porter, M.E. (1980) *Competitive Strategy: Techniques for Analysing Industries and Competitors.* New York: Free Press.

Porter, M.E. (1987) From competitive advantage to corporate strategy. *Harvard Business Review*, May–June: 43–55.

Porter, M.E. and Teisberg, E.O. (2004) Redefining competition in healthcare. *Harvard Business Review*, June: 65–76.

Saltman, B. and Figueras, J. (eds) (1997) *European Health Care Reform*. Copenhagen: World Health Organisation.

Secretary of State for Northern Ireland (2005) Speech on the outcome of the review of public administration. Belfast, 22 November.

Scottish Executive Health Department (2000) *Our National Health: A Plan for Action, a Plan for Change*. Edinburgh: Scottish Executive.

Scottish Executive Health Department (2003) *Partnership for Care*. Edinburgh: Scottish Executive.

Scottish Office Department of Health (1997) *Designed to Care: Reviewing the National Health Service in Scotland*. Edinburgh: Scottish Office.

Swayne, L.E., Duncan, W.J. and Ginter, P.M. (2006) *Strategic Management of Health Care Organisations*, 4th edn. Oxford: Blackwell.

Wanless, D. (2002) *Securing Our Future Health: Taking A Long-Term View*. London: The Stationery Office.

Webster, C. (1998) *National Health Service Reorganisation: Learning from History*. OHE annual lecture. London: Office of Health Economics.

Wigdahl, N. and Tomqvist, K. (2004) *Improving Efficiency in European Healthcare*. London: Applied Value LLC.

World Health Organization (WHO, 1996) *European Health Care Reforms. Analysis of Current Strategies*. Copenhagen: WHO.

Wortman, M.S. (1982). Strategic management and the changing leader-follower roles. *Journal of Applied Behavioural Science*, 18: 371–83.

Youngblood, M.D. (2000) Winning cultures for the new economy. *Strategy and Leadership*, November–December: 4–9.

Websites and resources

Healthcare regulation. Strategy for delivery: *www.healthcarecommission.org.uk*

Strategy implementation. *www.prospectus.ie*. *www.birnbaumassociates.com*. *www.centreforstrategyimplementation.com*

Systems thinking. Basic explanation: *www.harehall.co.uk/systems.html*. General papers: *www.systemsthinking.net/publications/*. Healthcare papers: *www.nelh.nhs.uk/quality/Process_and_system.asp*

Whole System Partnership: *www.thewholesystem.co.uk*.

12

Healthcare commissioning and contracting

Juliet Woodin

Introduction

Commissioning and contracting (also sometimes described as purchasing or procurement) are complex and much debated features of many healthcare systems today. This chapter initially explores commissioning and contracting through an account of the healthcare policy context within which they have developed, as a backcloth to understanding how the terms are commonly defined and understood. The key elements of commissioning and contracting will then be described, and the technical difficulties of implementing such systems in healthcare discussed. The chapter then considers how commissioning is organised to deliver this complex role. Finally, the chapter examines the evidence about the effectiveness and impact of commissioning in achieving health system goals.

The policy context

Organised healthcare systems are complex entities and include a number of fundamental functions and roles, which are shown in Box 12.1. In insurance-based systems, such as the United States of America (USA), Germany and the Netherlands, the insurance organisation (third party payer) is usually separate from the provider of services (although there are also examples of integration in the USA (Enthoven 1994). In tax funded, publicly run systems such as the United Kingdom, Sweden and New Zealand, third party payers and service providers have traditionally been largely within the same organisation.

During the last decades of the twentieth century healthcare reforms took place in many developed healthcare systems, which made changes to the third party payer role and its relationship with the provider role. These trends during the 1970s to 1990s can be seen as consisting of two phases: during the late 1970s and early 1980s a focus on cost containment

> **Box 12.1   Roles in the healthcare system – a conceptual framework**
>
> *Principal funder*   The citizen or consumer of healthcare who provides the funds
>   – directly or indirectly – to pay for healthcare.
> *Third party payer* The organisation that buys healthcare on behalf of the
>   individual citizen or consumer. This may be the government
>   itself, a public body such as a health authority, or an insurance
>   fund, an employer, or some other form of association. Where
>   the individual buys their own care direct from a healthcare
>   provider, there is no third party payer. This role is often
>   referred to as the 'commissioning' or 'purchasing' role.
> *Provider*   The organisation or clinician delivering care to the patient.
> *Government*   The generator of the national health strategy and priorities
>   which form the framework within which the healthcare system
>   operates.
>
> *Source:* Adapted from Figueras et al. (2005a)

at the macro level; then during the late 1980s and early 1990s, a focus on micro efficiency and responsiveness to users, including the introduction of market-like mechanisms, management reforms and budgetary incentives (Ham 1997). The development of purchasing as a function was a key part of this second phase and illustrates well the phenomenon known as the new public management (Ferlie 1996). NPM embodies the ideas of 'disaggregation of units in the public sector', 'greater competition in the public sector' 'explicit standards and measures of performance' and 'greater emphasis on output controls' (Hood 1991), all of which are features of a commissioning or contracting system.

In the UK an internal market was introduced into the formerly integrated, directly managed healthcare system (DH 1989). Health authorities and general practitioner (GP) fundholders took on a purchasing role and provision was strengthened through the creation of NHS trusts. After the devolution of political power to Scotland, Wales and Northern Ireland, the UK systems diverged somewhat, with Scotland returning to a more integrated system, but England developed the internal market even further (Ham 2004). Similar developments can be observed in the New Zealand health system (Ashton et al. 2004).

In Europe, there is considerable diversity amongst healthcare systems but purchasing or commissioning has become a feature of many (Dixon and Massialos 2002; Figueras, et al. 2005a; Saltman et al. 1998). In the USA, purchasing was well established in a system based predominantly on insurance arrangements and private provision, but many initiatives attempted to strengthen the purchasing function, through the introduction of health plans and managed care, and through experimentation with new funding and contracting mechanisms, such as capitation funding (Chambers et al. 2004; Enthoven 1994; Hughes et al. 1995; Hummel and Cooper 2005; Light 1998; Rodriguez 1990).

There were a number of drivers for these reforms. Most industrialised countries experienced economic crises during the 1970s and 1980s and public spending became a focus of attention. In addition, in economies such as the UK, the public sector (including the NHS) was seen as part of the problem in that its bureaucratic nature was perceived to cause inefficiencies and hold back economic recovery. Added to this there was a view, supported by survey evidence, that healthcare systems were unresponsive to the needs of patients and public and needed reform (Commonwealth Fund 2001). In some countries, political ideas were also a driver, with New Right politicians providing an ideological justification for a reform process which introduced market-type arrangements (Walsh 1995). Pollitt, in examining the drivers for NPM generally, argues that it was 'not so much caused as chosen', 'chosen by practitioners who have been less concerned with purity of theory than with solving (perceived) practical problems' (Pollitt 2003: 36–3).

Whatever the underlying drivers, there has been a burgeoning policy and academic interest in commissioning and contracting roles and processes, against the background of expectations that they will improve the efficiency and responsiveness of healthcare systems. The UK has introduced a number of experiments with commissioning and contracting, which have been studied and reported on, and this chapter will therefore draw on the UK literature to develop case study material and examples from other systems will also be used.

Definitions of commissioning and contracting

The increased interest in the role of the third party payer during the last two decades of the twentieth century has given rise to a vocabulary of terms such as commissioning, contracting, purchasing and procurement. The dynamic and evolving nature of the role has, unsurprisingly but confusingly, led to different terminology being used in different contexts, or the same terms being given slightly different meanings. These differences appear in policy documents and academic literature alike. This chapter will in the main use the terms commissioning, purchasing and contracting, and will define commissioning as the broadest and most strategic set of activities and contracting as the narrowest. These definitions accord with common usage in the UK NHS. The definitions are given in Box 12.2.

Commissioning is a term used most in the UK context and tends to denote a proactive strategic role in planning, designing and implementing the range of services required, rather than a more passive purchasing role. A commissioner decides which services or healthcare interventions should be provided, who should provide them and how they should be paid for, and may work closely with the provider in implementing changes. A purchaser buys what is on offer or reimburses the provider on the basis of usage.

> **Box 12.2   Definitions**
>
> • **Commissioning** is the set of linked activities required to assess the healthcare needs of a population, specify the services required to meet those needs within a strategic framework, secure those services, monitor and evaluate the outcomes.
> • **Purchasing** is the process of buying or funding services in response to demand or usage.
> • **Contracting** is the technical process of selecting a provider, negotiating and agreeing the terms of a contract for services, and ongoing management of the contract including payment, monitoring, variations.
> • **Procurement** is the process of identifying a supplier and may involve, for example, competitive tendering, competitive quotation, single sourcing. It may also involve stimulating the market through awareness raising and education.

Procurement and contracting focus on one specific part of the process – the selection, negotiation and agreement with the provider of the exact terms on which the service is to be supplied. Procurement usually refers to the process of provider sourcing and selection, and contracting to the establishment and negotiation of the contract documentation.

These definitions are similar to those offered by Øvretveit, although his definition of commissioning is even wider, incorporating activities which do not directly involve payment for services, such as influencing other agencies to promote the health of the population (Øvretveit 1995). These broader activities are indeed very likely to be undertaken by organisations designated as 'commissioners'. It is in their interests to encourage others to undertake health-promoting activities and thus contribute to the improvement of health and reduce the call on healthcare services. However, in this chapter the term 'commissioning' is reserved for those activities associated with securing healthcare services. This definition is illustrated in the three distinct functions given to primary care trusts (PCTs) when they were established in the NHS: improving the health of the population; commissioning secondary care services; and developing primary and community health services (NHS Executive 1999).

Finally, it should be noted that in much of the literature describing the US, European and New Zealand health systems the term most frequently used for third party payers is 'purchasing'. Yet the role described increasingly displays the more strategic proactive characteristics associated with 'commissioning' in the UK context. So inevitably when referring to international experience the term 'purchasing' will have a wider meaning.

Commissioning and contracting in theory and practice

As experience and evidence have accumulated about the implementation of health system reforms during the 1990s, a number of books have been published which provide a comprehensive analysis of the theory and practice of commissioning, contracting, primarily in the UK context (for example, Bamford 2001; Øvretveit 1995; Walsh 1995; Hodgson and Hoile 1996; Flynn and Williams 1997; Walsh and Spurgeon 1997). Practical guides to contracting were later produced by government to support commissioning organisations in developing their roles. (DH 2003; National Primary and Care Trust Development Programme 2004). There is not space in this chapter to cover the breadth and detail of these texts, but a brief overview of the tasks and processes involved in commissioning and contracting follows.

The commissioning cycle

As described above, commissioning consists of a set of linked activities. There are many ways of modelling the commissioning process, such as cycles, task lists and levels (Øvretveit 1995: 71–3). The presentation of commissioning as a cycle of activity has become well established, especially in the UK, so this will be adopted as the starting point for this section, as illustrated in Figure 12.1.

This cycle is a simplified model of a process which is in reality far more complex, containing many tasks and activities which cannot always be addressed sequentially as the cycle suggests, and often take place concurrently with each other. Box 12.3 illustrates the some of the more specific tasks that go to make up the main stages of the cycle.

Contracts

Contracts fulfil a number of functions within a commissioning or purchasing system: they incorporate details of the services required (the

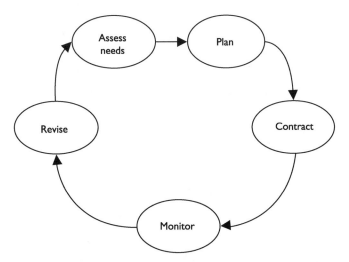

Figure 12.1 Adapted from the commissioning cycle (DH 2003)

Box 12.3   Commissioning and contracting activities

Main stage of cycle	Activities
Assess needs	• Quantification of need based on epidemiological studies, census data, mortality and morbidity rates and other population data • Quantification of need based on health records of registered population/members • Identification of evidence-based interventions • Patient surveys and focus groups • Professional and stakeholder views.
Plan	• Review of current provision • Gap analysis • Prioritisation • Assessment of market capacity • Specification of services required including quality standards
Contract	• Educating the market • Competitive tendering • Determination of contract currency • Negotiation with providers on volume quality and price • Terms and conditions of contract • Arrangements for variations • Determination of routine monitoring requirements.
Monitor	• Reconciliation of invoices • Payment • Analysis of information provided • Reporting and investigation of trends and variances • Contract monitoring meetings • Agreement to variations • Payment.
Revise	• Adjust contract volumes price and other aspects in accordance with terms and conditions • Feed trend and usage information through to longer term needs assessment and planning cycle.

---

specification), the price to be paid, the quality standards to be met, the information to be collected and supplied, the monitoring arrangements, the mechanisms for variation and review of the contract, the duration of the agreement and so on:

> Contracts are the most visible and practical part of purchasing. They are a key tool that defines the relationship between principals (purchasers) and agents (providers). They can be used to reflect the purchaser's health objectives and the health needs of the population, and to make clear what services are to be provided and under which

terms. They also have an important function in specifying the risk-sharing arrangements that apply to either the purchaser of provider in the event of unplanned events. (Duran et al. 2005: 187)

An example of the contents of a healthcare contract is given in Box 12.4. Healthcare systems use a range of contract types, and some of the commonest are shown in Box 12.5. Their use depends partly upon the degree of difficulty of specifying the service required, on the quality of information systems available to support the contracting process, and on the volume and cost of the relevant service or activity. While the theory of commissioning and contracting may suggest that it is a relatively straightforward process, experience has revealed a number of technical difficulties in implementing it in healthcare.

Box 12.4   Illustration of contents of a healthcare contract: the NHS Model Contract

 1 Definitions and interpretation
 2 Commencement and duration
 3 Review
 4 Services
 5 Quality
 6 Service improvement
 7 Service environment
 8 Emergencies and other referrals
 9 Information requirements
10 Access target management
11 Payment
12 Service variation
13 Serious untoward incidents and adverse patient incidents
14 Choice
15 Brokerage
16 Clinical audit
17 Information audit
18 Representatives
19 Dispute resolution
20 Termination
21 Discrimination
22 Data protection and freedom of information
23 Assignment
24 Legal status
25 Entire agreement
26 Schedules
27 Amendments

Source: DH (2003)

Box 12.5   Types of contract

Type of contract	Description	Use
Block	Like a budget for a service. The purchaser or commissioner agrees to pay a fee in exchange for access to a broadly defined range of services. Volumes may not be mentioned or may only be indicative	When costing and activity information is scarce
Cost and volume	Payment is related to treatment of a specified number of patients in a given specialty or service. Payment arrangements for activity above or below the specified volume are defined in the contract.	When reliable information is available to monitor activity and volumes are relatively high
Cost per case	A cost is set for an individual item of service or care package.	For high-cost care which occurs relatively infrequently.

Source: adapted from Savas et al. (1998)

How best should services be specified?

It is perhaps self-evident that in order to place a contract it is necessary to define the product which is to be purchased. The service specification sets out in writing the services required from suppliers, including volume and quality standards. The specification forms the basis of the contract and of monitoring of delivery. Designing service specifications is one of the most challenging parts of the commissioning cycle in healthcare because the healthcare product is in many cases difficult to define and describe in a precise way (Flynn and Williams 1997). These difficulties relate to:

- definition of services at a macro level
- the currency used to describe activity and interventions
- the pace of change of healthcare technology
- provider dominance.

The first difficulty is defining healthcare provision at a macro level. For the purposes of policy, strategy and planning, healthcare is traditionally subdivided or categorised largely on the basis of the professional expertise that delivers the services (e.g. by medical specialty such as general surgery, or ophthalmology, or professional group such as district nursing or physiotherapy). These descriptions reflect the way in which services are conventionally organised and delivered. They map against the supply side of healthcare very easily.

However, health system reform seeks to streamline patient care, removing inefficiencies that occur at organisational and professional boundaries and becoming more responsive to patient experience. Other ways of specifying services have become attractive to commissioners as they seek to pursue this objective; for instance, by reference to the client group to be served (e.g. mental health services, children's services, older people's services), or as disease or condition based (such as diabetes services, cancer services, coronary heart disease services, long-term medical conditions). These categorisations enable all the relevant service elements for that client or disease group to be included, whether they are supplied by primary, community, secondary or tertiary care organisations. However, specifying services in this way raises new boundary issues (many people, especially those who consume most health resources, experience multiple health conditions) and is also dependent upon the development of appropriate information systems and costing structures. Service definition needs to be resolved at this fundamental level for the purpose of designing appropriate specifications.

The second difficulty is in finding a common and meaningful currency in which service activity and interventions can be described. There are many options: diagnosis-related groups, consultant episodes, hospital stays, outpatient attendances, specific operations, complex care packages, capitation (that is the number of individuals for whom comprehensive care must be provided), patient pathways (where the specification describes the care process for a given condition which providers must follow), outcomes of care in terms of improved health status. Commentators have debated the merits and feasibility of some of these (Buckland 1994; Soderland 1994; Kindig 1997). It is generally agreed that some aspects of healthcare activity are more straightforward to specify than others; in particular, elective hospital inpatient activity as opposed to community health services, where interaction between professional and patient is key to the service (Atkinson 1990; Flynn et al. 1996).

The rapid pace of change of healthcare technology provides a further challenge for service specification. New drugs and medical technologies, research evidence about existing treatments and new disease patterns are all part of the fluid environment in which healthcare systems operate. It is not possible therefore to specify service requirements with certainty very far into the future. Service specifications date rapidly and this contains risks for the contracting parties. A further issue related to service specification, which probably compounds the difficulties referred to above, is that in many systems knowledge and expertise about healthcare provision are concentrated in the supplier organisations. Commissioners may not have the detailed understanding of services to specify them fully and incomplete or flawed contract documentation may result. Alternatively, as case studies of the early years of the internal market in the UK showed, purchasing organisations may rely upon providers to write their service specifications, which not only reinforces the tendency towards passive purchasing rather than active strategic commissioning but also undermines the credibility of the purchaser (Dopson and Locock 2002; Short and Norwood 2003).

Making contracts effective

The contract is a key part of any commissioning or purchasing process, but its value is not as an end in its own right but as a means of implementing the strategies and plans of the commissioner. Although contracts are in place in many healthcare systems today, they suffer from number of limitations (Ferlie and McGivern 2003). Amongst these are two areas which will be commented on here:

* information deficits
* enforcement issues.

The information deficits affecting contracts largely mirror those related to service specifications. The problem in many systems is that data collection systems are not developed sufficiently to support the monitoring of activity through contracts. Although some commentators argue that data is available but not systematically used (Soderland 1994), there is agreement that many aspects of healthcare are simply not covered by current systems in a meaningful way. Costing systems contain similar difficulties, especially in the tax-funded systems. A further issue is the management of risk within the contract. The introduction of formal contracts requires arrangements to be agreed about how increases in activity over and above the contracted volume are to be dealt with. The reduction of this risk through predictive modelling is an established technique in predominantly privatised insurance systems such as the USA (Chambers et al. 2004), but is only recently being considered for use in systems such as the UK (Roland et al. 2005).

Effective contracts contain mechanisms such as financial incentives and penalties and the ultimate possibility of termination, which can be used to steer the provider in the direction required or to move to an alternative supplier. Healthcare contracts may be commercial, legally enforceable contracts – as in the USA, New Zealand in the early years of the reforms there (Ashton et al. 2004) and between NHS commissioners and foundation trusts or independent providers – or may be internal service agreements (as within the UK NHS). In principle, both types are enforceable: the former with recourse to the courts if necessary and the latter through managerial action. However, there is evidence that in the UK at least commissioners have been discouraged from enforcement action that would destabilise an NHS provider and that this has impeded the use of contract-type instruments to achieve change (Walsh 1995). Finally, the extent to which a real market exists will affect a commissioner's scope to enforce contract penalties. If there are no alternative suppliers in the market the threat of termination is hollow.

Relational contracting

Although it can be argued that better constructed, written and legally enforceable contracts would have benefits for health systems (Ferlie and McGivern 2003), the real problems and constraints associated with formal or 'hard' contracting in a healthcare context suggest that there are likely to be ongoing obstacles to the achievement of this aim. In addition, there are significant transaction costs associated with establishing a contractual environment which must be set against any benefits gained (Light 1998).

These issues point to the importance of recognising the role that the wider context of relationships, including trust, common values and established and new networks, play in the operation of healthcare systems (Lapsley and Llewellyn 1997). Recognition of this dimension was illustrated in the moderation of the internal market at the start of the New Labour government in the UK, set out in *The New NHS, Modern, Dependable* (DH 1997) and in the development of new styles of agreement between commissioners and providers in Scotland (Deffenbaugh 1998).

Some writers identify the potential for conflict when commissioner–provider relationships and formal contracting are introduced into pre-existing trust-based relationships:

> The development of trust is central to the maintenance of social systems, and the danger of contract is that it undermines trust, through basing contracts on punishment for failure. If we undermine trust then we may find that the making of agreements, and ensuring that they are kept, will become very costly. The value of trust is that it is cheaper to trust people, and to develop institutions that will ensure trust, rather than to watch them. Control and influence over producers may go along with trust and the development of distrust make efficient public service impossible to attain. (Walsh 1995: 255)

However, a number of other writers (Bennett and Ferlie 1996; Ferlie 1996; Flynn et al. 1996; Hodgson and Hoile 1996; Forder et al. 2005; Dopson and Locock 2002; Ferlie and McGivern 2003; Ashton et al. 2004) have observed trust and informal contact continuing to play an important part in commissioner–provider relationships in healthcare alongside a formal contract or service agreement.

A caveat to the discussion about relational contracting is that such relationships cannot be understood without reference to the distribution of power within the system (Cox et al. 2003). Reference has already been made to the dominance of providers in the design of service specifications and this is a broader issue:

> Purchasing in health care is highly vulnerable to provider capture. After all, they control the technology, make the diagnosis, control what is ordered, and control the information that the buyers need.

Thus it has been a long struggle for American commissioning groups of employers to learn how to do it effectively. (Light 1998: 14)

The application of relational contracting ideas to healthcare is an interesting area but one which as yet has not been subjected to systematic analysis or development, taking account of the relative power of the parties.

The commissioning organisation

Discussion of the practical realities of commissioning and contracting for healthcare leads naturally to the question of who, or what type of organisation should be charged with this challenging and difficult role. There is considerable debate about the effectiveness of the variety of types of purchasing organisation that can be seen in different healthcare systems. Employers, commercial insurance companies, sick funds, mutual associations, groups of healthcare professionals and the national or local state in various forms all take on the purchasing or commissioning role (Dixon and Massialos 2002).

The UK has seen a vigorous debate about the appropriate organisational model for commissioning, which has been accompanied by frequent restructuring (Walshe et al. 2004). Locality-based models have been favoured since the mid-1990s, including small-scale, GP-led ones, largely because of the opportunities to build on the traditional strengths of UK primary care in demand management and the potential for joint commissioning with local government (Balogh 1996; Exworthy and Peckham 1998). However, the benefits of an approach based on programmes for specific client groups or conditions, which often need a larger population base, have also been argued (Dalziel 1990; Chappel et al. 1999). The evidence and arguments about the effectiveness of different organisational models are fully examined by Smith and colleagues (2004) who conclude that a mix of approaches is needed in each health economy in the light of the services involved and context.

The concept of the purchaser–provider split implies a clear separation of roles and functions. However, many systems display some degree of integration of the two. In the USA, the growth of managed care has resulted in organisational forms which provide some services in house and purchase others externally (Enthoven 1994). In the UK, GP fund holding, then primary care groups and trusts and now practice-based commissioning build on the gatekeeping role of primary care by giving general practitioners a central role in commissioning, and displaying only a partial separation of functions. Similar approaches were developed in Canada and New Zealand (Peckham 1999).

Linked with this debate about separation or integration is a related one about whether commissioning should be primary care led or not. In the UK the introduction of GP fundholding from 1991 onwards paved the way for further development of primary care led commissioning, so that by 2005 the majority of services were commissioned by primary care organisations. A number of studies of primary care led purchasing have identified an impact on services, albeit modest (Le Grand et al. 1998; Smith and Goodwin 2002; Smith et al. 2004). Internationally, though, this is not a common approach and Light (1998) commenting from a US perspective, has identified a number of drawbacks:

> Primary care lacks the clout to take on powerful specialty groups and hospitals; the technical skills and infrastructure to challenge ineffective or inefficient practices; the time and training to carry out this complex task; the ability to address inequalities and wasteful practices in primary care itself. (Light 1998: 72)

The debate about the extent of separation or integration of commissioning and provision reflects the tension between two principles: impartiality and independence of commissioning, versus integration of care. In a market situation independence is needed to ensure that the commissioner selects the most cost-effective service provision. On the other hand, managing some services directly (usually at the primary care end of the care pathway) may enable commissioners to improve micro-efficiency by integrating care for the patient, and better controlling demand and referrals (Forder et al. 2005).

Wherever commissioning is located, the organisation must possess sufficient capacity and capability to commission effectively. Mays and Dixon identify the following features which affect commissioners' ability to exert influence: holding a budget; 'voice'; pursuing an 'exit' strategy; size; detailed knowledge; personal characteristics; and the influence of the local environment and managerial culture (Mays and Dixon 1996: 24–5). Some of these characteristics are matters of policy (for example, whether or not a budget is held) but others flow from the characteristics of the commissioning organisation, particularly from the information at its disposal and the skills and capabilities of its staff.

Many commissioning organisations in tax-funded systems have evolved from their more bureaucratic and hierarchical predecessors with little attention paid to whether they are appropriately staffed or skilled for their new role. Light compares UK commissioners with US organisations:

> The best American commissioning groups have concluded that health care is far more complicated to purchase than anything else ... Their salary and bonus packages are designed to attract the best and the brightest. They require excellent data systems analysts and programmers, clinical epidemiologists, clinical managers, organizational experts, financial specialists and legal advisers. (Light 1998: 67)

Other writers have endorsed and added to this list of skills and competencies to include competencies such as negotiation, political sensitivity, knowledge of needs and demands of the population, quality management, service improvement, awareness of evidence on

effectiveness and cost effectiveness of different interventions, team working, understanding of ethics, and leadership (Mays and Dixon 1996; Jackson 1998; Bamford 2001; Kaufman 2002; Velasco–Garrido et al. 2005).
While some of these are general management skills, and not inherently
lacking in the evolving purchasing or commissioning organisations,
others are more commercially oriented and may not be present in public
sector bodies. Little investment has been made by governments into providing training and development which could ameliorate this. Ham concludes from his review of international experience that 'the importance
of the purchaser role was not fully appreciated at the outset of recent
reforms and only latterly has action been taken to rectify this' (Ham 1997:
137). In addition, some purchasing organisations have lacked the clinical
skills to engage credibly with providers, yet clinical engagement has been
identified as a key requirement for successful commissioning (Bhopal
1993; Siverbo 2005).

The frequent restructuring of commissioning organisations mentioned earlier has not been confined to the UK, and other systems such as
New Zealand and Sweden have experienced requirements to change
commissioning arrangements. Organisational restructuring has impeded
the development of a cohort of skilled and experienced commissioning
staff, changed the flow of information, and caused a loss of organisational
knowledge. All these factors have constrained the ability of commissioners to establish themselves as authoritative and effective bodies (Smith
et al. 2004; Walshe et al. 2004).

The impact of commissioning

Having considered the policy context for commissioning and contracting, the theory and the practice, this section discusses the evidence about
the strategic impact and effectiveness of commissioning.

The goals of commissioning reflect health system goals. Efficiency,
responsiveness, health improvement and quality, while not a comprehensive list and not always mutually compatible, are relevant to most systems
and form a basis for the evaluation of the effectiveness and impact of
commissioning (Figueras et al. 2005b; Le Grand et al. 1998).

Commissioning for efficiency

The evidence as to whether commissioning has improved system efficiency in any sense is mixed. The OECD states: 'In systems where both
financing and delivery of care is a public responsibility, efforts to distinguish the roles of health-care payers and providers, so as to allow
markets to function and generate efficiencies from competition, have
proved generally effective' (OECD 2004: 17). The purchaser–provider
separation appeared, in the 1990s, to be widely accepted and little

challenged in the UK NHS (Walsh 1995: 255). Le Grand and colleagues, examining the NHS internal market of the 1990s, noted an increase in efficiency as measured by the cost per unit of activity, but found little evidence to demonstrate whether this had been caused by the reforms or by other factors (Le Grand et al. 1998).

However, Ashton and colleagues (2004) found no evidence of major efficiency gains in the hospital sector following the introduction of market reforms in New Zealand. A review of purchasing in the US system in 1996 concluded that 'it is too soon to conclude that purchasers in every market are in the driver's seat guiding changes in the health market' and 'despite some impressive reductions in the rate of health care premium growth, it remains unclear whether these lower annual growth rates are the result of purchaser pressure or are due to exogenous factors at work in the health care market place' (Lipson and de Sa 1996: 75–6).

Several commentators identify the transaction costs incurred by the new system and Light points to a range of new inefficiencies, including 'managerialism, datamania, accountability as an end, disruptions and inefficiencies of underused losers and overused winners and an ethos of commercialism replacing ethos of service' (Light 1997: 322).

Commissioning for responsiveness

Purchasing or commissioning organisations are by definition third-party payers acting on behalf of a population or membership. Lupton and colleagues refer to the 'formal role of purchasers as champion of the people' (Lupton, et al. 1998: iii), within both collectivised and market health systems. Where purchasing or commissioning has been introduced as a system reform, there have been formal expectations that the commissioning organisations will engage with their populations or membership and demonstrate responsiveness to their requirements. The mechanisms for doing this can be categorised as 'voice' and 'exit' (den Exter 2005); the former broadly meaning the use of administrative and managerial techniques for hearing what patients and the public want, and the latter building in market-type mechanisms which give patients maximum opportunity to choose their care.

However, the evidence that exists on this topic suggests that practice has in most health systems been limited in scope and depth and often only occurred in relation to marginal investments or ad hoc issues (Lupton et al. 1998; Peckham et al. 1997). A review of international experience identified many examples of initiatives which facilitate patients or members of the public to influence purchasers, either through the exercise of 'voice' or 'choice'. However, it was not clear how far these mechanisms resulted in changes in the purchaser's policies or improvements in services in response to the issues raised (den Exter 2005). Similar conclusions were drawn in relation to the UK health reforms (Le Grand et al. 1998).

There are a number of reasons why this may be the case. Commissioning organisations in systems with strong national direction (such as the UK) are constrained by nationally determined policies and targets and the scope to respond to the priorities of local populations may be limited. Purchasers may have concerns about the legitimacy of the views of those members of the public who engage in consultation and involvement exercises, and there are costs involved in the proper organisation of patient and public involvement which purchasers may not consider justified (Lupton et al. 1998). The emphasis on clinical involvement in commissioning in many healthcare systems may be in tension with public involvement, in terms both of beliefs and understandings about what constitutes valid evidence of need and benefit, the clinical focus on the individual patient as opposed to the population or group focus, and in terms of established patterns of collaborative or non-collaborative behaviour (Peckham 1999). Finally, poor information systems impede the ability of commissioners to provide precise and meaningful accounts of their activities to the public on whose behalf they are acting.

Commissioning for health improvement

The tendency of contracting to focus on the available measures of activity, which are usually rather limited input measures as described earlier, has stimulated calls for a greater focus on the desired end product of health services: improved outcomes based on the commissioning of evidence-based services (Bhopal 1993; Milne and Hicks 1996; Kindig 1997). Studies of commissioning in the UK illustrate that in practice, however, there have been difficulties in translating strategies for health improvement into action through contracts. Case studies of the implementation of a strategy for stroke services (North 1998) and maternity services (Dopson and Locock 2002) demonstrate that in practice there has been a discontinuity between the needs assessment and planning stages of the cycle and the contracting stage. Contracts departments tended to focus on annual negotiation of volumes and prices of activity, while public health and planning functions considered the changes in services required in the longer term to meet the needs of the population (Milner and Meekings 1996). Implementing service change was not the main focus of contracting activity, and where it did occur, change tended to be at the margin. Studies of GP fundholding do show that fundholders used contracting to achieve service changes but again this tended to be small scale and localised rather than strategic (Le Grand et al. 1998; Smith et al. 2004).

Commissioning for quality

Improving the clinical quality of healthcare was not initially part of the European health system reform agenda, especially not in the case of the UK (Glennester 1998: 405). However, there has been a growing interest in this aspect. Reviews of quality in the early stages of the NHS internal market comment on the limited attention paid to quality in the purchasing process, as opposed to the focus on activity and price (Gray and Donaldson 1996; Thomson et al. 1996; Glennester 1998; BRI Inquiry Secretariat 1999). However, a later review of international experience identified a range of examples in France, Germany, Italy and the UK of quality being made an issue in contracts (Velasco-Garrido et al. 2005). The recent development in the NHS of the Quality and Outcomes Framework (DH 2004) as part of the new General Medical Services contract for GPs, provides a mechanism for linking payment to the achievement of defined quality standards, both clinical and organisational. In the USA, large employers have attempted to use quality standards as a contracting tool (Mello et al. 2003).

In terms of the effectiveness of commissioning in achieving the goal of improved quality, evidence is mixed. Le Grand and colleagues (1998) found some evidence that GP fundholders obtained greater provision of outreach services, quicker admission for their patients and generally more response from providers, compared with those non-fundholding GPs whose services were commissioned for them by health authorities. Despite a major focus on quality improvement in the USA, a review found little evidence of impact (Goldfarb et al. 2003). An international review of quality-based purchasing concluded that 'there is some evidence of public-sector purchasers acting as agents to improve quality, but there is almost no documentation of either formal-sector private insurers, or community-based health financing schemes promoting quality through purchasing' and highlighted the 'large knowledge gaps concerning the results of initiatives taken' (Waters et al. 2004).

Conclusion

Commissioning and contracting have been introduced into health systems comparatively recently against a background of high expectations and within an environment of significant social and economic challenge. There has been little systematic evaluation of their impact, and in any case evaluation of such policy interventions is fraught with difficulties (Le Grand et al. 1998). Such evidence as exists of the success or otherwise of commissioning and contracting is mixed. This is unsurprising given the complexity of the task, the relative youth of the roles and organisations and the limited attention paid to organisational development. What is clear is that commissioning organisations have struggled to assert their authority vis-à-vis provider organisations, which are able to exert influence through their detailed knowledge of services, their control of information, the power and influence vested in their medical staff and the public support which they enjoy. In the context of this imbalance of power, the commissioning role needs investment and development in order to realise its potential.

Summary box

- The separation of commissioning (or purchasing) and providing roles and the establishment of contractual relationships between health commissioners and providers has been a feature of healthcare system reform in many countries during the last two decades. They were expected to provide a means of controlling costs and generating greater efficiency and to make healthcare systems more responsive to public requirements.
- Commissioning and contracting are relatively straightforward concepts in theory, but there are technical difficulties associated with implementing contracting in the healthcare context. In particular, there are a number of problems with the design of meaningful service specifications and contracts.
- The constraints on formal contracting and other features associated with healthcare systems suggest that commissioning and contractual relationships in healthcare display many of the characteristics of relational contracting.
- The challenges of commissioning and contracting in all healthcare systems require strong and competent commissioning bodies. The development of such bodies has been slow, impeded, especially in the UK, by frequent restructuring.
- There has been little focus on the organisational development of the commissioning function.
- There is limited evidence that commissioning and contracting have successfully impacted on system efficiency and responsiveness. There has been considerable interest in their impact on other connected health system goals such as quality, and health improvement, but again evidence is limited.
- This is hardly surprising given the relative youth of commissioning and contracting for health, the lack of consistent attention to the development of the function, and the inherent difficulties of evaluation.

Self-test exercises

1 Obtain a copy of a health service specification. Review it with the following points in mind:

- How adequate is the description of services?
- Does it link to the strategic objectives of the commissioning body?
- Is the service's activity described in relation to inputs, outputs or outcomes?
- Will data be available with which to monitor whether the service is being delivered?
- Generally, do you feel this specification provides a satisfactory basis for a contract?

2 Imagine you are the chief executive of a healthcare commissioning organisation setting up a five-year prospective evaluation of the effectiveness of your commissioning process. Make a list of the

dimensions and indicators you would ask the evaluators to monitor in order to provide the evidence you require.

References

Ashton, T., Cumming, J. and McLean, J. (2004) Contracting for health services in a public health system: The New Zealand experience. *Health Policy*, 69: 21–31.

Atkinson, S. (1990) Commissioning community services. *British Journal of Hospital Medicine*, 44: 311.

Balogh, R. (1996) Exploring the role of localities in health commissioning: a review of the literature. *Social Policy and Administration*, 30(2): 99–113.

Bamford, T. (2001) *Commissioning and Purchasing*. London: Routledge.

Bennett, C. and Ferlie, E. (1996) Contracting in theory and in practice: Some evidence from the NHS. *Public Administration*, 74: 49–66.

Bhopal, R. S. (1993) Public health medicine and purchasing health care. *British Medical Journal*, 306: 381–2.

BRI Inquiry Secretariat (1999) *BRI Inquiry Paper on Commissioning, Purchasing, Contracting and Quality of Care in the NHS Internal Market*. London: The Stationery Office.

Buckland, R. W. (1994) Healthcare resource groups. *British Medical Journal*, 308(23): 1056.

Chambers, N., Kirkman-Liff, B. and Cassidy, M. (2004) Raising Arizona. *Health Service Journal*, 24–25.

Chappel, D., Miller, P., Parkin, D. and Thomson, R. (1999) Models of commissioning health services in the British National Health Service: A literature review. *Journal of Public Health Medicine*, 21(2): 221–7.

Commonwealth Fund (2001) *International Health Policy Survey*. New York: Commonwealth Fund.

Cox, A., Londsdale, C., Watson, G. and Qiao, H. (2003) Supplier relationship management: A framework for understanding managerial capacity and constraints. *European Business Journal*, 15(3): 135–45.

Dalziel, M. (1990) Who should purchase health services? *British Journal of Hospital Medicine*, 44: 381.

Deffenbaugh, J. L. (1998) Healthcare pacts to replace contracting. *Health Services Management Research*, 10: 266–74.

den Exter, A. P. (2005) Purchasers as the public's agent. In J. Figueras, R. Robinson and E. Jakubowski (eds) *Purchasing to Improve Health Systems Performance*. Maidenhead: Open University Press.

Department of Health (DH, 1989) *Working for Patients*. London: The Stationery Office.

Department of Health (DH, 1997) *The New NHS, Modern, Dependable*. London: Department of Health.

Department of Health (DH, 2003) *The NHS Contractors' Companion*. London: Department of Health.

Department of Health (DH, 2004) *Quality and Outcomes Framework Guidance*. London: Department of Health.

Dixon, A. and Massialos, E. (2002) *Healthcare Systems in Eight Countries: Trends and Challenges*. London: European Observatory on Healthcare Systems.

Dopson, S. and Locock, L. (2002) The commissioning process in the NHS. The theory and application. *Public Management Review*, 4(2): 209–29.

Duran, A., Sheiman, I., Schneider, M. and Øvretveit, J. (2005) Purchasers, providers and contracts. In J. Figueras, R. Robinson and E. Jakubowski (eds) *Purchasing to Improve Health System Performance*. Maidenhead: Open University Press.

Enthoven, A. C. (1994) On the ideal market structure for third-party purchasing of health care. *Social Science and Medicine*, 39(10): 1413–24.

Exworthy, M. and Peckham, S. (1998) The contribution of coterminosity to joint purchasing in health and social care. *Health and Place*, 4(3): 233–43.

Ferlie, E. (1996) *The New Public Management in Action*. Oxford: Oxford University Press.

Ferlie, E. and McGivern, G. (2003) *Relationships between Health Care Organisations. A Critical Overview of the Literature and a Research Agenda*. National Co-ordinating Centre for NHS Service Delivery and Organisation R&D.

Figueras, J., Robinson, R. and Jakubowski, E. (2005a) *Purchasing to Improve Health Systems Performance*. Maidenhead: Open University Press.

Figueras, J., Robinson, R. and Jakubowski, E. (2005b) Purchasing to improve health systems performance: Drawing the lessons. In J. Figueras, R. Robinson and E. Jakubowski (eds) *Purchasing to Improve Health Systems Performance*. Maidenhead: Open University Press.

Flynn, R. and Williams, G. (1997) *Contracting for Health. Quasi-Markets and the National Health Service*. Oxford: Oxford University Press.

Flynn, R., Williams, G. and Pickard, S. (1996) *Markets and Networks: Contracting in Community Health Services*. Maidenhead: Open University Press.

Forder, J., Robinson, R. and Hardy, B. (2005) Theories of purchasing. In J. Figueras, R. Robinson and E. Jakubowski (eds) *Purchasing to Improve Health Systems Performance*. Maidenhead: Open University Press.

Glennester, H. (1998) Competition and quality in health care: The UK experience. *International Journal for Quality in Health Care*, 10(5): 403–10.

Goldfarb, N. I., Maio, V., Carter, C. T., Pizzi, L. and Nash, D. B. (2003) *How Does Quality Enter into Health Care Purchasing Decisions?* New York: Commonwealth Fund.

Gray, J. D. G. and Donaldson, L. J. (1996) Improving the quality of health care through contracting: a study of health authority practice. *Quality in Health Care*, 5: 201–5.

Ham, C. J. (1997) *Healthcare Reform: Learning from International Experience*. Maidenhead: Open University Press.

Ham, C. J. (2004) *Health Policy in Britain*. Basingstoke: Palgrave Macmillan.

Hodgson, K. and Hoile, R. W. (1996) *Managing Health Service Contracts*. London: W. B. Saunders.

Hood, C. (1991) A public management for all seasons? *Public Administration*, 69: 3–19.

Hughes, D., Stolzfus Jost, T., Griffiths, L. and McHale, J. V. (1995) Health care contracts in Britain and the United States: A case for technology transfer? *Journal of Nursing Management*, 3: 287–93.

Hummel, J.R. and Cooper, S.J. (2005) The managed care contract: The blueprint for monitoring agreements. *Healthcare Financial Management*, 55(6): 49–52.

Jackson, S. (1998) Skills required for healthy commissioning. *Health Manpower Management*, 24(1): 40–43.

Kaufman, G. (2002) Investigating the nursing contribution to commissioning in primary health-care. *Journal of Nursing Management*, 10: 83–94.

Kindig, D.A. (1997) *Purchasing Population Health*. Ann Arbor: University of Michigan Press.

Lapsley, I. and Llewellyn, S. (1997) Statements of mutual faith: Soft contracts in social care. In R. Flynn and G. Williams (eds) *Contracting for Health. Quasi-Markets and the National Health Service.* Maidenhead: Open University Press.

Le Grand, J., Mays, N. and Mulligan, J.-A. (1998) *Learning from the NHS Internal Market. A Review of the Evidence.* London: King's Fund.

Light, D.W. (1997) From managed competition to managed cooperation: Theory and lessons from the British experience. *Milbank Quarterly*, 75(3): 297–341.

Light, D.W. (1998) *Effective Commissioning: Lessons from Purchasing in American Managed Care.* London: Office of Health Economics.

Lipson, D. J. and de Sa, J. M. (1996) Impact of purchasing strategies on local health care systems. *Health Affairs*, 15(2): 62–76.

Lupton, C., Peckham, S. and Taylor, P. (1998) *Managing Public Involvement in Healthcare Purchasing.* Maidenhead: Open University Press.

Mays, N. and Dixon, J. (1996) *Purchaser Plurality in Healthcare: Is A Consensus Emerging and Is It the Right One?* London: King's Fund.

Mello, M. M., Studdert, D. M. and Brennan, T. A. (2003) The leapfrog standards: Ready to jump from marketplace to courtroom? *Health Affairs*, 22(2): 46–59.

Milne, R. and Hicks, N. (1996) Evidence-based purchasing. *Evidence-Based Medicine*, 1(4): 101–102.

Milner, P. and Meekings, J. (1996) Failings of the purchaser-provider split. *Journal of Public Health Medicine*, 18(4): 379–80.

National Primary and Care Trust Development Programme (2004) *The Commissioning Friend for PCTs. Whole System Commissioning of Acute Services.* London: NHS Modernisation Agency.

NHS Executive (1999) *Primary Care Trusts. Establishing Better Services.* London: NHSE.

North, N. (1998) Implementing strategy: The politics of healthcare commissioning. *Policy and Politics*, 26(1): 5–14.

OECD (2004) *Towards High Performing Health Systems.* Paris: OECD.

Øvretveit, J. (1995) *Purchasing for Health. A Multidisciplinary Introduction to the Theory and Practice of Health Purchasing.* Maidenhead: Open University Press.

Peckham, S. (1999) Primary care puchasing: Are integrated primary care provider/purchasers the way forward? *Pharmacoeconomics*, 15(3): 209–16.

Peckham, S., Macdonald, J. and Taylor, P. (1997) *Towards a Public Health Model of Primary Care.* Birmingham: Public Health Alliance.

Pollitt, C. (2003) *The Essential Public Manager.* Maidenhead: Open University Press.

Rodriguez, A. R. (1990) Directions in contracting for psychiatric services managed care firms. *The Psychiatric Hospital*, 21(4): 165–70.

Roland, M., Dusheiko, M., Gravelle, H. and Parker, S. (2005) Follow up of people aged 65 and over with a history of emergency admissions: Analysis of routine admission data. *British Medical Journal*, 330(7486): 289–92.

Saltman, R. B., Figueras, J. and Sakellarider, C. (1998) *Critical Challenges for Health Care Reform in Europe.* Maidenhead: Open University Press.

Savas, S., Sheiman, I., Tragakes, E. and Maarse, H. (1998) Contracting models and provider competition. In R. B. Saltman, J. Figueras and C. Sakellarider (eds) *Critical Challenges for Health Care Reform in Europe.* Maidenhead: Open University Press.

Short, D. and Norwood, J. (2003) Why is high-tech healthcare at home purchasing underdeveloped and what could be done to improve it? *Health Services Management Research*, 16(2): 127–35.

Siverbo, S. (2005) The purchaser–provider split in principle and practice: Experiences from Sweden. *Financial Accountability and Management*, 20(4): 401–20.

Smith, J. and Goodwin, N. (2002) *Developing Effective Commissioning by Primary Care Trusts: Lessons from the Research Evidence*. Birmingham: Health Services Management Centre, School of Public Policy, University of Birmingham.

Smith, J., Mays, N., Dixon, J., Goodwin, N., Lewis, R., McClelland, S. and Wyke, S. (2004) *A Review of the Effectiveness of Primary Care-Led Commissioning and its Place in the NHS*. London: Health Foundation.

Soderland, N. (1994) Product definition for healthcare contracting: An overview of approaches to measuring hospital output with reference to the UK internal market. *Journal of Epidemiology and Community Health*, 48: 224–31.

Thomson, R., Elcoat, C. and Pugh, E. (1996) Clinical audit and the purchaser–provider interaction: Different attitudes and expectations in the United Kingdom. *Quality in Health Care*, 5: 97–103.

Velasco-Garrido, M., Borowitz, M., Øvretveit, J. and Busse, R. (2005) Purchasing for quality of care. In J. Figueras, R. Robinson and E. Jakubowski (eds) *Purchasing to Improve Health Systems Performance*. Maidenhead: Open University Press.

Walsh, K. (1995) *Public Services and Market Mechanisms: Competition, Contracting and the New Public Management*. Basingstoke: Macmillan.

Walsh, K. and Spurgeon, P. (1997) *Contracting for Change*. Oxford: Oxford University Press.

Walshe, K., Smith, J., Dixon, J., Edwards, N., Hunter, D. J., Mays, N., Normand, C. and Robinson, R. (2004) Primary care trusts. *British Medical Journal*, 329(7471): 871–2.

Waters, H. R., Morlock, L. L. and Hatt, L. (2004) Quality-based purchasing in health care. *International Journal of Health Planning and Management*, (19): 365–81.

Websites and resources

Care Services Improvement Partnership, Better Commissioning Network. The Better Commissioning Learning and Improvement Network was established in April 2004 under the auspices of the Health and Social Care Change Agents Team, part of the English Department of Health. It now forms part of the national networks of the Care Services Improvement Partnership. Its main focus is on commissioning social care but its web pages also provide resources which are relevant to health care: *http://www.changeagentteam.org.uk/index.cfm?pid=7*

Commonwealth Fund. A private foundation supporting independent research on health and social issues. While US focused, it conducts and publishes international comparative surveys of health systems performance and policy approaches: *www.cmwf.org*

Department of Health. Official UK government site. The commissioning pages provide access to policy documentation, guidance and resources for the National Health Service on commissioning and contracting: *http://www.dh.gov.uk/PolicyAndGuidance/OrganisationPolicy/Commissioning/fs/en*

National Committee for Quality Assurance. The NCQA accredits US Health Plans for quality. The website explains the quality rating system, the Health Plan Employer Data and Information Set (HEDIS) which is the NCQA's data collection tool, and provides information about the quality ratings of individual health plans. It gives a useful insight into the US health system of managed care: *www.ncqa.org*

National Electronic Library for Health Specialist Health Management Library. Official electronic library for the English NHS. Produces hot topic guides which include a number on commissioning and contracting related topics: *http://libraries.nelh.nhs.uk/healthManagement/*

National Primary and Care Trust Development Programme. An official government programme linked to the Department of Health. This is an archived site but its commissioning page gives access to key documents supporting primary care-led commissioning such as the PCT Commissioning Friend: *http://www.natpact.nhs.uk/cms.php?pid=99*

Organisation for Economic Co-operation and Development. Health pages give access to key statistics and publications about the health systems of the OECD's 30 member countries: *http://www.oecd.org/topic/0,2686,en_2649_37407_1_1_1_1_37407,00.html*

World Health Organisation Regional Office for Europe. Health systems pages provide details of WHO projects and programmes on all aspects of health systems, and access to publications and reports: *http://www.euro.who.int/healthtopics/HT2ndLvlPage?HTCode=health_systems*

13

Information technology and information systems: so beguiling, so difficult

Justin Keen

Introduction

Electronic services are all around us. Millions of us use the internet, the mobile phone and the many services that they have spawned. Yet peer into any healthcare system and it will still be awash with paper. The technologies and services will be there in the form of email and pagers and sometimes clinical systems, but the relative lack of penetration is very striking.

This chapter argues that electronic services are now very appealing to politicians and policymakers, but they remain difficult to develop and implement in practice. In spite of the ubiquity of electronic services in our everyday lives, policymakers do not have convincing strategies to promote cost-effective solutions in healthcare settings. The next section sets out some of the reasons why IT and electronic services are attractive to politicians and policymakers. The following sections review the current state of implementation, offer a political explanation for this state of affairs and argue that a radically different approach to policymaking is required in order to develop an environment where electronic services can be properly integrated into the fabric of health and social care delivery.

Why is IT so beguiling?

As with many new technologies, IT has long been associated with a number of bold claims. In the 1970s and 1980s these claims focused on the capacity of IT to generate cash savings by reducing the numbers of staff needed for administrative tasks, and quality improvements that would be achieved through increased standardisation and reliability of data processing. In the 1990s the technologies changed and new claims came to the fore. One was that IT was a panacea for a range of management ills, notably in business process re-engineering (Hammer and Champy 1993). IT was a new tool for tackling an age-old problem, namely facilitating the coordination of activities within and between firms. In the expansive language of the business world, the claim was that IT would 'transform' business (Scott Morton 1991). Another, following the arrival of the internet and mobile telephony as social and economic forces, was that technologies and the services they enabled would fundamentally change our private and social lives (Castells 2001).

These developments increased expectations that IT would soon be used extensively in public services, including health services. After all, if we all use them at home, why not at work as well? They were already used in 'back office' functions in the great majority of finance departments and for patient administration. But in all developed countries IT had only penetrated a short distance into the working lives of clinicians. The high penetration of general practice computing in the UK, the extensive networking of healthcare organisations in Denmark and the computerisation of the US Veterans' Administration hospital network were among the few exceptions that proved the general rule. In the UK the problem was compounded because perceptions of IT projects in public services were negatively influenced by a string of high profile failures (Inquiry into the London Ambulance Service 1993; National Audit Office 1996, 1998). Understandably, health service managers and many clinicians were wary of the bolder claims.

But from the late 1990s onwards, politicians and civil servants worldwide bought into the claims. They believed that IT and electronic services would increase the efficiency of public services, partly through service redesign, and would help to improve service quality. They also realised that core government policies would depend for their success on IT implementation in a way they never had done before. For example, it is difficult to imagine delivering choices to consumers of healthcare without real time information systems that show availability and allow people to book their preferred options.

From claims to policies

The bold claims about the transformational potential of IT would, of course, only be fulfilled if 'front office' usage in clinical practice, and the networking of systems to facilitate the exchange of data between services, could be achieved. The main policy response was to publish IT strategies reflecting acceptance of the claims. In many countries – though not the USA – these policies were funded particularly for the development of national or regional network infrastructure and for shared electronic health records.

It is useful to think of the network infrastructure as the spinal cord of an IT infrastructure. In any healthcare system, including centrally funded systems such as the NHS, individual medical centres, hospitals and other organisations purchase their own systems from suppliers. Having done so, organisations can link to the spine and use it to send data to one another. Governments have found themselves funding the spines, principally because no single healthcare organisation has sufficiently strong incentives or the necessary funding; that is, government funding of these network spines solves a 'first mover' problem.

In a few countries elements of this infrastructure have been in place for some years. The NHS and the Danish health services began development of national networks in the mid-1990s. The NHS network, NHSnet, was little used initially but carried substantial volumes of email traffic – up to one million emails on a working day – by 2002. It was not used to exchange clinical information though, partly due to a recommended boycott of NHSnet by the medical profession (Anderson 1995), and partly due to the realisation by civil servants that data within NHSnet were – as doctors' representatives claimed – not secure. The Danish network, in contrast, carried both clinical and administrative data so that by 2002 the majority of prescriptions, as well as hospital referrals, were handled electronically.

It only makes sense to finance a network infrastructure if there are data that can usefully be sent over it. For many policymakers, the key data are in personal electronic health records; that is, the networks and the records systems are really two elements of a single policy idea. Australia, for example, is implementing Health*Connect* (Department of Health and Ageing 2004). The federal government is providing funding – equivalent to around £50 million at 2005 prices – to develop a national network infrastructure. This is happening in parallel with the development of the technical infrastructure for electronic records. Following a series of trials the Australian government has decided, largely on the basis of data protection considerations, to create health summaries which will be shared across the new network. The intention is that these summaries will contain current information needed to treat someone, including their 'live' prescriptions, wherever they happen to access healthcare. Full patient records will not be shared, but kept by the people who treat patients on a regular basis.

Many other countries are pursuing strategies which combine the use of networks and personal records (Gunter and Terry 2005). In his State of the Union address in 2004, President Bush stated: 'By computerizing health records, we can avoid dangerous medical mistakes, reduce costs, and improve care.' His address was accompanied by statements that set a target of access to complete health records for everyone in the USA, anywhere, anytime within ten years (i.e. by 2014). This announcement followed a series of reports from influential bodies, including *The Computer-Based Patient Record* (Institute of Medicine 1997) and *Crossing the Quality Chasm* (Institute of Medicine 2001). Detmer (2003) provides an overview of these developments. One key difference, compared to Australia, is the intention to make complete personal records universally accessible. Another difference is that the fragmented structure of US healthcare creates serious coordination problems, which are perhaps more evident in electronic services than in other spheres. The US federal government is temperamentally averse to solving the 'first mover' problem by funding the network infrastructure directly itself, and prefers exhortation of the healthcare sector and the IT industry to develop and implement the new infrastructure.

Shared health records have a similar place in policymaking in the Department of Health's National Programme for IT in England. It will come as little surprise to English readers to hear that the National Programme, which was formally launched in 2002, is hedging its bets and following Lindblom's (1959) famous dictum – it is muddling through. Building on experience with NHSnet, the National Programme now supports its successor, called N3, which policymakers hope and expect will be used to carry clinical as well as administrative data. In the first instance, summary patient data will be held in something called the 'Spine', a central database connected to N3, in a model broadly similar to Australia's. The long-term aspiration, and one long desired by policymakers, is to build up lifetime medical records and make all records available 'anywhere, any time'. On the face of it this would move England closer to the US proposals, but it remains unclear what data will be available to clinicians operationally. For example, it is not unusual for three different clinicians to see a patient on the same day. It does not make much sense if all three only have access to summary data, when the three of them may need to share vital, detailed contextual information. But there are as yet no formal policies that suggest that this more detailed data will be available, either via local systems or the Spine.

In Denmark, Australia and England, the governments have brought together healthcare organisations and suppliers and provided funding. This said, the National Programme in England is being funded far more generously than initiatives in other countries. Contracts have been awarded for the development of the infrastructure for the NHS Care Records Service to a value of over £4 billion over 10 years from 2004. Further contracts have been awarded for three national initiatives, including N3, hardware and software for booking of appointments (called Choose and Book) and for the electronic transmission of prescriptions, to a combined value of £2 billion. That is, over ten years the additional investment will run at around £600 million per year. It is also significant that the Programme in England is placing its faith squarely with commercial contractors, albeit in an arrangement where they have been set stringent, legally binding performance targets.

The current situation: the evidence base

The policy environment is now encouraging investment then, but what is the state of affairs on the ground? Two types of evidence are available on this question, one conventional, the other less so. The conventional source is the published evidence on the costs and effects of IT and electronic services. The news is dispiriting. Systematic reviews of evidence about electronic health records suggest that there is little evidence of positive effects of records on the working practices of clinicians or administrative staff (Ross and Lin 2003; Delpierre et al. 2004; Poissant et al. 2005). Even where there is evidence of positive change, it tends to be associated with countervailing negative changes. For example, some well-conducted studies show that electronic records reduce the time costs of administrative staff – but the same studies show they simultaneously increase doctors' time costs. For all practical purposes, there is no evidence about cost changes associated with electronic health records.

Casting the net wider, there is little positive evidence about the costs or effects of other information technologies, including communications technologies (Whitten et al. 2002), or large-scale network infrastructure, where there does not appear to be any empirical evidence at all. As a result, there is no evidence that the various claims, such as reduction of medical errors and increased efficiency, will be substantiated in practice. In short, policies around the world are based on beliefs about information technologies and services, not evidence.

Man cannot live by experimental evidence alone, however, and it would be a brave person who suggested that hospital finance departments could be run without the aid of computers, or that no electronic service will ever prove to be effective. Indeed, one possible explanation for the depressing state of the evidence is that academics are guilty of designing the wrong studies. For example, it is possible that the main effects of modern electronic services is structural – that is, experienced across hundreds or thousands of users – and that even large effects of this kind will never be detected using conventional health services research methods. There is indirect evidence that this may be the case, in studies which suggest that differences in IT investment appear to explain differences in economic growth rates for a range of countries during the 1990s (Pilat and Wyckoff 2005). High investment in IT, particularly in the USA, does seem to have led to structural changes in several sectors of the economy, which are in turn now being reflected in productivity gains in those sectors.

The current situation: diffusion

The second type of evidence about the current state of affairs comes from evidence on the diffusion of technologies and services in healthcare systems. Keen and Wyatt (2005) make two observations about diffusion that appear to be borne out in many developed countries. First, there are stark differences between the diffusion of IT across economies in general and in healthcare settings. Second, within healthcare settings it is possible to identify distinct patterns of diffusion for different technologies:

- *No diffusion*: many technologies and services have never progressed beyond the research and development (R and D) phase.

- *Extensive diffusion for networked activities*: for example, for accessing health information on the internet.
- *Extensive diffusion within any one function*: most hospitals in developed countries now have financial management systems and patient administration systems (PAS).
- *'Polynesian' patterns of diffusion within any one function*: for example, some radiology departments have picture archiving and communication systems (PACS) but the majority still do not.

Various explanations can be offered for these different diffusion patterns (Rogers 1995; Van de Ven et al. 1999), but Keen and Wyatt (2005) argue that a political model offers the most convincing explanation. The argument is most easily understood by starting with Moran's (1999) technology policy framework. Moran argues that the state, clinicians (particularly doctors) and technology suppliers are locked into a long-term triangular relationship with one another. The arrangement has been stable over long periods and in many countries because each party derives benefits from the relationship. For example, in the pharmaceutical industry firms have access to markets to sell their products, doctors can use those products to treat people, and governments benefit by being perceived to have paid for a valued service.

In the case of IT and electronic services the same three groups all have interests but, crucially, they have not been able to form stable, long-term relationships with one another. There are two distinct reasons for this. First, the technologies and services are immature and relatively poorly understood: electronic health records are just not as well developed as modern pharmaceuticals, or medical devices. Second, the arrival of the new technologies creates tensions in a system in which working relationships between doctors, other clinicians and managers are often problematic. Examples such as Kaiser Permanente in the USA notwithstanding, it is typical for healthcare delivery to be riddled with coordination problems.

Historically, IT did not pose any new problems because systems were developed initially by small groups of people interested in a particular technology, often together with a relatively small supplier company. This led to the 'cottage industry' feel of IT solutions in many countries. Now, as we have seen, government policies reflect the creation of new, formal alliances between the state, suppliers and other key interests such as large private healthcare providers or insurers. Doctors and other clinicians are faced with a challenge rather than a cosy political alliance.

The problem for clinicians is that, unlike pharmaceuticals or medical devices, electronic services are double-edged. The positive edge is that new services promise plausible sounding quality improvements; for example, in allowing clinicians to access a patient's records in any location and at any time – in someone's own home at 2am, for example – and hence make better diagnosis and treatment decisions. The negative edge is that the same services seem bound to lead to fundamental changes in the nature of clinical work. One does not have to be a disciple of electronic services to believe this claim. By their nature, new services necessitate greater standardisation and greater transparency – transparency being the natural consequence of improved coordination of services. To give a simple example, at the moment there is at best limited cross-over between primary care and hospital patient records. In the future, when all clinicians can access a single patient record, the record will only make sense to readers if everyone agrees to use common terms, but by definition many clinicians will be able to see the decisions and actions taken by all clinicians. While some clinicians are used to working in teams and sharing patient records, this represents a major change for many. It is therefore unrealistic to imagine that all clinicians will immediately welcome the changes.

The extent of this change cannot be overstated and is perhaps best understood using cultural theory, developed originally by the anthropologist Mary Douglas (1987) and since applied to problems of public administration by Christopher Hood (1998). Figure 13.1 shows a 2*2 grid, defined by the dimensions 'grid' and 'group'. Hood explains them in the following way:

> 'Grid' denotes the degree to which our lives are circumscribed by conventions or rules, reducing the area of life that is open to individual negotiation. . . . 'Group', by contrast, denotes the extent to which individual choice is constrained by group choice, by binding the individual into a collective body. For example, if we live in a community which involves common pooling of resources and is differentiated from the world outside – as in a monastic community, a hippy commune, or even some types of exclusive 'clubland' environment – we are operating in high-group mode. (Hood 1998: 9)

Using the grid–group distinction, we can say that doctors have historically been individualists, located in the bottom left-hand corner.

'Group'	Low	High
'Grid'		
High	*The Fatalist Way* Low co-operation, rule-bound approaches	*The Hierarchist Way* Socially cohesive, rule-bound approaches
Low	*The Individualist Way* Atomised approaches stressing local bargaining	*The Egalitarian Way* High participation structures where every decision is 'up for grabs'

Figure 13.1 Four styles of public management organisation
Source: Adapted from Hood (1998).

Electronic services, as in the example of shared electronic records, tend to increase the pressures to coordinate their activities, particularly with other clinical professionals, and thus move from the low to the high group. Because they require standardisation of descriptions of health events, they also imply the need for a move from a low to a high grid environment: electronic services imply compliance with routines, at least in respect of record keeping, but this seems likely to influence clinical behaviour more generally. In short, electronic services require doctors to change along both key dimensions of public administration.

Turning to nurses, we can say that they have historically been located in the fatalist quadrant, at the top left of Figure 13.1. As they are already used to rule-based working, particularly in relation to key aspects of their record keeping, they are likely to have to move along the group dimension, joining many doctors in the high grid–high group quadrant. This said, there is unlikely to be a uniform response and some doctors and nurses will find themselves closer to the bottom right-hand quadrant, particularly in contexts where local discretion remains important, for example, in a range of emergency care contexts. It is also very likely that individual clinicians will respond to these pressures in different ways. Some will judge that the improved coordination and the standardisation are welcome, possibly even overdue, developments. Others will feel threatened by the changes and be inclined to resist them.

The overall result is that IT and electronic services in many countries now have a high political profile and committed public funds, but in a context of immature relationships between the key stakeholders, and where clinicians are likely to respond in different ways to policies reflecting the interests of governments and suppliers.

The politics of IT and electronic services seem set to be further complicated by the emergence of patients as active participants. Policy documents in many countries emphasise the importance of moving from producer-driven to consumer-driven models of healthcare – or put another way towards more person-centred care. This is important in the context of electronic services because increasing numbers of patients, quite reasonably, want to have access to their records and indeed to enter data themselves. In England there is a plan to formalise this arrangement. The NHS has a website called Healthspace (*https://www.healthspace.nhs.uk/*) where individuals can enter their own details. In time, individuals' Healthspace sites will be linked to their NHS records (although again detailed policies are not available at present).

Many readers might view this as an obvious and positive development, but again it is worth emphasising its political dimension. The co-production of care, where doctors and others work collaboratively with patients during diagnosis and treatment, would be a natural consequence of working in a 'high-group' environment. Some clinicians, particularly in primary care, could reasonably be said to do this already, but it will be an unfamiliar way of working to many others. So, this further emphasises the point that many clinicians are facing a fundamental shift in their working practices.

Towards better regulation

The political account of IT and electronic services highlights two key challenges for policymakers. One is to ensure that suppliers operate in a competitive market. The other is to improve the coordination of services, in order to provide a more conducive environment for R and D, and for the implementation of systems and services.

There are compelling reasons to focus on competition, over and above the general point that competition will tend to encourage an efficient (and therefore keenly priced) market and product innovation. One is that the letting of large contracts creates natural monopolies for some services, and monopolies always need watching. A second is that e-government policies also encourage monopolies because they tend to recommend the creation of single channels of communication, for example, individual tax returns filed via a single website such that whoever controls the website has a natural monopoly on that service. A third reason is that the health-care IT market seems to have unusual features, and has historically been filled with niche firms operating on small margins, and consequently investing little in R and D and offering uninspiring products. (These niche players are important because national policies are concerned mainly with infrastructure, and organisations will continue to have to purchase their own systems for internal purposes.) In short, markets seem to have a natural tendency to inefficiency, including low investment in R and D.

A fourth reason concerns ownership arrangements, particularly in countries like England where there is a shift from state-owned to a 'mixed economy' of publicly and privately owned organisations provid-ing services. In a mixed economy the state may have relatively limited control over either the supplier or the healthcare provider – as is the case already in countries with more extensive private or voluntary sector ownership of health organisations. If a government wants private or voluntary providers to adhere to its policies, then it needs a strategy for ensuring proper commercial relationships between them and IT suppliers.

Turning to implementation, there is a key problem of coordination. Whereas healthcare organisations used to be able to purchase systems on their own behalf, electronic services will be used by clinicians across many organisations, so that purchasing decisions and implementation need to be coordinated. Even though governments are contributing to the infrastructure, local organisations will continue to need to purchase and maintain their own systems, and any one organisation will therefore be dealing with many suppliers for the foreseeable future.

In practice, the coordination and competition problems are linked. Two examples help to clarify the nature of the regulatory challenge. First, it is tempting to think that 'Choose and Book' policies in England which allow patients a choice of secondary care providers at the point of referral will be successful if targets set in the national contracts are met. In a regulatory environment, though, the government's task should be to encourage the development of a healthy market for booking services. Bearing in mind the potential for technological monopolies, it might decide to offer different ways of booking appointments, for example, using software in a GP surgery, using alternative software for booking from home and by telephone. There could thus be competition between different communication channels.

Second, there will be some natural monopolies whatever governments do, most obviously in the management of the network infrastructure. Again, it may be tempting to steam ahead and try to fulfil the contracts. A regulator could, though, devise a number of strategies for limiting the deleterious effects of any monopoly, for example, by enforcing quality of service standards and by encouraging a number of firms to stay in the market, even though they do not currently hold contracts. In both cases, the regulator's behaviour would be determined by its view of its own role.

It seems reasonable to argue that these two major issues, both concerned with the regulatory environment, should be the main focus of policies in this area. As we have already seen, governments are seeking to address the large-scale coordination problems through the funding of IT infrastructure. It is striking, though, that there is relatively little in the way of strategies for encouraging the necessary coordination of implementation between individual healthcare organisations beyond the (sensible) identification of standards for exchanging data. Indeed, a fairly laisser-faire approach seems to be the order of the day. If the earlier political analysis is even partially accurate, then this looks like an oversight in policymaking. Neither is there much comment on the need to ensure proper competition in the healthcare IT sector: there is no policy statement on this issue at all in England.

This line of argument has implications for the triangular relationship described earlier. It could be argued that the biggest single regulatory risk lies in the alliance of the state and the suppliers. Conflicts of interest could easily arise because both of them want clinicians to use the new services – even though there is scant evidence of their effectiveness. Governments therefore need to appoint regulators with a formal remit to act as referees in the relationship between suppliers and healthcare organisations, partly to ensure that the supplier–clinician relationship works efficiently, but also to avoid conflicts of interest. There are plenty of precedents for this sort of role. Regulators might, for example, develop a role similar to that of OFCOM, the regulator of telecommunications, wireless services, television and radio in the UK: that is, regulators would need to be able to influence all aspects of the market for IT services, ranging from key data and technical standards, through software marketing regulation to rules for accessing patient records.

Conclusion

The argument in this chapter is that IT and electronic services in health-care systems are intuitively attractive and appealing, but difficult in practice. There is very little empirical evidence that investments are worthwhile, and to date diffusion of systems into clinical work has been patchy. Current policies, around the world, are designed to embed IT and electronic services into clinical work and thereby 'transform' it. The political analysis and the argument about the need for a new approach to policymaking suggest that the bold claims about system reform are unlikely to be substantiated in the short term. A radical rethink of the focus of policies is a priority if governments are to avoid problems of monopoly and market failure in this sector, and provide an environment where organisations can coordinate their implementation efforts. This is not to say that current policies will fail, but is to say that diffusion of the use of shared electronic services will be subject to the vagaries of organisational politics, and likely to proceed in fits and starts.

Summary box

- IT and electronic services are attractive to politicians and policymakers.
- There is scant evidence that investments in IT and electronic services are cost effective.
- On the ground, implementation has historically been patchy, with far greater penetration of IT in 'back office' functions than in clinical practice. Looking at the international picture, general practice computing in the UK is a rare example of high penetration into clinical work.
- Current patterns of diffusion of IT and services are best explained within a political framework.
- Government policies tend to underplay or ignore the political dimension of IT and electronic services. They also ignore a number of problems inherent in the structure of the healthcare IT market. A radical rethink of policies is required, which would involve governments moving towards a more overtly regulatory role.

Self-test exercises

1 What is the ratio of paper and electronic transactions in your own work? In answering the question you should include all communication channels, including post, telephone and email.
2 Why do so many clinicians continue to rely on paper rather than electronic records? What are the arguments in favour of retaining paper records?

3 How do you think doctors' and nurses' work will change when they eventually begin to share personal electronic health records?

4 How can governments ensure that private healthcare organisations are able to generate and share patient health data electronically with one another? Think of ways in which governments can influence organisations in other sectors, such as the television industry, where there are rules governing the technologies that organisations can use and the content of programmes.

References and further reading

Anderson, R. (1995) NHS-wide networking and patient confidentiality. *British Medical Journal*, 311: 5–6.

Castells, M. (2001) *The Internet Galaxy*. Oxford: Oxford University Press.

Danish Centre for Health Telematics (2006) *http://cfstuk.temp.fyns-amt.dk/wm150976* (accessed January 2006).

Delpierre, C., Cuzin, L., Fillaux, J., Alvarez, M., Massip, P. and Lang, T. (2004) A systematic review of computer-based patient record systems and quality of care: More randomized clinical trials or a broader approach? *International Journal of Quality Health Care*, 16: 407–16.

Department of Health and Ageing (2006) *http://www.healthconnect.gov.au/pdf/overviewDec04.pdf* (accessed January 2006).

Detmer, D. (2003) Building the national health information infrastructure for personal health, health care services, public health and research. *BMC Medical Informatics and Decision Making*, 3: 1–18.

Douglas, M. (1987) *How Institutions Think*. London: Routledge.

Gunter, T. and Terry, N. (2005) The emergence of national electronic health record architectures in the United States and Australia: Models, costs and questions. *Journal of Medical Internet Research*, 7(1): e3.

Hammer, M. and Champy, J. (1993) *Reengineering the Corporation*. London: Allen and Unwin.

Hood, C. (1998) *The Art of The State*. Oxford: Oxford University Press.

Inquiry into the London Ambulance Service (1993) *http://www.cs.ucl.ac.uk/staff/A.Finkelstein/las/lascase0.9.pdf* (accessed January 2006).

Institute of Medicine (1997) *The Computer-Based Patient Record: An Essential Technology for Health Care*. Washington, DC: National Academy Press.

Institute of Medicine (2001) *Crossing the Quality Chasm: A New Health System for the 21st Century*. Washington, DC: National Academy Press.

Keen, J. and Wyatt, J. (2005) The social epidemiology of information technologies. In S. Dawson and C. Sausman (eds) *Future Health Organisations and Systems*. Basingstoke: Palgrave Macmillan.

Lindblom, C. (1959) The science of 'muddling through'. *Public Administration Review*, 19: 79–88.

Moran, M. (1999) *Governing the Health Care State*. Manchester: Manchester University Press.

National Audit Office (1996) *The Hospital Information Support Systems Initiative*. HC 332, Session 1995–1996. London: The Stationery Office.

National Audit Office (1998) *NHS Executive: The Purchase of the Read Codes and the Management of the NHS Centre for Coding and Classification.* HC 607, Session 1997–1998. London: The Stationery Office.

Pilat, D. and Wyckoff, A. (2005) The impacts of ICT on economic performance: An international comparison at three levels of analysis. In W. Dutton et al. (eds) *Transforming Enterprise: The Economic and Social Implications of Information Technology.* Cambridge, MA: MIT Press.

Poissant, L., Pereira, J., Tamblyn, R. and Kawasumi, Y. (2005) The impact of electronic health records on time efficiency of physicians and nurses: A systematic review. *Journal of American Medical Information Association,* 12: 505–16.

Rogers, E. (1995) *Diffusion of Innovations,* 5th edn. New York: Free Press.

Ross, S.E. and Lin, C.T. (2003) The effects of promoting patient access to medical records: A review. *Journal of American Medical Information Association,* 10: 129–38.

Scott Morton, M. (1991) *The Corporation of the 1990s.* New York: Oxford University Press.

Shapiro C, Varian H. (1999), *Information Rules.* Boston MA, Harvard Business School Press.

Van de Ven, A. et al. (1999) *The Innovation Journey.* Oxford: Oxford University Press.

Varian H, Farrell J, Shapiro C. (2004), *The Economics of Information Technology.* Cambridge, Cambridge University Press.

Whitten, P.S., Mair, F.S., Haycox, A., May, C.R., Williams, T.L. and Hellmich, S. (2002) Systematic review of cost effectiveness studies of telemedicine interventions. *British Medical Journal,* 324: 1434–7.

Websites and resources

Australian policy. Department of Health and Ageing: *http://www.healthconnect.gov.au/pdf/overviewDec04.pdf*

US Institute of Medicine. Reports can be found at: *http://www.iom.edu/CMS/8089.aspx*

National Programme for IT *http://www.connectingforhealth.nhs.uk/*

Denmark. For developments see: *http://cfstuk.temp.fyns-amt.dk/wm150976*

14 Human resource management in healthcare

Anne McBride and Paula Hyde

Introduction

Healthcare delivery relies upon the ability of healthcare organisations to train and develop, then deploy, manage and engage their workforce. Challenges to healthcare managers are demonstrated through difficulties involved in getting good staff to provide high quality services as efficiently as possible. These challenges remain critical to healthcare management as significant staff shortages are predicted, exacerbated by increasing demand for services. Managers around the world, therefore, share a common desire to manage people in ways that enable the workforce to perform at their best.

There is a range of approaches to managing the healthcare workforce for high(er) performance. In the UK, two streams of activity are evident: the first focuses on making the NHS a 'good employer' thereby recruiting and retaining 'good staff', which could be called human resource (HR) management; the second approach concerns rethinking how to provide 'high quality services' as 'efficiently' as possible, which could be called 'different ways of working'. Such approaches are often referred to as 'modernisation' (see Bach 2002). However, Seifert and Sibley's argument that ' "modernisation" is not a neutral step forward but a highly coloured version of progress rooted in market-style efficiency' (2005: 226) indicates the contentious nature of such terminology. 'Different ways of working' is an attempt to avoid value judgements on the process and outcome of the different ways of working for employees, employers and service users. Given that the UK NHS is the third largest employer in the world, employing 1.3 million staff in 2004, it provides a useful case study to illustrate the processes, outcomes and questions raised by both streams of work.

The chapter begins by outlining characteristics of the healthcare workforce in the UK and the challenges raised for managers. Against this background, the chapter reviews the rationales put forward for HR management and different ways of working, providing recent UK examples of both types of initiatives. The authors then use the Changing Workforce

Programme as an example to provide an illustration of some issues which should be of particular concern to managers endeavouring to get the best from their healthcare workforce.

Characteristics of the UK healthcare workforce

Healthcare organisations are characteristically made up of a large proportion (around 50%) of professionally qualified staff providing frontline services to recipients of healthcare. Table 14.1 gives the proportions of clinical and support staff groups in the NHS. This type of organisational arrangement has been called a 'professional bureaucracy' (Daft 1992). Such organisations are characterised by having high proportions of professionally qualified staff organised around clients or services. Decision making takes place around the operating core (professional frontline staff) and management and administration take place by mutual agreement.

Healthcare is a rapidly growing industry sector. A combination of rapid expansion, high staff turnover and an increasingly ageing workforce has contributed to significant projected staff shortfalls of registered professionals and other skilled staff in countries such as the USA, UK and Australia (Wanless 2002; National Center for Workforce Analysis 2004; Australian Government Productivity Commission 2005). The NHS workforce has experienced an annual staff growth rate in the UK of around 3.5% per year since 1997 (DH 2005a). Doctors and other professionals traditionally work long hours and absence rates in the NHS are high. The average time lost per year in the health service is around 5%, compared to 3.1% elsewhere. Furthermore, management style, poor communication, poor working conditions and stress are cited as reasons for nurse exit or intention to leave (Levell and Jones 1996; Cangelosi et al. 1998; Newman and Maylor 2002). Successful recruitment has been hampered by poor public perceptions of the NHS as an employer because of poor pay, lack of flexible hours and pressures associated with low staff numbers (Arnold 2004).

In this context, healthcare managers face particular challenges not only of recruitment but also of improving working conditions in order that absenteeism reduces and staff retention improves. Managers are challenged with overcoming skills shortages and reducing labour costs. A

Table 14.1   Professionally qualified and support staff in the NHS, 2004

Staff Group	Percentage of NHS workforce
Professionally qualified clinical staff	49.7
Support to clinical staff	34.7
Infrastructure support	15.9

Source: Adapted from Department of Health (2005a).

frequent panacea offered up to address such challenges is workforce 'modernisation'. This can refer to a range of changes to working practices, but within the health service attention has often been focused on challenging professional demarcations. Professional staff groups have distinctive characteristics which include a commitment to a distinct body of knowledge, restrictive entry and peer group evaluation, control and promotion (Dawson 1992). *The NHS Plan* (DH 2000a) and subsequent materials imply that there is a greater scope for overlapping responsibilities, flexibility, multi-skilling and generic work – none of which fits easily with the aforementioned characteristics of professionals. The UK is involved in two streams of activity with the healthcare workforce – HR management and different ways of working.

Why HR management?

There is a substantial body of work supporting the claim that HR management contributes significantly to improved organisational performance (Guest and Peccei 1994; Huselid 1995; Pfeffer 1998; Ulrich 1998). For example, within the UK, a link has been reported between human resource management (HRM) and patient mortality (West et al. 2002) and within the US health sector research has shown that hospitals able to attract and retain good nursing staff (Magnet Hospitals) demonstrate lower mortality rates (Aiken et al. 1994). The exact nature of this HR–performance relationship, however, remains unclear. Common sense suggests that there must be a link between good employment practices and improved performance, but some authors claim that more practices are better; others that specific bundles of practices are more effective and others that the link between HR management and performance is indirect and that there are no clearly identifiable bundles of effective HR practice.

Since linkages between HR management and performance were identified, much has been written about the form HR management should take. These can be broadly categorised into three approaches: 'best practice', 'resource based', and 'best fit'. Each approach implies different means of improving organisational performance through the management of the workforce. For competitive advantage HR practices also aim to improve employee attitudes such as motivation and commitment. Hutchinson and Purcell (2003) illustrate the vital role that frontline managers play in converting HR policies to meaningful action for staff. The following commentary on these three approaches is derived from Boxall and Purcell 2003; Marchington and Wilkinson 2005; Hyde et al. 2006; McBride et al. 2006.

Best practice HR management

Best practice HR management is a universalistic view that the adoption of sets (or bundles) of HR practices will improve performance and benefit organisations and employees. This approach suggests that the closer an organisation gets to applying best practice HR and the more they apply, the better their performance will be. Advocates of this approach stress the importance of mutual goals, a climate of respect, ability of employees to influence decisions, adequate reward structures and shared responsibility.

Although the 'best practice' HR management literature unquestionably flags up key priorities in areas of HR management activity and draws attention to areas where synergy or complementarity between HR management practices are likely to be important in influencing organisational performance, there is no universally accepted list of best practices. Some models involve four or five key practices while others have a dozen or more (Boxall and Purcell 2003: 62). Table 14.2 contains a list of eight HR practices (adapted from Hyde et al. 2006) and will be referred to again later.

Because of its unitary view of the organisation, the best practice approach is likely to create tensions in complex, pluralist healthcare organisations. This is likely to render the unilateral implementation of a single management vision impractical. The constituent organisations that make up healthcare systems will have their own priorities which may constrain implementation of broader policy objectives, and failure to appreciate potentially divergent interests of management and employees could prove costly.

Resource-based HR management

A second approach to HR management is the 'resource-based view' (RBV). This model derives from ideas of 'sustained competitive advantage'; such advantage arising from 'firm resources that are valuable, rare, imperfectly imitable and non-substitutable' (Barney 1991: 116). This model emphasises the role of managers in generating competitive advantage through the development of human capital (see Colbert 2004). Under the RBV, 'core competencies' form the focus as sources of unique competitive advantage, with a priority placed on knowledge within the organisation and developing a focus on 'knowledge management' in order to build on these competencies (Boxall and Purcell 2003: 82). The emphasis here is on competition, with a focus on external factors in determining which resources have value and are worth developing. This approach assumes a competitive environment so would not be suitable for the NHS in its current form. The universal nature of provision that NHS organisations are obliged to provide make it impossible for them to focus only on what they are 'good' at. This approach may, however, be useful to organisations in other countries that do need to develop competitive advantage in the healthcare market place.

Table 14.2   HR practices and NHS policies

HR practice	Purpose and illustration	NHS policy or initiative
Recruitment and selection	*Means of hiring new staff* Techniques can include assessment centres, interviews, psychometric tests, reference checks and work sampling.	Productive Time Efficiency Map
Pay and rewards	*Means of compensating worker* Extrinsic or monetary rewards include: wages, salaries, bonuses, health insurance, company cars and occupational pensions. Intrinsic or non-monetary rewards include: recognition, personal development and social status.	Agenda for Change and HR in the NHS Plan
Appraisal and career development	*Means of assessing performance and offering new opportunities* Evaluation of performance according to managers, work colleagues and/or employees own assessment. Career development may take the form of mentoring, training, career tracking and be linked to appraisal.	NHS Career Framework, Knowledge and Skills Framework, Skills Escalator, and HR in the NHS Plan
Learning and development	*Education and training opportunities* On-the-job training: training on how to do the job within the place of work. May include observation and trial and error. Off-the-job training: takes place away from the place of work and may be based on theory. Examples include: competency training, management development, graduation schemes.	Career Framework, Knowledge and Skills Framework, and Skills Escalator
Employment security	*Means of retaining workers* Making use of internal labour markets through internal promotion.	HR in the NHS Plan
Employee involvement and communication	*Means of communicating between managers and staff* Downwards communications from management to workers including briefing groups, town hall talks and informal communications. Upwards communication including quality circles, attitude surveys, suggestion schemes, problem-solving groups.	Improving Working Lives
Team working and task-based participation	*Means of increasing worker participation* Task-based participation – enlarged or enriched jobs in terms of widening skills or having greater responsibility for organising and managing work.	Changing Workforce Programme
Work–life balance	*Means of improving working conditions* May include crèche facilities, job sharing, parental leave or flexible working hours.	Improving Working Lives

Source: Adapted from Hyde et al. (2006)

Contingency HR management

Contingency or best-fit models (from here referred to as contingency models) offer an alternative model. These approaches advocate the tailoring of HR practices based on contingent factors and the principle that such practices must also complement one another. Boxall and Purcell (2003) identify two main groupings of factors affecting management choices of HR strategy. The first grouping consists of economic and technological factors including sector and competitive strategy, the nature of the dominant technology, size and structure of the firm and stage in the industry life cycle, whether the organisation is well funded or under-capitalised, and general economic conditions. The second grouping of factors is social and political, including labour scarcity, expectations and power of employees, including union strategies, managerial capabilities and politics, labour laws and social norms and general education levels and vocational training systems.

There is a risk that this model is too complex and that at least the 'best practice' model suggests a clear policy focus. However, this approach is more pragmatic and contextually based than the 'one size fits all' approach of the best practice model, in that it considers the range of external and internal factors affecting an organisation when deciding which HR policies to implement. This creates a very flexible framework for analysis that can be applied by managers in any organisational circumstances. (See Self-test exercise 1.)

Why different ways of working?

There is a growing trend across the globe towards changes in workforce configuration and skill mix in healthcare that has been driven by a range of environmental pressures and challenges (Davies 2003). These drivers include: the need to respond to skills shortages; pressure for better management of labour costs (which account for much of overall healthcare cost); a desire to enhance organisational effectiveness; and changes in professional regulation (Adams et al. 2000; Sibbald et al. 2004). Central to such initiatives have been ideas borrowed from two overlapping traditions: first, business process re-engineering, which includes emphasis on worker responsibility, multi-skilling and job variety (Leverment et al. 1998; McNulty and Ferlie 2002); second, role redesign, which focuses on skill variety, task identity and significance, autonomy and feedback (Parker and Wall 1998).

Role redesign 'concerns the way jobs are designed or configured within the overall organization of production' (Bélanger et al. 2002: 17) and dates back to the 1960s. Such initiatives took place against a background of trade union activism and labour shortages and were part of an attempt to deal with rising absenteeism and high staff turnover often linked with Taylorist production systems (Payne and Keep 2003). Role redesign initiatives were claimed to improve outcomes by increasing the meaningfulness of work whilst encouraging employees to experience responsibility for outcomes and to have active knowledge of the results of work activities. Moderating factors included knowledge and skills of the workers and motivation to adapt the role (Parker and Wall 1998).

In the 1980s with labour surpluses and declining union power, role redesign was focused on improving organisational performance. Kelly (1992) proposed that role redesign led to improved performance through: employees negotiating changes in content (and increased output) in exchange for increased pay; employees perceiving closer links between effort, performance and valued rewards; increased goal setting motivating better performance; and improved efficiency of work methods leading to performance improvements. However, improved efficiency can come at a price. Within the NHS, work by Thornley (1996: 165) illustrates how 'the state was able to play on the nebulous character of "skill" in nursing' and substitute cheaper labour for more expensive grades in a process that Thornley calls 'grade dilution'.

The UK policy context

In recent years government policy has moved away from restructuring and reorganising health services towards modernising working practices in particular, and systems and processes of care generally. These policies – aimed at tackling skills shortages and reducing labour costs – originated with *The NHS Plan* which presented a ten-year plan of investment in the NHS (DH 2000a). Furthermore, it laid out two objectives for the work-force: first, specified increases in staff numbers; second, major redesign of roles for NHS staff. Although emanating from the same policy document, in effect these have become two streams of activity.

The HR management approach

The policy document *HR in the NHS Plan* underpins much of the HR management activity in the NHS. Officially launched in 2003, it set out 'a comprehensive strategy for growing and developing the NHS work-force to meet the challenges in the NHS Plan' (DH 2002). The strategy involved four 'pillars' of activity with associated measures to enable staff to redesign jobs around the patient:

1 Making the NHS a model employer by creating an environment conducive to healthy work–life balance, a diverse workforce, job security,
   fair pay, lifelong learning and staff involvement and partnership
   working. Measured through a national target called *Improving Working
   Lives*.
2 Providing model careers through the 'skills escalator', pay modernisation,

learning and personal development, professional regulation and work-force planning.

3 Improving staff morale, recognising that staff attitudes and behaviours impact on patient care.

4 Building people management skills through leadership development programmes and national HR networks.

Development of the strategy as a whole has been underpinned by a national HR in the NHS conference, and the development of leadership development programmes and national HR networks. Progress is measured against annual national targets, for example, *Improving Working Lives*, which contributed to the overall performance rating of each NHS organisation. As noted earlier, Table 14.2 illustrates a range of HR practices (adapted from Hyde et al. 2006). Against each practice is an example of an NHS HR policy initiative, which demonstrates the comprehensive nature of the NHS HR approach. Whilst some policy initiatives have multiple aims, for example, the *HR in the NHS Plan* focuses on HR as a whole, others, like *Agenda for Change*, focus on pay.

This example of a 'best practice' approach managing the workforce, with the NHS endeavouring to become a good employer, was an explicit attempt to address labour market challenge and overcome negative attitudes to working in the NHS noted above. However, this approach has been criticised as its emphasis on national, short-term targets preclude longer term, locally adapted developments. It is therefore possible to see the downside of a best practice approach, which assumes one approach fits all organisational circumstances. National policies and targets have been criticised for diverting manager's attention away from local (rather than national) priorities onto short-term (rather than long-term) developments (Bach 2004). In addition, McBride and Shephard (2006) note that the *HR in the NHS Plan* neglects to focus on the development of line managers, which they note is a serious omission, given the raft of policies they are required to implement and the need to involve line managers in implementing policies (Procter and Currie 1999; Hutchinson and Purcell 2003).

Although the *HR in the NHS Plan* emphasised 'more people, working differently', which infers different ways of working, the HR approach has tended to dominate. Indeed, *New Ways of Working* was a separate stream of activity developed under the Modernisation Agency.

Different ways of working

The policy document *A Health Service of all the Talents* (DH 2000b) underpins much of the NHS work encouraging different ways of working. It argues for an emphasis on 'maximising the contribution of all staff to patient care, doing away with barriers which say only doctors or nurses can provide particular types of care' (original italics; DH 2000b: 5). In particular, professional staff groups are being challenged to change traditional roles, conventional team structures and hierarchies and existing care processes. The example given in the following section examines one attempt to introduce different ways of working (other examples are available at *www.wise.nhs.uk*).

Introducing different ways of working: the CWP example

One of the key mechanisms employed to move towards a patient-centred health service was the NHS Modernisation Agency. This agency was established in 2001 and absorbed into a new NHS Institute for Improvement and Innovation in July 2005. The Modernisation Agency's *New Ways of Working* team was given a remit that involved the revision of pay and staff structures and introduction of new and redesign roles. Introducing the latter was the responsibility of the Changing Workforce Programme (CWP).

Beginning in 2001, 13 CWP pilot sites were established within NHS organisations or health economies around England. The intention was that roles would be redesigned locally under the guidance of CWP who provided project managers and workforce designers to each pilot site for the period of the pilot programme. Potential roles were identified and redesigned through the Role Redesign Workshop (a set of materials aimed at supporting local staff in redesigning their own roles) where local stakeholders came together to redesign roles around a particular patient pathway. A phase of testing was planned to precede anticipated implementation and national spread throughout the NHS, should the redesigned role be judged a success.

CWP employed a contingent, emergent approach to workforce design that could be adapted and used locally. Project managers and workforce designers worked locally, with staff from organisations to initiate role redesign. Nationally, the CWP team worked with professional bodies and education institutions to overcome barriers to change. CWP established a national database of information on new and redesigned roles in health and social care and printed materials and guides (Modernisation Agency 2002a, 2002b). They established Accelerated Development Programmes to support speedier implementation of new roles in areas where the benefits had been tested and proven models were available to guide implementation (Hyde et al. 2005).

Hyde et al.'s (2004) evaluation of CWP led them to conclude that nationally CWP played a key role in developing capacity in the health service for workforce modernisation through role redesign – providing training across the UK, national level support to 'join up the dots' between different initiatives and bodies, and disseminating learning. Locally, CWP led to personal development and job satisfaction for staff; service improvements and strengthened organisational partnerships through the development of roles that involved cross-boundary working.

However, Hyde et al. (2004) indicate that notes of caution were sounded. Questions were raised about how far the new role would free up specialist time. Some CWP participants raised doubts about how radical the redesign roles had been. The researchers also noted that a number of roles were stalled at the funding stage, with neither the organisation nor the funders being prepared to underwrite roles that were in effect additional to previously agreed workforce quotas. The authors also noted that line managers were not easy to involve as they often felt they had more pressing issues to deal with.

Economic and technical factors

Attention to this set of factors means looking at the economic position of the organisation and making decisions based on its organisational strategy and where it stands within the sector/industry. As noted above, a number of roles were not funded beyond the testing stage. This was despite the roles being effective, addressing patient needs and giving staff high levels of job satisfaction and greater commitment to the organisation. McBride et al. (2005) argue that this is explained by the competing logics within the NHS that are geared around the needs of the customer at the same time as being geared around the need for rationality and efficiency. These logics are frequently in contradiction such that a nurse (taking over a task from the junior doctor and thereby saving 20 hours per week) may wish to spend (more) time taking consent from a patient commensurate with patient need, not productivity concerns. If this additional time cannot be absorbed into the overall workforce plan, or become part of a new 'premium fee' business strategy, then such role redesign will not proceed past the testing stage. As noted by one interviewee, 'Directorates are very good at saying they want more, but not that good at saying we are going to fund it by stopping doing Y' (Hyde et al. 2004: 66). Attention to the interface between the economic status of the organisation, organisational strategy, workforce planning and workplace development would be one way of counteracting the tensions between providing patient-centred care and being as efficient as possible. (See Self-test exercise 2.)

Social and political factors

Peck observes (Chapter 19) that power is an underplayed theme in discussions about leadership. Power is also an underplayed theme in discussions about HR and different ways of working and certainly an important feature of the nurse–doctor relationship (Wicks 1998). As noted earlier, CWP was explicitly attempting to challenge profession role demarcations, conventional team structures and hierarchies and established health/social care divides. Parker and Wall (1998) stress the need to involve stakeholders. In complex healthcare organisations there are many to consult: senior managers, line managers, professional groups, unions, users/carer groups. A number of CWP role redesigns required agreement from a number of different stakeholders to a transfer or delegation of duties, and gaining this agreement often took considerable time and expertise.

It is suggested that clear routes for management and accountability should be established prior to the introduction of new roles as failure to provide clear systems can amplify existing professional tensions (Parker and Wall 1998). Generally, within CWP, there were fewer problems of management and accountability when redesigned roles could draw upon existing lines of control. Where organisational or professional boundaries were crossed, responsibility often remained with the delegating professional group who needed to be convinced that appropriate clinical governance procedures were followed. (See Self-test exercise 3.)

Links between HR approach and different ways of working

Hyde et al. (2004) indicate important issues for the manager of the healthcare workforce by illustrating the inextricable links between HR management and different ways of working. Remuneration provides one such illustration.

A large number of redesigned roles were staffed through extensions of existing staff roles (53%). This testing of extended roles through existing staff raised concerns about future recognition and remuneration. For example, one role redesign was delayed because the staff group 'wouldn't do it without remuneration'. Settling pay in advance was an important factor. Not discussing pay in advance of role development led to limitations in the numbers involved (Hyde et al. 2005). Difficulties were also found in roles that crossed professional boundaries where there were existing pay disparities. One example of this was the emergency care worker who could be a paramedic or a nurse who were performing the same new role but who received substantially different remuneration. Difficulties in determining pay settlements faced by healthcare organisations are not unique to this programme (see Bach 1998) and the importance of pay for successful policy implementation has already been noted (Sibbald et al. 2004: 34). Parker and Wall (1998) argued that remuneration should be settled prior to implementation of role redesign and some pilot sites managed this whilst others did not. Increased pay has been linked to increased performance, especially where the employee is involved in negotiating changes of role (Kelly 1992).

Where the links between HR management and different ways of working operate successfully, new practices may become embedded in the organisation. Successful role redesign, whilst developed at a service delivery level, was successful only where strong, explicit support of senior managers was obtained along with associated funding. This meant that roles that had been redesigned by the frontline staff providing the service could be examined at a higher level in the organisation for sustainability by addressing a series of key questions:

- Could the role be financed if expanded to include other workers?
- What arrangements were needed for managerial accountability of roles that crossed traditional boundaries?
- Would it be possible to offer the necessary training and development to a wider group of staff?
- Would the role fit with organisational strategy?

Each of these questions involves an HR management approach in understanding different ways of working. CWP roles that did not continue beyond the testing phase were often impractical in terms of one of the questions above and had proceeded without explicit involvement or commitment of senior managers. Although not stated explicitly, Hyde et al. imply that lack of HR involvement made it more likely that role redesigns would be singular examples, for one or two people, and that they would not be fully funded on a permanent basis. However, Bach (2004) noted that HR management already has numerous and conflicting objectives.

Conclusion

We would argue that HR managers stand in a good position to link HR management to different ways of working as illustrated in successful CWP role redesigns. Indeed, at the time of writing the Department of Health appear to be aligning these two streams of activity by indicating job and service redesign as one of their recommended high impact HR changes (DH 2005b). HR staff have a background in staff involvement and change management as well as an understanding of workforce planning and development, although implementation may be delegated to others.

The example of Changing Workforce Programme suggests that an appropriate role for HR management would be to apply a contingency approach to different ways of working. This approach emphasises the need to understand the economic and technological, and the social and political. (See Self-test exercise 4.)

Summary box

- Approximately 50% of healthcare workforce is professionally qualified.
- Managers challenged with overcoming skills shortages and reducing labour costs often focus on professional demarcations.
- There are links between HR management and improved organisational performance that seem to operate through the employee and line manager, making workforce management an important area for attention.
- There are three different approaches to HR management: best practice, resource-based view and contingency.

- Different ways of working can lead to improved performance, but care must be taken that improved performance is through working smarter rather than harder (since this will only be a short-term gain).
- Considerable recent investment in workforce development in NHS UK through two streams of activity (HR management and different ways of working).
- Using a best practice approach, the UK has focused significant attention on a number of HR practices, but sometimes 'one size does not fit all'.
- Using a contingent approach, the NHS has developed a number of new roles across the UK which has enabled tasks to be delegated to other staff groups to the mutual satisfaction of all stakeholders.
- Critical success factors in long-term workforce development are an awareness of economic and technical and social and political factors of organisation.

These practices are more likely to be embedded in organisations if there are links between HR management and different ways of working.

Self-test exercises

1 Consider the three HR management models (best practice, resource based and contingency). Consider the circumstances of your organisation. Which of these models do you think best suits your organisation? Why do you think this? Which model, or combination, applies to your organisation at the moment? What could you do differently? What benefits would this change bring?

2 Consider the economic and technical factors facing your organisation. What is the level of competition within your healthcare sector? What is the position of your organisation within this environment? Is your organisation well funded or under-capitalised? What is the dominant technology in your organisation? What are the implications of this for developing different ways of working across the organisation?

3 Consider the social and political factors facing your organisation. Is labour scarce? What are the expectations of employees, unions and professional staff groups? What are managerial capabilities? Does the organisation have a workforce plan? What are the politics of the organisation? Is there senior commitment to developing the workforce? What is line management capability and capacity? What is the general level of education of employees? What does the vocational training system provide? What lines of accountability exist within the organisation? What are the implications of this for developing different ways of working across the organisation?

4 In your organisation, consider the extent to which HR are involved in the introduction of different ways of working. Could HR be involved more? If so, what could facilitate this change? What is your role in building these links?

References

Adams, A., Lugsden, E., Chase, J. and Bond, S. (2000) Skill–mix changes and work intensification in nursing. *Work Employment and Society*, 14(3): 541–55.

Aiken, L., Smith, H. and Lake, E. (1994) Lower medicare mortality among a set of hospitals known for good nursing care. *Medical Care*, 32: 771–87.

Arnold, J. (2004) Cut to the chase. *Health Service Journal*, 22: 36–7.

Australian Government Productivity Commission (2005) *Australia's Health Workforce*. Melbourne: Productivity Commission.

Bach, S. (1998) NHS pay determination and work re-organization: Employment relations reform in NHS trusts. *Employee Relations*, 20(6): 565–76.

Bach, S. (2002) Public-sector employment relations reform under Labour: Muddling through on modernization? *British Journal of Industrial Relations*, 40(2): 319–39.

Bach, S. (2004) *Employment Relations and the Health Service: The Management of Reforms*. London: Routledge.

Barney, J. (1991) Firm resources and sustained competitive advantage. *Journal of Management*, 17(1): 99–120.

Bélanger, J., Giles, A. and Murray, G. (2002) Towards a new production model: Potentialities, tensions and contradictions. In G. Murray, A. Giles and J. Bélanger (eds) *Work and Employment Relations in the High performance Workplace*. London: Continuum.

Boxall, P. and Purcell, J. (2003) *Strategy and Human Resource Management*. New York: Palgrave Macmillan.

Cangelosi, J.D., Markham, F.S. and Bounds, W.T. (1998) Factors related to nurse retention and turnover: An updated study. *Health Marketing Quarterly*, 15(3): 25–43.

Colbert, B.A (2004) The complex resource-based view: implications for theory and practice in strategic human resource management. *Academy of Management Review*, 29(3): 341–58.

Daft, R. (1992) *Organization Theory and Design*, 4th edn. New York: West Publishing Company.

Dawson, S. (1992) *Analysing Organisations*. London: Macmillan.

Davies, C. (2003) *The Future Health Workforce*. London: Palgrave Macmillan.

Department of Health (DH, 2000a) *The NHS Plan*. London: DH.

Department of Health (DH, 2000b) *A Health Service of all the Talents*. London: DH.

Department of Health (DH, 2002) *HR in the NHS Plan*. London: DH.

Department of Health (DH, 2005a) Staff in the NHS 2004: An overview of staff numbers in the NHS. *http://www.dh.gov.uk/PublicationsAndStatistics/Statistics/StatisticalWorkAreas/StatisticalWorkforce/fs/en* (accessed 20 June 2005).

Department of Health (DH, 2005b) A national framework to support local workforce strategy development: A guide for HR directors in the NHS and social care. *http://www.dh.gov.uk/PublicationsAndStatistics/Publications/PublicationsPolicyAndGuidance/PublicationsPolicyAndGuidanceArticle/fs/en?CONTENT_ID=4124746&chk=iv8Gmm* (accessed 3 January 2006).

Guest, D. and Peccei, R. (1994) The nature and causes of effective human resource management. *British Journal of Industrial Relations*, 32(3): 219–41.

Huselid, M. (1995) The impact of human resource management practices on turnover, productivity, and corporate financial performance. *Academy of Management Journal*, 38: 635–72.

Hutchinson, S. and Purcell, J. (2003) *Bringing Policies to Life. The Vital Role of Front Line Managers in People Management.* London: Chartered Institute of Personnel and Development.

Hyde, P., McBride, A., Young, R. and Walshe, K. (2004) *A Catalyst for Change: The National Evaluation of the Changing Workforce Programme.* Manchester: Manchester Centre for Healthcare Management, Manchester Business School.

Hyde, P., McBride, A., Young, R. and Walshe, K. (2005) Role redesign: Introducing new ways of working in the NHS. *Personnel Review*, 34(6): 697–712.

Hyde, P., Boaden, R., Cortvriend, P., Harris, C., Marchington, M., Pass, S., Sparrow, P. and Sibbald, B. (2006) *Improving Health Through HRM: Mapping the Territory.* London: Chartered Institute for Personnel and Development.

Kelly, J.E. (1992) Does job re-design theory explain job re-design outcomes? *Human Relations*, 45: 753–74.

Kendall, L. and Lissauer, R. (2003) *The Future Health Worker.* London: IPPR.

Levell, M. and Jones, C. (1996) The nursing practice environment, staff retention and quality of care. *Research in Nursing and Health*, 19(4).

Leverment, Y., Ackers, P. and Preston, D. (1998) Professionals in the NHS – a case study of business process re-engineering. *Work and Employment*, 13(2): 129–39.

McBride, A., Hyde, P., Young, R. and Walshe, K. (2005) Changing the skills of front-line workers: The impact of the embodied customer. *Human Resource Management Journal*, 15(2): 35–49.

McBride, A., Cox, A., Mustchin, S., Antonacopoulou, E., Hyde, P. and Walshe, K. (2006) *Developing Skills in the NHS: Literature Review.* Manchester: Manchester Business School.

McBride, A. and Shephard, A. (2006) HR in the NHS Plan: The perfect plan? A critical appraisal of the HR in the NHS Plan. In M. Tavakoli and H.T.O. Davies (eds) *Reforming Health Systems: Analysis and Evidence.* St Andrews: Tavakoli and Davies.

McNulty, T. and Ferlie, E. (2002) *Re-engineering Healthcare: The Complexities of Organizational Transformation.* Oxford: Oxford University Press.

Marchington, M. and Wilkinson, A. (2005) *Human Resource Management at Work*, 3rd edn. London: Chartered Institute of Personnel and Development.

Modernisation Agency (2002a) *Workforce Matters: A Good Practice Guide to Role Redesign in Primary Care.* London: Department of Health.

Modernisation Agency (2002b) *Workforce Matters: A Guide to Role Redesign for Staff in the Wider Healthcare Team.* London: Department of Health.

National Center for Workforce Analysis (2004) *Effects of the Workforce Investment Act of 1998 on Health Workforce Development in the States.* Washington, DC: Department of Health and Human Services. *http://bhpr.hrsa.gov/healthworkforce/reports/factbook.htm* (accessed 5 December 2005).

Newman, K. and Maylor, U. (2002) The NHS Plan: Nurse satisfaction, commitment and retention strategies. *Health Services Management Research*, 15: 93–105.

Parker, S. and Wall, T. (1998) *Job and Work Redesign: Organizing Work to Promote Well-being and Effectiveness.* London: Sage.

Paauwe, J. (2004) *Human Resource Management and Performance.* Oxford: Oxford University Press.

Payne, J. and Keep, E. (2003) Revisiting the Nordic approaches to work re-organization and job redesign: Lessons for UK skills policy. *Policy Studies*, 24(4): 205–25.

Pfeffer, J. (1998) *The Human Equation: Building Profits by Putting People First.* Boston: Harvard Business School Press.

Procter, S. and Currie, G. (1999) The role of the personnel function: roles, perceptions and processes in an NHS Trust. *International Journal of Human Resource Management*, 10(6): 1077–91.

Purcell, J., Kinnie, N., Hutchinson, S., Rayton, B. and Swart, J. (2003) *Understanding the People and Performance Link: Unlocking the Black Box*. London: Chartered Institute of Personnel and Development.

Seifert, R. and Sibley, T. (2005) *United They Stood: The Story of the UK Firefighters' Dispute 2003–2004*. London: Lawrence and Wishart.

Sibbald, B., Shen, J. and McBride, A. (2004) Changing the skill mix of the healthcare workforce, *Journal of Health Service Research and Policy*, 9(1): 28–38.

Thornley, C. (1996) Segmentation and Inequality in the nursing workforce: Re-evaluating the evaluation of skills. In R. Crompton, D. Gallie and K. Purcell (eds) *Changing Forms of Employment*. London: Routledge.

Ulrich, D. (1998) A new mandate for human resources, *Harvard Business Review*, January–February: 124–34.

Wanless, D. (2002) *Securing our Future Health: Taking a Long-term View – The Wanless Report*. London: HM Treasury.

West, M., Borrill, C., Dawson, J., Scully, J., Carter, M., Anelay, S., Patterson, M. and Waring, J. (2002) The link between the management of employees and patient mortality in acute hospitals. *International Journal of Human Resource Management*, 13(8): 1299–1310.

Wicks, D. (1998) *Nurses and Doctors at Work*. Maidenhead: Open University Press.

Websites and resources

Australia Industries Skills Council. Details from industry skills council for community services and health industry, Australia: *http://www.cshisc.com.au/load_page.asp*

Changing Workforce Programme (UK). Also role redesign more generally: *http://www.wise.nhs.uk/cmsWISE/default.htm*

Chartered Institute of Personnel and Development. Includes information about human resource management and development: *http://www.cipd.co.uk/default.cipd*

Future Health Worker project. Details and reports: *http://www.ippr.org.uk/research/teams/project.asp?id=913&tID=100&pID=913*

Healthcare People Managers Association (UK). Provides a network for healthcare managers: *http://www.hpma.org.uk/*

Healthcare Workforce. UK healthcare workforce planning information and details about National Workforce projects: *http://www.healthcareworkforce.org.uk/default.aspx*

King's Fund. Publications and resources on workforce issues: *http://www.kingsfund.org.uk/health_topics/workforce.html*

National Center for Health Workforce Analysis (US). health workforce trends and reports: *http://bhpr.hrsa.gov/healthworkforce/reports/factbook.htm*

Skills for Health. Details of skills development in the UK health sector: *http://www.skillsforhealth.org.uk*

UK workforce development. For details of UK national policy covering workforce development: *http://www.dh.gov.uk/PolicyAndGuidance/HumanResourcesAndTraining/MoreStaff/fs/en*

15 | Working with healthcare professionals

Carol Brooks

Introduction

The relationship between managers and doctors is pivotal to the effective delivery of healthcare services. Healthcare organisations can succeed or fail as a consequence of the nature of this relationship. Edwards et al. (2003) comment on the risks of not allowing medicine and management to come together in the organisational setting. They illustrate that there is a 'mounting body of evidence that badly managed organisations fail patients, frustrate staff, deliver poor quality care, and cannot adapt to the rapidly changing environment in which they operate' and go on to suggest that 'poor management practice is at least as lethal as poor clinical practice'.

This chapter seeks to explore the nature of this relationship between managers and doctors, both from an interpersonal perspective and an organisational perspective as illustrated in Figure 15.1. Although the discussion will focus primarily on the manager–doctor relationship, it is clear that many of the themes and frameworks can be extrapolated and transferred to other relationships between managers and the wider clinician community in healthcare organisations. This chapter particularly explores the changing nature of the relationship between doctors and managers over the last 30 years within the context of National Health Service changes and reforms in the United Kingdom, but it is fair to say that the issues faced by managers and doctors in the UK are found in many other countries globally, particularly in the United States and Europe.

It is critical for managers to understand the impact of professional and organisational cultures on the relationship they have with doctors, particularly in terms of behaviours displayed at an organisational level. The design and implementation of specific types of organisational structures will also affect behaviours within the relationship. This chapter illustrates how the organisational forms prevalent in healthcare have a significant impact on how doctors and managers work together. The overarching aim of the chapter is to provide both managers and doctors with the

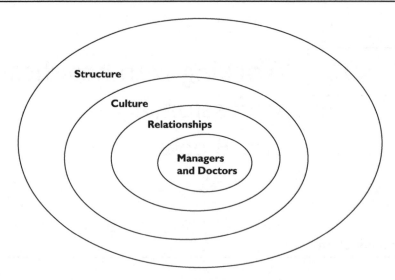

Figure 15.1   Relationships between managers and doctors

awareness, information, knowledge and frameworks to facilitate the development of positive and productive relationships, which in turn are crucial to the successful delivery of healthcare to patients.

The historical context: the changing relationship between managers and doctors in the uk

Before the 1980s, healthcare services in the UK's National Health Service were dominated by doctors in terms of both influence over decision making about the distribution of resources and the control of the day-to-day running of healthcare establishments. Doctors managed with a senior nurse or matron at their side, with administrators providing the third member of the triumvirate, and taking primary responsibility for non-clinical support services and for general administration and coordination. Hospital doctors exercised their professional autonomy and used their professional power base to achieve the outcomes they thought were best for the service they provided (Davies and Harrison 2003).

The Griffiths Report in the 1980s (Griffiths 1983) introduced the concept of general management to the NHS – a single person with overall managerial responsibility at each level within the organisation, to replace the triumvirate of doctor, nurse and manager. These reforms both reflected and promoted a move towards a more managerial and business-like culture in the National Health Service, particularly within hospitals. Although the reforms did create a new cadre of identified senior leaders with whom 'the buck' stopped (in terms of financial decision making), doctors still remained entirely responsible and accountable for their own clinical practice. However, the new managerial structures did serve to break up the old triumvirate structure for decision making and created a career management structure for healthcare managers. The introduction of general management signalled the future drive for closer parallels with private and commercial organisations' structures and governance arrangements. In the early 1990s, the internal market was introduced and provider and purchaser organisations, marketing and strategy departments, chief executives and boards were all the paraphernalia of the commercial sector. Small 'business units' were created in healthcare organisations, manifesting themselves as directorates arranged around clinical areas. The dynamic between managers and doctors shifted again, with doctors being asked to lead and manage directorate areas, working with a senior nurse and a manager, usually a business manager. This relationship was reminiscent of the pre-1980s triumvirate arrangements. However, there were some fundamental differences in that arguably doctors in these positions had less freedom as they were now a part of a corporate management structure, and were expected to contribute to the development of the whole organisation. Business managers (usually from a general management background) were expected to support the lead clinician, but were also expected to challenge and facilitate service development, rather than reinforce the status quo. The place of the doctor within the corporate management structure was reinforced by having a place for a lead doctor, or medical director as a part of the management executive.

In today's healthcare organisations, the legacy of this history can still be seen within hospital structures. Most hospitals still arrange the services around specific clinical or disease areas. However, the trend more recently has been to further enhance the significance of the doctor in the management and leadership of the organisation, played out through the role of clinical director. There has been increasing importance attached to these roles, with a gradual shift from doctors being voted into the role by their peers, or simply taking on the role as part of a rotation of responsibilities, to chief executives running recruitment more formally and recruiting to the role against a job description and person specification. These job descriptions often have an emphasis on management and leadership which goes beyond the professional world of doctors. Examples from a 'live' job description (in 2006) are given in Figure 15.2.

General managers are still working alongside clinical directors to manage the operational aspects of the service, and in some hospitals a general manager takes overall responsibility for the performance within the service. This is a move on from the clinical directorate structures of the 1990s when the most senior person within the service team was always the lead doctor. The continuing engagement and direct involvement of doctors in management will remain central to the public sector reform agenda around choice, empowerment and personalised care (DH 2005a, 2005b, 2006). Doctors working as equals to managers, working in partnership, will be required to lead huge strands of the organisational

---

OPERATIONAL DELIVERY

The post holder is accountable for

Overall responsibility and leadership for operational management of services

Effective and efficient business management and planning for group services

MODERNISATION AND SERVICE IMPROVEMENT

The post holder is accountable for

Leading the strategic development, modernisation and improvement of group services

Developing partnerships in the public and independent sectors

CORPORATE RELATIONSHIPS

The post holder will

Act as senior member of the team taking responsibility for setting and delivering corporate objectives

PEOPLE AND RESOURCE MANAGEMENT

The post holder is accountable for

Effective delivery and management of all human resource functions

CLINICAL CARE AND MANAGERIAL DELEGATION

The delivery of the role will be achieved through effective team working and through clear and effective communication.

Figure 15.2   Examples from a job description
Source: reproduced with permission from Airedale NHS Trust (2006)

development agenda in order to successfully implement policies and achieve the reform agenda.

Working with doctors in management and leadership roles

Understanding the historical context and development of the changing relationship between doctors and manager is important if the attitudes and viewpoints of doctors in leadership roles in modern healthcare organisations working in the twenty-first century are to be explored. Managers have a responsibility to draw on their own professional skills and expertise to encourage and support doctors in these leadership roles, which are so important to the effective delivery of health services.

The leadership roles occupied by doctors in hospitals are distributed throughout the organisation. At board level it is a statutory requirement to appoint a medical director as a part of the executive team. This individual will have a challenging role in that they are expected to provide leadership to their medical colleagues, but are also required to take a corporate stance whilst being a member of the executive team and a member of the trust board. The medical director can be viewed as a conduit between the body of medics working in the hospital and the board. This leadership role often requires degrees of diplomatic and political skills that the role holder has not been required to deploy in any other arena. The leap from a clinical director role to medical director needs to be managed carefully, or the risk of failure in the role increases. Ferlie and Shortell (2001) explore the concept of leadership within the context of improving quality of healthcare in the UK and USA. They write of the importance of distributing leadership throughout the different levels of the healthcare system; the individual, the team, the organisation and the wider environment in which healthcare organisations exist. It is therefore of limited effectiveness to focus leadership development solely at the individual clinicians or individual managers. Instead, a 'whole system' approach should be taken, with managers, doctors and other professional groups participating together in leadership activities.

Clinical directors, as noted earlier, are often in position because it happens to be their turn, or they have been voted into the position by other doctors. Sometimes they are in the role because there is no one else willing to take it on, and sometimes it can be that managers (the executive team and chief executive) see the person as the one least likely to cause tensions and trouble for the organisation. For managers, this is a tempting route to take in appointing clinical directors, as it then means that the managers are likely to have more relative control and influence in the organisation. However, this approach carries its own risks in that inept and unassertive clinical directors are very unlikely to become significantly involved in leading their medical colleagues (they are likely to lack the necessary credibility), shaping services and leading organisational change. Somehow, managers have to find the right balance so that doctors and managers, as far as possible, both play their part within the organisational setting. Chief executives shape the organisational culture and climate in which these roles of medical director and clinical directors are played out, and so have a considerable influence on (and responsibility for) the way things work.

The transition from consultant to clinical director (still usually encompassing the consultant's clinical responsibilities) presents some similar challenges to the individual occupying the role. In the majority of organisations, a move into the clinical director post is not usually accompanied by any structured development programme to facilitate the acquisition of skills and knowledge needed to carry out the job. It is often the case that consultants do not have a shared concept with managers as to what 'management' means as an activity. If this is so, there is little likelihood of any shared concept of how 'leadership' is played out in the organisation in terms of behaviours and activities. It can be observed that doctors embarking on their career as a new consultant often see management narrowly as a matter of sorting out rotas and dealing with other administrative tasks, and do not immediately see the role of clinical managers as leading and motivating teams of people, or having to be a part of a change management process. Most junior doctors have actually participated in these types of activity when questioned, but this perception of what management and leadership is may not change very much over time without some organisational effort to provide development opportunities for doctors and a recognition that doctors in managerial or leadership roles do not necessarily start with the same understanding as career managers. The ideal scenario is for doctors and managers to participate in facilitated development opportunities together in order to identify common perceptions and understandings and acknowledge differences in fundamental beliefs and viewpoints.

Transition across different work roles for individuals is common in all healthcare organisations, and partly reflects societal expectations that people do not necessarily choose a career path and remain in the same role and organisation for the entirety of their working life. Such expectations have become more dominant within the medical profession since the end of the 1990s. These days new consultants are much less likely to expect that they are entering a 'job for life'. They accept that there will be changes and choices presented to them throughout their career as a doctor, some of which may well relate to embarking on more specific management or leadership roles, such as clinical director or medical director. However, this does not mean that they are particularly well prepared to deal with such personal transitions in the workplace. The organisation and its leaders need to recognise that, as with any change in job role, the transitions from specialist registrar to consultant, from consultant to clinical director and from clinical director to medical director should be approached from a change management perspective. Nicholson (1990) has examined this work role transition and how it is managed. His work shows how organisations can either support or fail individuals, in this case doctors who are experiencing work role transition. This is a practical framework that managers (both within the generalist and human resource fields) can adopt to ensure that they are supporting individuals effectively during the key career transitions, and it can encompass people development initiatives such as mentoring, appraisal and induction. Nicholson identifies four key stages to any work role transition, and these are summarised in Table 15.1. An important aspect of Nicholson's approach is the link he makes between each of the stages. If the transition process begins in a negative manner, then it will be difficult to break out of the negative cycle and the situation is likely to feel increasingly worse for the doctor concerned. However, if the transition is actively managed within the organisation, a positive cycle is stimulated, which is clearly desirable for the doctor, work colleagues and the organisation. For managers and doctors working in leadership roles, it can be helpful to understand the nature of work role transitions so that there can be support for each other within the organisational context.

Table 15.1 The transition cycle

Stage in Cycle	Positive cycle Feelings/ reactions	Negative cycle Feelings/ reactions	Practical support
Preparation (before the role change)	Anticipation. High expectations. Excitement.	Fear. Anxiety. Reluctance to move	Continuous communication, provide written documents, face-to-face discussion, begin to involve.
Encounter (first few weeks into new role)	Coping well. Confident. Enjoying the move.	Shock. Regret.	Induction. Intense one-to-one support.
Adjustment (first year of new role)	Developing new role. Building new networks. Developing culture.	Grieving for what used to be. Not appearing to 'fit in'.	Frequent one-to-one discussion. Frequent appraisal. Positive feedback and reinforcement.
Stabilisation (after first year of new role)	Performing job well. Committed to people and tasks.	Failure to perform. Possibly leave.	Continue to reinforce commitment. Appraisal. Mentoring. Possibly manage exit from the organisation.

Source: Nicholson (1990).

Working within doctor and manager cultures

Mintzberg (1998: 265) refers to an organisation's culture as 'collective cognition' or the 'organisation's mind'. If this is the case, then it is reasonable to describe the NHS and other healthcare systems as having more than one mind, all of which happen to come together in sharing fundamental beliefs and principles. In the NHS this would be about healthcare being a service that should be provided free at the point of contact, based on need, and irrespective of an individual's level of wealth. If doctors and managers were to be observed working together over a substantial period of time, then these differences in 'mind' would become obvious. The two groups would work partly within a context of a shared values and beliefs system, but also from within cultures typical of their own profession.

Degeling et al. (2003) provide evidence to suggest that 'understanding different professional cultures is crucial for understanding each profession's response to . . . reforms'. For example, they illustrate how managers tend to systematise organisational activities, whilst doctors in management roles tend to start with an individualist perspective. Clearly, it is possible to make links back to the training and culture of the two professions. Career managers will have been exposed to management training starting with an organisational perspective, whilst doctors have been trained to focus on the individual presenting to them at a particular point in time. Simply beginning to understand and acknowledge differences, however, can significantly help to reduce and manage any potential conflict between the two groups, as behaviours demonstrated can usually be rationalised within the context of differing cultures.

Ferlie and Shortell (2001) also examine the differences in manager and doctor cultures as a way to aid understanding of behaviours in organisations. They suggest that doctors will resist managerial efforts to impose systems for achieving organisational perspectives, arguing that 'while managers view physicians and other professionals as a means for achieving the organization's overall patient care goals, physicians view organizations as a means for achieving their goals for individual patients'.

The nebulous and sometimes ambiguous nature of the concept of organisational culture may make it difficult to operationalise, but there are frameworks available that can help to bring some structure to the analysis of organisational culture. Johnson and Scholes (2002) describe the activity of cultural mapping, where a cultural 'web' is developed under six headings: symbols, power structures, organisational structures, control systems, rituals and routines, stories and paradigm. For each group, at a very general level, the cultural web is illustrated in Table 15.2.

For managers and doctors who are working together in an organisation, a useful activity would be to create this cultural web from each group's perspective, compare and contrast the outputs, agree to acknowledge differences, and agree any actions that could bring the two 'webs' closer together, so reducing the potential for conflict (see Johnson and Scholes 2002). This can be the first step towards achieving some bringing

Table 15.2   The cultural web

	Doctors	*Managers*
Symbols	Stethoscope, stereotypical attire for specialty, titles, colleges, terminology	Reserved parking, dark suits, language/jargon, laptops
Power structures	Negotiating committees, cliques of 'political' doctors	Executive management team
Organisational structures	Hierarchy based on seniority and respect for longevity/experience	'Macho' behaviours, fluid, project based
Control systems	Who knows who, audit	Financial/activity reporting, targets
Rituals and routines	Patient consultations, merit awards	Board meetings, long hours in the office, meetings and committees
Stories	'Us and them', heroes, mavericks, 'in the old days'	'Us and them', things have to change, change is for the best
Paradigm	NHS a 'good thing', should be free at point of delivery, desire to be the best	NHS a 'good thing', should be free at point of delivery, desire to be the best

Source: Johnson and Scholes (2002).

together or synthesis of cultures. Belasen (2002) sees this as a challenge for organisations attempting to strive for 'high-performance leadership'. He writes that where cultures are 'separated by contradictory values and realities' then the organisation's leaders (and this would be both doctors and managers in healthcare organisations) have a responsibility 'to foster loyalty and facilitate the assimilation process to reduce cultural clash and resistance'.

It is probably not possible or even desirable for there to be a total merger of managerial and medical cultures, or indeed any other professional culture within healthcare. There should perhaps be more focus on achieving what Nahavandi and Malekzadeh (1995) refer to as assimilation, as opposed to full integration. This could mean that the different cultures do not become fully merged, but rather retain the identity of the profession, but organisational structures strive to disperse and interweave the cultures throughout the organisation by design. Current organisational structures which aim to bring doctors into management structures are probably an acceptable way to try and achieve this. However, reciprocal arrangements tend not to exist to the same extent with career managers becoming an integral part of the clinical structures.

One of the key domains of organisational culture is power (as illustrated in the cultural web), and how power is played out in terms of organisational activities and, more importantly, individual behaviours. Managers and doctors have sources of power available to them which can be used in a positive or negative manner in the organisational setting. Understanding each other's power sources can aid negotiation between the groups and provide a route into resolving conflict. Hellriegal et al. (1992) and Makin and Cox (1994) refer to the French and Raven classification of power developed 40 years ago, but which still has resonance in the twenty-first century organisation. At a basic level, this classification identifies five sources of interpersonal power: reward, coercive, legitimate, expert and referent. In the NHS, doctors and managers have each of these at their disposal. It is useful to demonstrate how each of these sources of power is displayed in the organisational setting. Reward power is displayed when a manager or doctor offers a staff member or colleague promotion, a reference or more money in return for compliant behaviours. Coercive power can be identified in the disciplinary procedures used by both doctors and managers, or at a more general level it is a source of power which simply threatens that something bad and awful will occur as a consequence of not complying with desired behavioural codes. Legitimate power refers to the use of a person's position in the organisational structure, so the fact that someone is a manager or doctor should give at least some leverage in achieving compliance. Expert power is demonstrated when doctors attempt to influence outcomes by referring to their medical knowledge base, whilst managers could refer to their broader and more detailed knowledge about healthcare, policy initiatives and government directives. Finally, referent power is displayed in organisations when individuals use force of personality to gain compliance from others. At various junctures during a doctor's or manager's career, the strength of each of these sources will be variable. For example, as doctors progress up the medical career pathway they will have increasing expert power at their disposal. For managers, one of the most significant sources of power to increase as their career progresses is legitimate power, as they acquire more status from their job title and role in the organisation.

Another perspective to consider when examining sources of power is the situational source of power (external as opposed to interpersonal). Hellriegal et al. (1992) identify four such sources of power: knowledge, resources, decision making and networks. Knowledge power refers to knowing information about the strategy and direction of the organisation. Clearly, unless doctors decide actively to increase their personal knowledge outside their own speciality area, there will be an imbalance of power between doctors and managers in this sphere. Power related to resources can be seen around organisations when individual departments choose to allow others to have some of their resources at their discretion. This might include money equipment or information. Basically, individuals have this type of power at their disposal if they have a resource someone else wants or needs. The most obvious resource to impact on the relationship between doctors and managers is finance. Usually, managers have the funding and the doctors need it or want it to purchase equipment, support posts or develop services. Within all healthcare settings, there will be a plethora of meetings, committees, working parties, or similar decision-making fora. The individuals who attend and belong to such groups are building up their decision-making power base. It is likely that the majority of these decision-making groups sit at or near to corporate decision-making structures, and will be heavily populated by managers. Again, if doctors wish to distribute or build their power base within the organisation, there is an argument for them becoming more involved in corporate decision-making structures. Finally, the fourth external source of power, as identified by Hellriegal et al., is networking power. This could be viewed as the informal source of power from within an organisation. If a doctor or manager has this power at their disposal, then they are likely to engage in the behaviour of building networks and relationships quite intensely, so that when needed there will be an army of allies prepared to support their actions. Both doctors and managers can be observed engaging in this type of behaviour. Unfortunately, the networks of both groups do not always overlap or join forces. This can lead to tensions and conflicts between the two groups. Similar to interpersonal sources of power, doctors and managers can choose to deploy the situational sources of power in either a positive or negative manner. Conflict can arise between the two groups when there is a clash of the different power bases. For example, if the board and executive team are attempting to deploy a legitimate source of power in order to achieve compliance to an organisational policy, but the consultant body is ignoring this and using its network and expert sources of power, it is likely that tension will be the outcome. Both parties will need to respect and understand the power bases being used. To ignore each other's power bases is a risky business for the organisation and patients.

Working with doctors in different organisational structures

Managers are usually responsible in organisations for designing and changing organisational structures and systems. Such activities tend to be related to the requirement to implement national policies and initiatives. With every major reform in healthcare, there has been a parallel change in organisational structures. Indeed, during the last ten years it has been possible to observe an increasing trend within healthcare to redesign the shape of organisations to best reflect the trend towards more collaboration and partnership working, both within the healthcare sector and across health and social care. Such redesign exercises have demanded that managers think beyond the traditional hierarchical structures of traditional organisations.

The traditional shape of organisations (which can still be seen in healthcare organisations across the globe) is one which reflects Taylorism or a scientific management approach from the nineteenth century. The emphasis is on the division of labour and having well-defined role and job boundaries. Belasen (2002) refers to Perrow (1986) in explaining how such organisations 'are geared toward maximising efficiency'. He continues to describe how these traditional organisations 'adopt a strategy of centralised control through vertical hierarchies and functional departments'. Communication is expected to flow up and down the hierarchical structures, as opposed to across or around the organisation. This bureaucratic organisational shape depends heavily upon the respect of status and seniority in order to be successful. In fact, such respect is an integral part of culture within the medical profession itself and has underpinned medical training and development for many years, still having the same significant impact today. It could be argued that the organisational shape of the medical profession is bureaucratic, driven by the need and necessity to have rules, compliance and monitoring, to ensure quality and safety for the public. All bureaucratic organisations would be peppered with committees and structures required to give permission for organisational activities. It is in fact incredibly difficult for large organisations to avoid adopting some of the characteristics of the bureaucratic organisation. Belasen (2002) states that in the bureaucratic organisation 'managers rely heavily on rules and quantitative skills to generate compliance and achieve desired results'.

Referring back to the preceding reference to medical culture, it is understandable if doctors have a preference for working within a traditionally designed organisation with little ambiguity and a high degree of predictability. Their profession is based on science and rationality, whilst the profession of management, although underpinned by research and an attempt at order and discipline, is basically less deterministic and more open to interpretation. In today's healthcare organisation (and indeed in most other sectors) managers are being placed in roles which are an antithesis to doctor roles. They are increasingly being expected to lead the way in breaking up the traditional organisational shape and creating organisations which are arguably less certain, have more ambiguity and more complexity. It is easy to see how these contradictions between the roles will potentially raise tensions for managers and doctors as they work together to implement major policy reforms. Managers have a challenge and responsibility to lead, motivate and inspire doctors to fully participate and engage in major organisational change initiatives.

The 'new' organisational structures appear to take two particular forms. First, traditional hierarchy is being replaced by flatter, more fluid structures. Matrix structures, where linear superior–subordinate relationships have less significance for achieving outputs, and where communications can flow across the organisation as well as vertically, are becoming the norm. Doctors and managers can find themselves working increasingly in teams, but in a growing number of teams, each with a different 'raison d'être'. It is becoming more common for individuals to be accountable to more than one person and to be responsible for staff who may have roles within structures outside of the department, or even the organisation. Shortell et al. (2005) identify the challenge of developing effective teams in healthcare both in the UK and USA, showing that there is increasing evidence that effective teams are associated with a higher quality of healthcare. However, they also suggest that insufficient attention is being given to the interactions and relations between different teams in healthcare. This point can only be of growing importance as the provision of healthcare becomes integrated across organisational boundaries and sectors. Teams of doctors and other healthcare professionals will increasingly find themselves having to work in matrix or virtual type organisational structures.

Second, we are seeing the growing use of networks or virtual organisations. These organisations break down all traditional organisational barriers, with individuals working across large geographical areas, or across different health, social and government agencies, and they may be more difficult or demanding to manage in some respects. For example, a key organisational change challenge is achieving excellent communication, and the network organisation compromises the traditional way of communicating in bureaucratic structures. Managers and doctors will need to identify and agree new methods of communicating in order to avoid a communication vacuum, or inefficient communication. Yet another challenge is achieving best fit between organisation design and styles of working. Styles of working and behaviours are challenged in networks because there has to be less dependence upon hierarchy to achieve results and far more emphasis on developing partnerships and working in a collaborative manner. Managers and doctors will need to develop partnership working between themselves as two distinct groups, focusing on some of the success factors of building partnerships as outlined by Belasen (2002). First, it is crucial to identify the critical drivers for working together, or reasons for the two groups having to work together. There is also a need to develop what Belasen refers to as 'strategic synergy', which would mean doctors and managers striving to use their complementary strengths to achieve an excellence that could not be achieved by one group alone. Clearly, if it is possible to create a win–win situation where both groups perceive that they are benefiting from partnering and that the relationship is fair, this will also increase the probability of successful working together. However, none of this is likely to work unless there is top-level commitment to building partnerships within the organisation and a desire and spirit to behave in a cooperative manner (Belasen 2002).

Observing behaviours in healthcare organisations, there are in fact many contradictions that have to be dealt with by managers and doctors in relation to organisational structures. Board structures tend to reinforce the bureaucratic decision-making processes associated with traditional organisations and a command and control approach to achieving goals and objectives. There can be tension between this approach and the desire to stimulate more flexible, innovative organisations through having flatter organisational shapes at sub-board level and encouraging doctors and managers to become involved in activities external to the organisation. A leaner, flatter, more flexible organisational shape is indeed desirable in an increasingly complex healthcare environment. Belasen (2002) writes that organisations must 'adopt decentralised structures of decision-making' in an organisational world full of complexity. This would ensure that the new organisational shape is supported through the infrastructures. However, the willingness and desire to create new infrastructures does not guarantee an easy route through the transition from working in a bureaucratic manner to working more flexibly. If it is assumed that medicine tends to reflect a bureaucratic approach towards service delivery, then managers must acknowledge that 'bureaucratic organisations have limited capacity to change due to inertia and preservation of the status quo, and also due to systemic barriers such as limited resources, high specialisation, and such formal constraints as rules and standardised work processes' (Belasen 2002: 228).

It is then the responsibility of managers from their professional perspective, knowledge and understanding to illustrate these potential tensions to medical colleagues, so that practical solutions can be identified to reduce conflict and maximise effectiveness in service delivery.

Conclusion

There will always be potential for tension and conflict between doctors and managers in healthcare. The challenge of facing this and then dealing with it in a constructive manner is an integral part of the organisational landscape. Dukerich et al. (2002) argue that managers are challenged to 'elicit cooperative behaviours from professionals in organisations'. If the context, history and interpersonal factors are understood clearly, then neither doctors nor managers should be striving to become dominant over the other group. Both groups have a responsibility to develop awareness and understanding of individual behaviour within professional cultures, the impact of organisational structure on behaviours and attitudes, and the opportunities for joint professional and personal development. Huge untapped and undeveloped potential exists to maximise the partnership between doctors and managers to stimulate and implement service changes that will benefit patients.

Summary box

1 The relationship between doctors and managers has a historical context that impacts on organisations and individuals today. The role of doctors in management is central to the effective delivery of healthcare services and doctor–manager posts can be found dispersed across organisational structures.

2 Managers have a role and responsibility to support doctors progressing into management roles. More attention should be given to initiatives such as succession planning, coaching and mentoring. There is also an argument to suggest that leadership training and development would be best delivered to multi-professional groups, including doctors and managers, who then learn together.

3 Managers and doctors inhabit different cultural worlds that cannot and should not be totally merged. Both groups have been trained from different professional perspectives, namely the individual versus the organisation. It is probably not desirable to merge both cultures, but there is a need to understand the two and to be aware of how different sources of power are played out through behaviours observed in organisations.

4 Organisational structures present challenges for working style and behaviours. The transformation from essentially bureaucratic organisational structures to flatter, less hierarchical structures presents challenges for doctors and managers in organisational activities such as communication and team working.

5 Partnership working is the way forward to ensure the strengths of both groups are deployed effectively to implement change and achieve excellence. Currently, the emphasis appears to be on managers stimulating appropriate organisational behaviours from doctors. There is a need for both groups to understand the huge untapped and undeveloped potential that could be used to continually improve patient care, if working more closely to some shared explicit agenda could be achieved.

Self-test exercises

1 Consider the current practice in your organisation in supporting doctors experiencing the work role transitions of:

- new consultant (first post)
- becoming clinical director (or equivalent)
- becoming medical director (lead doctor at board level).

Use the Nicholson framework to identify what improvements might be introduced to ensure a positive transition cycle, that is:

- preparation
- encounter
- adjustment
- stabilisation.

2 Identify a small group of doctors and a small group of managers you could work with to explore organisational/professional cultures. Using the cultural web framework of Johnson and Scholes (2002), brief the two groups to:

- map out each other's culture as they perceive it
- map out their own professional culture as they perceive it
- compare and contrast the outputs of the discussions highlighting potential areas of tension and conflict, highlighting strengths and opportunities.

3 Identify a number of doctors you work with on a regular basis. Reflect on your interactions with them:

- What sources of power are you drawing on during these interactions?
- What sources of power do the doctors you know tend to use?
- Do your respective sources of power ever lead to tension and conflict?
- Are there different sources of power you could deploy in order to reduce the likelihood of tension and conflict?

References and further reading

Belasen, A. T. (2002) *Leading the Learning Organisation. Communication and Competencies for Managing Change.* New York: State University of New York Press.

Davies, T. O. and Harrison, S. (2003) Trends in doctor–manager relationships. *British Medical Journal*, 326: 646–56.

Degeling, P., Maxwell, S., Kennedy, J. and Coyle, B. (2003) Medicine, management and modernisation: A 'danse macabre'? *British Medical Journal*, 326: 649–52.

Department of Health (DH, 2005a) *Commissioning a Patient-Led NHS*. London: DH.

Department of Health (DH, 2005b) *Creating a Patient-Led NHS*. London: DH.

Department of Health (DH, 2006) *Health Reforms in England: Update and Next Steps*. London: DH.

Dukerich, J. M., Golden, B. R. and Shortell, S. M. (2002) Beauty is in the eye of the beholder: The impact of organizational identification, identity, and image on the cooperative behaviours of physicians. *Administrative Science Quarterly*, 47: 507–33.

Edwards, N., Marshall, M., McLellan, A. and Abbasi, K. (2003) Doctors and managers: A problem without a solution? *British Medical Journal*, 326: 609–10.

Ferlie, E. B. and Shortell, S. M. (2001) Improving the quality of healthcare in the United Kingdom and the United States: A framework for change. *Milbank Quarterly*, 79: 281–315.

Griffiths, R. (1983) *NHS Management Enquiry: Report*. London: Department of Health.

Hellriegal, D., Slocum, J. W. and Woodman, R. W. (1992) *Organizational Behaviour*. St. Paul, MN: West.

Johnson, G. and Scholes, K. (2002) *Exploring Corporate Strategy*. Harlow: Prentice Hall.

Makin, P. and Cox, C. (1994) *Managing People at Work*. London: British Psychological Society.

Mintzberg, H. (1998) *Strategy Safari. The Complete Guide through the Wilds of Strategic Management*. New York: Prentice Hall.

Nahavandi, A. and Malekzadeh, A. (1995) Acculturation in mergers and acquisitions. In T. Jackson (ed) *Cross-Cultural Management*. Oxford: Butterworth Heinemann.

Nicholson, N. (1990) The transition cycle: Causes, outcomes, processes and forms. In S. Fisher and C. L. Cooper (eds) *On the Move: The Psychology of Change and Transition*. Chichester: Wiley.

Perrow, C. (1986) *Complex Organisations*. New York: Random House.

Shortell, S. M., Schmittdiel, J., Wang, M. C., Li, R., Gillies, R. R., Casalino, L. P., Bodenheimer, T. and Rundall, T. G. (2005) An empirical assessment of high-performing medical groups: Results from a national study. *Medical Care Research and Review*, 62(4): 407–34.

Websites and resources

BAMM. Provides support to doctors in all management and leadership roles across the UK and guides medical managers through the complex changes as the service moves towards a truly patient-led NHS, with clinicians and managers working together to a single set of ideals and values: *www.bamm.co.uk*

British Medical Journal. The general medical journal website offering best treatments evidence for patients from the *British Medical Journal*: *www.bmj.com*

General Medical Council. Website promoting and protecting the health of the public by ensuring proper standards in medicine. *www.gmc-uk.org*

16

Governance and the work of health service boards

Naomi Chambers

Introduction

The term governance has only relatively recently gained currency as a distinct entity within the study of the management of organisations. The development of the debate around governance can be largely traced to incidents relating to the high profile organisation failures of the early 1990s (Maxwell, Polly Peck, Barings Bank), the US corporate scandals (Enron, WorldCom) a few years later and which have continued on into this decade (Equity Life, Parmalat). These examples demonstrate that the problem is international. The responses to these events have provided much of the impetus for clarifying concepts of 'good' governance and have also framed the discussions around the management of corporate risk. This chapter examines the impact of the governance debate on the management of health services, outlines different board models and analyses the evolving role of boards of health organisations. Many examples used relate to the English NHS but reference is also made to other health systems, and the discussion is in addition framed within the wider context of debates around the role of boards.

Three main strands of argument will be developed; first that the governance debate is largely overshadowed by notions of control and that this impacts significantly on health service governance; second, that there is some consensus that board structures and forms matter less than choices around behaviours and clarity of purpose; third, that despite extensive elaborations of the roles of boards there are enduring concerns about board performance. A putative framework will be outlined for developing effective boards, based on a study in the English NHS but with relevance for other types of boards and other health systems. The chapter will end by arguing that boards do matter, but we need better ways of expressing why this is the case, and that research is required to find out exactly how they make a difference to organisational performance.

Evolving trends in health governance

A number of different elucidations of the term 'governance' exist and it is worth examining these in order to arrive at a working definition for the purposes of this discussion. Within a political science paradigm, Pierre and Peters argue that at a state level governance revolves around the capacity of government to make and implement policy – in other words, to steer society (Pierre and Peters 2000). A recent OECD review identified six levers in modernising governance at state level, comprising open government, performance management, restructuring, marketisation and new forms of employment (OECD 2005). Within healthcare, Davies (2005) examines markets, hierarchies and networks as the main contrasting forms of governance, relating these to different incentives and hence to different outcomes. At an institution level, the Cadbury Report describes corporate governance as a system by which an organisation is directed and controlled (Cadbury 1992). This is amplified by a subsequent OECD definition of corporate governance as 'the structure through which the objectives of the company are set, and the means of attaining those objectives and monitoring performance are determined' (OECD 2004:11). The Langlands Review of governance for public services in the UK outlines the following as the function of governance: 'to ensure that an organisation or partnership fulfils its overall purpose, achieves its intended outcomes for citizens and service users, and operates in an effective, efficient and ethical manner' (Independent Commission 2004: 7). Beyond the notion of governance as steering society, four clear generic strands, which are all non-country or sector specific, emerge from these statements: the need for direction, the importance of control, the relevance of an underpinning set of values and the requirement to demonstrate accountability. These strands are also, as we shall see, embedded within the health sector. It is interesting to note that governance discussions are dominated more by terms relating to control and accountability than by those relating to renewal and entrepreneurship. This has implications for priorities in the management of health services: one of the consequences is that lapses of control are more likely to be deemed governance failures rather than lack of attention to innovation. We can track this in the development of and the focus of attention paid to governance arrangements in the English NHS over the past 15 years.

Having adopted a private sector business model in place of the stakeholder model for its local bodies (about which more below) in 1990, the English NHS, via guidance from HM Treasury, moved quickly to embrace lessons from the corporate failures of the 1990s. A number of reports emanating from these failures were used to strengthen corporate governance in the NHS. Key recommendations from the Cadbury Report (1992) to separate roles of chair and chief executive and to strengthen audit and establish remuneration committees were swiftly adopted. One of the products of the Nolan Committee report on standards in public life, the Code of Conduct, with its crucial public sector values of accountability, probity and openness, first issued in 1994, remains – with some updating – in force (NHS 2004). The Turnbull Report (1999) on internal control resulted in the development of a controls assurance framework for the NHS (DH 2002) itself superseded by a move towards integrated governance, the latest manifestation of which is encapsulated in Standards For Better Health (DH 2004).

Despite the plethora of guidance, challenges remain. The documents outlined above imply that the existence of frameworks and audit trails will suffice: for example, the Foreword to *The Good Governance Standard for Public Services* argues: 'Good governance leads to good management, good performance, good stewardship of public money, good public engagement and, ultimately, good outcomes' (Independent Commission 2004: v). The evidence from financial and wider organisational failings in the NHS suggests that this is somewhat wishful thinking. On the financial side, one of the first significant failures was at North Bristol NHS Trust, which forecast a deficit of £11.6 million in November 2002, rising to an end-of-year position in March 2003 of £44.3 million. External consultants reviewed the case and pointed to failings within the finance directorate, internal audit, executive management team and the board (Avon 2003). In November 2005, the NHS was forecasting a deficit of £1 billion with 43 trusts having to make cuts in clinical services (*Health Service Journal* 2005). Reasons – or excuses – for the shortage of cash in the system range from the financial turbulence caused by the introduction of the new funding system (Payment by Results), the cost of the new consultant and GP contracts, the implementation of the new staff pay system (Agenda for Change) and shorter waits for care (Plumridge 2005).

On the clinical and reputational side, organisational failures in the NHS over the past 15 years, referred to in more detail elsewhere in this book, have arguably matched or surpassed those in the UK commercial sector. NHS organisations have successively failed to protect children with heart problems in Bristol, elderly patients who were registered with GP Harold Shipman, babies in the care of nurse Beverley Allitt and parents whose deceased children's organs were removed without their consent at Alder Hey hospital. The question has to be asked about who is responsible for this apparent unevenness of quality and assurance within a dense architecture of corporate governance arrangements and within a 'national' health service: it is not unreasonable to suggest that local boards which have ultimate control for what goes on in their organisations bear at least some of that responsibility.

Forms of health boards

Boards, as Pointer (1999) has pointed out, are late nineteenth-century inventions. They were developed as a result of the industrial revolution and the growing commercial complexity of business. Boards, as agents of the owners, represented absent shareholders' interests, and management became the agents of the board. Today the function of the board in the commercial and the non–profit and state sectors is essentially the same – the main difference being that shareholders are replaced by 'stakeholders' (Pointer 1999). The term 'board' itself is not universal. In different parts of the public sector in the UK, for example, in school education, the equivalent is the governing body; within the voluntary sector it might be the trustees; in local government it is the council. The term 'council' is used in different countries to denote the body that oversees the management or procurement of local health services.

Local boards in the English NHS are derived in structure from the Anglo-Saxon private sector unitary board model which predominates in UK and US business (Ferlie et al. 1996; Garrett 1997). The unitary board typically comprises a chair, chief executive, executive directors and independent (or non–executive) directors. All members of the board bear the same responsibility, individually and collectively, for the performance of the enterprise. In the English NHS, local provider boards (hospital trusts) and commissioning bodies (primary care trusts) consist typically of 11 people: five executive directors (including the chief executive and finance director), five non–executive directors and a non–executive chair. Until 2001, chairs and non–executive directors were appointed by the Secretary of State for Health, but they are now selected on behalf of parliament by the independent NHS Appointments Commission. This method of appointment (instead of via local elections for example) has led to criticisms of a 'democratic deficit' in the local NHS (Ferlie et al. 1996). But despite successive reorganisations and reconfigurations of clinical services this model has survived more or less intact since 1990, although an alternative governance model is now being developed with the introduction of NHS foundation trusts.

NHS foundation trusts are independent public benefit corporations modelled on cooperative and mutual traditions which by the end of 2005 were providing acute hospital care to about one quarter of the population in England (*www.dh.gov.uk/PolicyandGuidance*). Although subject to national targets and standards, they have greater freedoms than other types of NHS hospitals. The financial regime underpinning foundation trusts is significantly more rigorous and the consequent expectations by the regulator, Monitor, of board performance in ensuring financial control are also therefore markedly enhanced.

The governance structure of foundation trusts is also quite different: there are two boards – a board of governors (up to about 50) made up of people elected from the local community membership, and representatives of other stakeholders such as primary care trusts, education bodies and local authorities, and a board of directors (around 11 people) made up of a chair and non–executive directors appointed by the governors, and a chief executive and executive directors, appointed by the chair and approved by the governors. This whole structure resembles the Anglo-Saxon unitary board model we have seen adopted by the English NHS but nested within a two-tier European or Senate model, commonly found in the Netherlands, France and Germany. Here there is a lower tier operational board which deals with management and strategic issues and an upper tier supervisory board which ratifies certain decisions taken by the operational board, sets the direction and represents the different interests in the company, particularly those of shareholders and employees (Johnson et al. 2005).

In a variant of the English NHS structures and an example of a non-executive board, New Zealand has 21 district health boards tasked with strategic oversight of local health services, but in this case all 11 people on the board are non-executive directors: seven are elected at the time of local government elections and four are appointed by the Ministry of Health; the chief executive is appointed by and accountable to the board but is not a board member (www.moh.govt.nz/districthealthboards).

From the US perspective, Pointer outlines four types of boards commonly found within US healthcare. Parent boards govern free-standing independently owned institutions; subsidiary boards are local boards of large enterprises; advisory boards provide steer and guidance without a formal corporate governance role; affiliate organisation boards serve their members' interests. There are 7500 hospital and health system boards in the US – part of an economic and social system which supports 5.5 million boards altogether or one for every 45 citizens (Pointer 1999).

Within the UK itself with the advent of devolution there have been deepening policy differences (for example, in the role of the market) and an increasing divergence in the structures for managing health services. Wales has separated commissioning from providing functions but its local health board model is stakeholder based with up to 25 members on each board, resembling the English NHS pre-1990. Scotland has an integrated health model and a unified board structure with strong local authority representation.

The above illustrates the broad range of board structures and models in use in health services and demonstrates the highly contextual nature of the board form chosen. There are non-executive boards, executive boards, two-tier boards and unitary boards. There are models for different health service purposes: for insurers, commissioners, providers and for partnerships (cross public sector and public/private). Board membership is achieved through different processes of nomination, appointment and election and can be paid or unpaid.

What is the evidence around the relative effectiveness of these different board models? In his review of public sector boards, Cornforth argues that searching for an idealised board model and membership is ultimately futile, but that boards can work on enhancing their legitimacy and effectiveness (Cornforth 2003). Carver and Carver (2001) argue that key governance principles can work with whatever structural arrangements have come about as a result of a board's composition, history, and particular circumstances. There is more evidence available about the conditions under which boards preside over organisation failures. Inquiries and reviews have repeatedly pointed to a lack of challenge by the board at critical junctures. In his examination of US corporate failures, Makosz points out the importance of board members in asking the tough questions and reviewing the effectiveness of internal controls (*www.csa-pdk.com*). In the case of the financial meltdown at North Bristol NHS Trust in 2003, Deloitte and Touche reflect on relationship difficulties at board level and a failure to probe the financial situation and to put in place risk management processes (Avon 2003). A review of inquiries over the past 30 years into failures of care in the UK demonstrated a remarkable consistency in key recurring themes which include inadequate systems and processes, lack of leadership, isolation, disempowerment of staff and patients and poor communications (Higgins 2001). Echoes of these themes are also found in a study relating cultures to performance, in which low performing acute hospital trusts in England were found to be characterised by charismatic leaders with poor transactional skills and a tendency to cliques, confused internal lines of accountability and under-developed external relationships (Mannion et al. 2003). There is also a growing literature on failure and turnaround, some of which is health related (for example NHS Confederation 2003; Walshe et al. 2004). The literature suggests that the challenge for health service boards is not therefore to embark upon a quest for the perfect structure or model but to acknowledge the need for clarity of purpose in order to steer high performing organisations towards providing or securing safe and high quality healthcare for patients.

Roles of boards

The Langlands Review produced six core principles for good governance to guide the work of public service boards (see Figure 16.3 in Self-test Exercise 2). These comprise a focus on purpose and outcomes, clarity about functions and roles, promotion and demonstration of values, transparent decision making whilst managing risk, developing the capacity and capability of the governing body itself and engaging stakeholders and making accountability real (Independent Commission 2004). This 'good governance standard' indicates both core style and key content for board work in the public sector and comes closest to the iterative and cyclical framework advocated by authors working from the commercial sector.

Turning now to some of these authors who work within the private sector, Garratt (1997) has developed Tricker's (1983) model of four principal board roles into a board tasks model reproduced in a simplified form in Figure 16.1. Garratt emphasises the importance of Revans' axiom that for organisations to survive and grow, their rate of learning has to be equal to or greater than the rate of change in their environment. Drawing also from the Institute of Directors publication *Standards for the Board* (IOD 2005), Garratt argues that boards have to pay attention to both the conformance (accountability and supervision of management) and to the performance (policy formulation and strategic thinking) aspects of their role, and in turn to the iterative cycle of policy development,

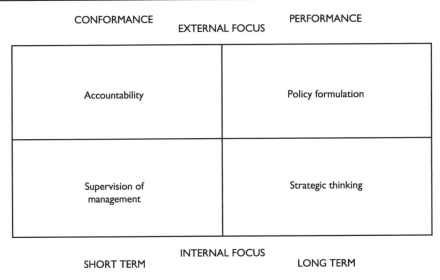

Figure 16.1   Board tasks model
Source: Adapted from Garratt (1997).

strategic formulation, supervision/monitoring and accounting to key stakeholders. Within these cycles, boards need to be sensitive to the well-being of their own organisation and attuned to the external environment, and to take into account both short-term pressures and longer term trends in making their decisions. The conclusion appears to be that there is a need to pay appropriate attention to activities in all four quadrants, to face inwards and outwards and to find a balance between short-term and long-term thinking, but how easy is this to achieve?

High profile corporate failures in the UK and US have, as we have seen, prompted stricter rules around conformance through tighter corporate governance arrangements and clearer controls assurance frameworks. As organisations are subjected to ever more rigorous risk management, is 'performance' being subjugated to 'conformance'? Power (1999) warns against the growing influence of the audit society, reward systems which pay checkers more than doers and the rituals of verification: 'Does the rustle of paper systems . . . provide only slogans of accountability and quality which perpetuate rather than alleviate organ-isational rigidity? (p. 123) Pollitt (1999) suggest that audit itself is undergoing a transformation, with auditors developing performance audit programmes in addition to traditional financial audit. These programmes have the potential to add managerial effectiveness to the traditional values of prudence and procedural correctness and could in themselves help to swing the pendulum back to 'performance'. At best they could exert pressure and provide an evidence base for policymaking and strategic choice. Taylor (2001) further argues that the time has now come to move from the current corporate governance paradigm with its emphasis on controls and restraint to corporate entrepreneurship, creating the conditions for corporate renewal, encouraging the development of new activities and the elimination of old ones.

In another framing of the conformance/performance dichotomy, Hodgkinson and Sparrow argue that organisations depend for their survival on developing strategic competence. This is defined as an ability to acquire, store, recall, interpret and act upon information of relevance to the longer term survival and well-being of the organisation (Hodgkinson and Sparrow 2002: xiv-xv). Strategic competence comes from organisational memory, learning, knowledge management, creativity, intuition and use of knowledge elicitation techniques. The authors warn against the competency trap ethos where there is no place for devil's advocates or court jesters and where organisations always favour exploitation (of existing expertise and knowledge base) over exploration (search for new knowledge).

How can we place the work of health service boards within these discussions? The unitary learning board model described by Garratt has clear resonances with the NHS where board structures and modus operandi are heavily drawn from the private sector business model. NHS boards are expected to operate along all four of Garratt's quadrants from developing a clear vision, to clarifying strategic direction, and also to monitoring performance and accounting to local communities and to government. These map onto the principles of good governance advocated in the Langlands Review for the public sector (Independent Commission 2004). The key challenges for NHS boards can therefore be segmented into these four quadrants and existing guidance reinforces this.

There is indeed plenty of guidance available to support NHS boards in their work. In *Governing the NHS* the NHS Appointments Commission outlines the duty of NHS Boards to 'add value . . . . by providing a framework of good governance within which the organisation can thrive and grow' (NHS Appointments Commission 2003: 9). The Commission divides the role of boards into four main areas: collective responsibility for adding value, leadership and control, looking ahead by setting strategic aims and reviewing performance, and setting and maintaining values. The part played by individual members, including the chair, non-executive directors and the role of board committees is also given much attention. The overall tone is one of exercising control rather than of setting direction, and this is reinforced by additional mandatory guidance from the Department of Health and HM Treasury issued for the NHS in order to to ensure that statements of internal control can be signed by the chief executive of each NHS organisation. The more recent guidance on integrated governance, the new suite of healthcare standards and the annual healthcheck required and vetted by the Healthcare Commission offers little relief. This does provide substance for the argument that current conformance requirements are acting as 'dead weight' against carefully considered risk taking, innovation and entrepreneurship. The counter-argument is that, given the recent examples of high-profile clinical, financial and organisational failures in the NHS, it is irresponsible not to have in place controls (and assurances about those controls) against the risks of these occurring. The solution may be to find new ways of thinking and doing within the processes of establishing and verifying controls; for example, by using Hodgkinson and Sparrow's (2002) knowledge elicitation techniques, or performance, programme and policy audit as suggested by Pollitt (1999).

The added value of boards mentioned by the NHS Appointments Commission is questioned in a couple of papers. The NHS Confederation has identified four key characteristics of effective boards: a focus on strategic decision making, trust and corporate working, constructive challenge and effective chairs. In their examination of boards at work, however, the authors found that 'the daily grind' often obscured strategic decision making, and whilst there was often a good deal of trust between board members, there was too little constructive challenge and therefore some missed opportunities (NHS Confederation 2005). Peck argues, on the other hand, that even as a mainly ratifying body the board ritual has some value in itself as a way of according significance to important decisions (Peck et al. 2004).

As significant players within a country's social and economic system, boards of local health services face continuing challenges in setting strategy, monitoring performance and in balancing tensions between risk management and innovation, and governance duties versus entrepreneurship. But their sphere of influence is also limited. In the UK, for example, local boards are constrained by operating within a 'national' health service. In other countries, the power of professional accrediting bodies and national regulators is significant. There is also the emergence of shadow boards without formal or statutory authority but with immense power; for example at a local level in the UK a health community chief executives group, and at a national level the NHS chief executive Top Team meetings. As state sector health services across the OECD countries shift from being providers to commissioners (OECD 2005), there has been a proliferation of different types of boards to direct, approve and monitor developments which cross institution or sector boundaries. One example of this is the partnership boards for joint commissioning of those services which are typically provided by a combination of health and social care staff. A second example is the private-public joint venture boards (e.g. controlling capital developments in primary care in England via the LIFT companies). These may at present be 'mini boards', but the formalisation of inter-organisational and inter-sectoral working both in the UK health sector and elsewhere (analysed in more detail in Chapter 17) suggests these types of boards will have an increasing influence.

The perspectives provided above indicate that the current environment in which health service boards operate is both complex and febrile. Advice on the role of boards is not wanting but organisations are pulled and pushed in different directions and their boards need to face at least four ways in order to remain standing. How can boards proactively perform these delicate balancing acts and how can they know when they are about to fall from the wire?

Making a difference: developing effective boards

Over recent years there has been a particular focus on the role of the non-executive director. The Higgs Report (2003) into this role within the UK commercial sector called for greater clarity around responsibilities, induction, development and performance. In the US there is a focus on developing governance tools for boards – for example, by the Center for Healthcare Governance (*www.americangovernance.com*). Following a commissioned survey of NHS non-executive directors (MCHM 2002), the NHS Appointments Commission has developed a training and development programme at national and regional levels for non executive directors. Extensive guidance about the work of board committees is also available, for example, from the Audit Commission. In the NHS the Clinical Governance Support Team has reported on its work with many boards to improve the quality of constructive challenge (NHS Confederation 2005). Less guidance is available for board secretaries and a deep ambiguity about the nature of their role (are they silent servants or corporate guardians?) may be hampering the work of boards (Chambers and Smith 2004). As we have seen from the litany of past failures and the complexity of present challenges facing health service governance across the world, there remains a way to go. An exploratory study outlined below attempts to construct a systematic method for developing health boards utilising a synthesis of theoretical frameworks.

Although arguing from different perspectives, Cornforth and West both emphasise the need for reflexivity. Cornforth suggests that reflexivity compensates for the impossibility of achieving an 'ideal' board structure and defines reflexivity as the process of achieving a better understanding of behaviours, roles, teamworking and impact of the board (Cornforth 2003). West proposes that reflexivity provides the space to promote team health, creativity and robust challenge to the existing ways of doing things (West 1997) that is essential for innovation. Boards sometimes seek external support to help them in this task and may also embark on a wide-ranging organisation development programme of which development of the board is only a part.

Patching offers a two-by-two grid to understand the range of different interventions for effective organisation development (Patching 1999). His argument is that the choice of interventions should depend on what the organisation's main concerns are around organisation development (OD). One half of the grid comprises achieving success through alignment (divided into OD activities for enhancing *specific* and *generic* *capabilities*, for example, by implementing an agreed organisation-specific strategy, or embedding industry-wide best practice). The other half of the grid comprises success through change (divided into OD activities which are *transformational* and *exploratory*, for example, developing a new vision or testing new ideas and challenging the status quo).

Cockman et al. (1999) describe four distinct consulting styles or facilitator modes. The acceptant mode involves listening actively, encouraging 'story telling', and is particularly helpful in revealing the impact of emotions in shaping organisational life. The catalytic mode comprises collecting, shaping and rearranging information, for example, through forcefield analysis, multi-voting, flowcharts, staff/customer interviews and surveys, and is essential in helping the client to take decisions and move forward. In the confrontational mode the consultant highlights discrepancies, for example, in behaviours, decisions, espoused values, and offers both challenge and support. Finally, the prescriptive mode involves the provision of expert advice and depends on the consultant's technical or content expertise in the client's area, for example, his or her knowledge of comparable organisations.

Using Patching and Cockman's frameworks together with Garratt's board tasks model (see Figure 16.1) it is possible to construct a framework for board development which has a degree of relevance for all boards and in different kinds of health systems. An exploratory study to determine the utility of this for NHS boards revealed that, with three refinements, the framework had both resonance and relevance (Chambers and Higgins 2005). In the first main refinement, the study found that the board development cycle needs a further iteration to reflect different levels of maturity, depending on the newness of whole boards and individual new appointments to boards. Second, as it stands, the framework omits sufficiently to acknowledge the need for boards to do work around the identification, articulation, espousal and demonstration of a set of core values for the organisation. These values inherently imbue all parts of the board cycle of work; for example, from the principles agreed which underpin policy development, the range of legitimate strategic choices and tactics employed, the monitoring of organisation behaviours and the style of accounting to stakeholders. Recent work from the public sector perspective, for example, the Langlands Review, has emphasised the importance of this area of work. A third proposed refinement is the fifth facilitator approach identified by participants in the course of this study. In addition, therefore to the acceptant, confrontational, catalytic and prescriptive styles, we would now add 'reflective' as an alternative facilitator approach. This encapsulates the role of the facilitator who is grounded in wider health policy and culture to provide understanding and insight about the context in which the board is operating and knowledge of health 'realpolitik'.

There is a final lesson for boards in this study about the commissioning of external facilitators to support their development. Boards need to have clarity around their own expectations and should understand the potential of upstream diagnostic work before awayday events. Proper attention also has to be paid to the processes for securing facilitators to ensure that the recruitment results in support which is appropriate for the work that is required.

The framework for NHS board development incorporating Garratt's board tasks, Patching's organisation development schema and Cockman's facilitator modes, and refinements arising from the Chambers and Higgins (2005) study are outlined in Figure 16.2. Further work is now

EXTERNAL FOCUS

CONFORMANCE	PERFORMANCE
Board focus: Accountability (*explaining*) Requires exploratory OD activities and generic and specific induction and skills development programmes (e.g. training on patient and public involvement). Acceptant, catalytic and prescriptive consulting styles.	Board focus: Policy formulation, establishing core values (*what*) Requires exploratory and transformational OD activities (e.g. awaydays, visioning) & 'new board' work. Reflective, acceptant and confrontational consulting styles.
SHORT TERM	LONG TERM
Board focus: Monitoring of progress and behaviours (*monitoring*) Requires generic and specific induction and skills development programmes (e.g. briefings, seminars, board director induction programmes, clinical governance training). Catalytic and prescriptive consulting styles.	Board focus: Strategic thinking and key principles (*how*) Requires exploratory and transformational OD activities (e.g. awaydays, workshops, teambuilding) and 'new board' work. Reflective and catalytic consulting styles.

INTERNAL FOCUS

Figure 16.2   Framework for NHS board development
Source: Adapted from Chambers and Higgins (2005)

needed to test a revised framework with a wider group of boards and in other health systems. Equally important, there is a need to examine through empirical research the relationship between high performing organisations, the attention they pay to board development and the balance they strike between the board tasks described above. Like all other forms of organisational life, boards benefit from attention being paid to their development. There is evidence of an association between organisational cultures and performance, but the precise positive impact of boards is less clear and it is here also that further research is required.

Conclusion

How much does any of this matter? A key challenge in debates about governance at state and institutional level is how to engage a wider audience beyond those immediately engaged in, affected by or intellectually interested in the topic. One way of doing this is to demonstrate how decisions about governance issues can directly affect people's lives. We have traced the development of the 'audit society' and demonstrated how the impact of organisation failures across the world has influenced how health service organisations are governed. Issues of control are arguably accorded more weight than those of renewal. Put simply, we might be in danger of continuing to do the same thing better at times when we should be trying out new things. This can occur at an international, state and institution level. Within organisations, boards are responsible for making these kinds of choices. This means that within health services, deep-seated beliefs and values which boards espouse will guide decisions affecting staff performance and behaviours and the kinds of care and treatments provided to patients. The issue of board competence is equally important and, deservedly, under scrutiny. As well as a need to articulate more clearly the point and purpose of governance and the work of boards, the evidence shows that proper attention to developing the effectiveness of boards is also required.

Summary box

- Ideas about governance in public sector are evolving and are particularly affected by high-profile organisation failures across the world.
- Health service boards have a range of key roles in directing organisations but there are also limits to their influence.
- There are many different board models; the perfect model may not be attainable and is less important than positive behaviours and clarity of purpose.
- Boards and board members need structured development in order to be more effective.
- There is a need for better articulation about the point and purpose of governance and the work of boards.

Self-test exercises

1 How well do you know the work of the board/council/governing body of your organisation?
2 How far does the board of your organisation meet the tests of the Good Governance Standard? (See Figure 16.3.)
3 Ask to attend a board meeting (many are held in public anyway), reflect on content and behaviours and examine how much attention is paid to the four areas of board focus in the four quadrants in Figure 16.2.

1 **Good governance means focusing on the organisation's purpose and on outcomes for citizens and service users:**

- What is this organisation for?
- What is being done to improve services?
- Can I easily find out about the organisation's funding and how it spends its money?

2 **Good governance means performing effectively in clearly defined functions and roles:**

- Who is in charge of the organisation?
- How are they elected or appointed?
- At the top of the organisation, who is responsible for what?

3 **Good governance means promoting values for the whole organisation and demonstrating the values of good governance through behaviour:**

- According to the organisation, what values guide its work?
- What standards of behaviour should I expect from the organisation?
- Do the senior people put into practice the 'Nolan' principles for people in public life (selflessness, integrity, objectivity, accountability, openness, honesty and leadership)?

4 **Good governance means taking informed transparent decisions and managing risk:**

- Who is responsible for what kinds of decisions?
- Can I easily find out what decisions have been taken and the reasons for them?
- Does the organisation publish a clear annual statement on the effectiveness of its risk management system?

5 **Good governance means developing the capacity and capability of the governing body to be effective:**

- How does the organisation encourage people to get involved in running it?
- What support does it provide for people to get involved?
- How does the organisation make sure that all those running the organisation are doing a good job?

6 **Good governance means engaging stakeholders and making accountability real:**

- Are there opportunities for me and other people to make our views known?
- How can I go about asking the people in charge about their plans and decisions?
- Can I easily find out how to complain and who to contact with suggestions for changes?

Figure 16.3   How far does the board of your organisation meet the tests of the Good Governance Standard?

Source: Adapted with kind permission from Good Governance Standard for Public Services, the report of the Independent Commission on Good Governance in Public Services CIPFA/OPM (2004)

References

Avon, Gloucestershire and Wiltshire NHS Strategic Health Authority (2003) *North Bristol NHS Trust – Financial and Governance Review*. London: Deloitte and Touche.

Cadbury, Sir A. (1992) *Report of the Committee on the Financial Aspects of Corporate Governance*. London: Gee.

Carver, J. and Carver, M. (2001) *Carver's Policy Governance Model in Non Profit Organisations*. www.carvergovernance.com (accessed January 2006).

Chambers, N. (2003) Non-executive decisions. *Health Service Journal*, 30 October: 12–13.

Chambers, N. and Higgins, J. (2005) *Building a Framework for Developing Effective NHS Boards*. Manchester: University of Manchester.

Chambers, N. and Smith, E. (2004) *The Role of NHS Board Secretaries: Report for Network Meeting*. 29 November. Manchester: MCHM, University of Manchester.

Cockman, P. et al. (1999) *Consulting for Real People*. Maidenhead: McGraw-Hill.

Cornforth, C. (2003) *The Governance of Public and NonProfit Organisations*. London: Routledge.

Davies, C. et al. (2005) *Links between Governance, Incentives and Outcomes: A Review of the Literature National Co-ordinating Centre for NHS Service Delivery and Organisation R&D*. London: The Stationery Office.

Department of Health (DH, 2002) *Assurance: The Board Agenda*. London: DH.

Department of Health (DH, 2004) *Standards for Better Health*. London: DH.

Ferlie, E., Ashburner, L., Fitzgerald, L. and Pettigrew, A. (1996) *The New Public Management in Action*. Oxford: Oxford University Press.

Garratt, B. (1997) *The Fish Rots from the Head*. London: HarperCollins.

Health Service Journal (2005) News. 17 November: 5.

Higgs, D. (2003) *Review of the Role and Effectiveness of Non Executive Directors*. London: The Stationery Office.

Higgins, J. (2001) Adverse events or patterns of failure? *British Journal of Health Care Management*, 7(4): 145–7.

Higgins, J., Bradshaw, D. and Walshe, K. (2005) *The Developing Role of Strategic Health Authorities: Summary Report*. Manchester: University of Manchester.

Hodgkinson, G. and Sparrow, P. (2002) *The Competent Organisation*. Maidenhead: Open University Press.

Independent Commission for Good Governance in Public Services (2004) *The Good Governance Standard for Public Services*. (The Langlands Review.) London: OPM and CIPFA.

Institute of Directors (IOD, 2005) *Standards for the Board*. London: IOD.

Johnson, G., Scholes, K. and Whittington, R. (2005) *Exploring Corporate Strategy*. Harlow: Pearson.

Mannion, R., Davies, H.T.O. and Marshall, M. (2003) *Cultures for Performance in Health Care*. York: Centre for Health Economics, University of York.

MCHM (2002) *Report on a Survey of the Training and Development of Chairs and Non Executives in England*. Manchester: University of Manchester.

NHS Appointments Commission (2003) *Governing the NHS: A guide for NHS Boards*. London: Department of Health.

NHS Appointments Commission (2004) *Code of Conduct/Code of Accountability*. London: Department of Health.

NHS Confederation (2003) *Failure and Turnaround*. London: NHS Confederation.

NHS Confederation (2005) *Effective Boards in the NHS?* London: NHS Confederation.

OECD (2004) *Principles of Corporate Governance*. Paris: OECD (www.oecd.org).

OECD (2005) *Modernising Government: The Way Forward*. Paris: OECD (www.oecd.org).

Patching, K. (1999) *Management and Organisation Development*. Basingstoke: Macmillan.

Peck, E., Perri, T., Gulliver, P. and Towell, D. (2004) Why do we keep on meeting like this? The board as ritual in health and social care. *Health Services Management Research*, 17: 100–109.

Pierre, J. and Peters, B.G. (2000) *Governance, Politics and the State*. Basingstoke: Macmillan.

Plumridge, N. (2005) Opinion. *Health Service Journal*, 3 November: 17.

Pointer, D. (1999) *Board Work: Governing Health Care Organisations*. New York: Jossey-Bass.

Pollitt, C. (1999) *Performance or Compliance?* Oxford: Oxford University Press.

Power, M. (1999) *The Audit Society*. Oxford: Oxford University Press.

Taylor, B. (2001) *From Corporate Governance to Corporate Entrepreneurship* Henley-on-Thames: Henley Management College.

Tricker, R.I. (1983) *Corporate Governance*. Aldershot: Gower.

Turnbull Report (1999) *Internal Control Guidance for Directors on the Combined Code*. London: Institute of Chartered Certified Accountants in England and Wales.

Walshe, K., Harvey, G., Hyde, P. and Pandit, N. (2004) Organisational failure and turnaround: Lessons for public services from the for-profit sector. *Public Money and Management*, August: 201–208.

West, M. (1997) *Developing Creativity in Organisations*. Leicester: British Psychological Society.

Websites and resources

Center for Healthcare Governance. US membership organisation with aims to promote innovation and accountability in healthcare governance: *www.americangovernance.com*

Department of Health. Information and guidance including information for NHS Boards: *www.dh.gov.uk*

Governance. Monthly newsletter on issues of corporate governance and boardroom performance and useful links: *www.governance.co.uk*

Institute of Directors. Factsheets, policy papers, information about corporate governance initiatives and views on the economic outlook: *www.iod.com*

New Zealand District Health Boards. Information about the boards which were established in 2001: *www.moh.govt.nz/districthealthboards*

NHS Alliance. Represents NHS primary care organisations and issues reports and policy briefings: *www.nhsalliance.org*

NHS Appointments Commission. Details of vacancies, information about the work of local NHS boards, and guidance on the roles of boards, chairs and non-executives: *www.appointments.org.uk*

NHS Confederation. NHS employers organisation representing PCTs and trusts with a focus on influencing health policy and providing information and support to NHS organisations: *www.nhsconfed.org*

OECD. Organisation for Economic Development and Co-operation including full-text documents relating to corporate governance initiatives: *www.oecd.org*

PDK Control Consulting International. Canadian website with practical information about corporate governance tools, workshop presentations, references and a control self assessment process for companies to use: *www.csa-pdk.com*

17

Managing in partnership with other agencies

Jon Glasby

Introduction

In almost every country of the world there are problems of fragmentation and a lack of continuity in services for frail older people and other groups with complex, multiple needs (for examples see Glasby 2004 for a summary; see also Banks 2004; Leichsenring and Alaszewski 2004; Nies and Berman 2005). Almost irrespective of language, culture, structure, context and funding, there are different services responsible for different aspects of service provision and with different financial and regulatory systems, roles and responsibilities, and organisational and professional cultures. Making sense of this in a way that leads to joined up and well-organised experiences for service users and their families is a difficult political, managerial and practical task. Put simply, people do not live their lives according to the categories we create in our welfare services, and any holistic response to health needs will have to link to and be coordinated with the responses of other agencies if it is to be successful.

In pursuit of more effective inter-agency working, a number of countries have sought to develop more formal partnerships between local organisations. These tend to share a number of characteristics such as a focus on a particular at risk group and a defined catchment area, overall responsibility for arranging and/or delivering comprehensive services, the active involvement of primary care services and a focus on multidisciplinary teamwork at ground level. Such an approach is a powerful idea and intuitively seems like a sensible way forward. In theory, such integration could lead to more seamless services, user-centred care, an emphasis on prevention and rehabilitation, greater continuity of care, improved access to services, more integrated primary and secondary care and a reduction in inappropriate service use. However, key concerns include the difficulty of combining medical and social models and the risk of acute care (and the high cost of such services) distorting priorities.

There is a range of different models in different countries – each with strengths and limitations. Examples include the Program of All-Inclusive Care for the Elderly (PACE) and Social Health Maintenance Organisations in the USA; the SIPA project in Canada; the Rovereto Project in Italy; and Co-ordinated Care Trials in Australia (see Kodner and Kay Kyriacou 2000 for a summary). However, in a UK context, partnership working between health and social care is a central feature of current government policy and the focus of a significant range of activities at a local level. Although there has long been a recognition of the need for inter-agency collaboration to provide seamless services for users and carers (see, for example, Means and Smith 1998; Glasby and Littlechild 2004), this has acquired increasing impetus following the commitment of the New Labour government to achieving 'joined-up solutions' to 'joined-up problems'. Responding to the emphasis of central government on part- nership working, a large number of different partnership arrangements are being developed in different parts of the country, including Care Trusts, use of the Health Act flexibilities, joint appointments, and the use of staff secondments/joint management arrangements (see below for further discussion).

Against this background, the chapter reviews the rationales put for- ward for partnership working, summarises the history of recent partner- ship initiatives and provides brief discussion of some key theoretical models that managers can use to conceptualise and develop working relationships with other agencies. While this discussion focuses on UK approaches to health and social care, reference is also made to inter- national models, and many of the key issues may well be applicable to other contexts and to other types of partnership. Finally, the conclusion challenges healthcare managers to reflect on the skills that have tradition- ally been valued in their profession, and consider the extent to which new values, skills and approaches may be required in order to work effectively in partnership.

Why work in partnership?

Although there is a substantial and growing literature on partnership working (see, for example, Hudson 2000; Payne 2000; Rummery and Glendinning 2000; Balloch and Taylor 2001; Sullivan and Skelcher 2002; Glendinning et al. 2002a), there are a number of limitations to our exist- ing knowledge. In particular, much of the current literature is very descriptive and sometimes very 'faith based', emphasising the perceived virtues of partnership working without necessarily citing any evidence for the claims made. Moreover, as a recent literature review suggests, most studies focus on the process of partnership working (how well services are working together), not on the outcomes of partnerships (whether they make a difference to services or to outcomes for users and carers; Dowling et al. 2004).

As a result of these shortcomings, many accounts provide long lists of potential benefits, but are less clear about the extent to which these benefits are realisable in practice or about how to achieve such desired outcomes. Thus, the Audit Commission (1998) suggests that partnership working can help to deliver coordinated packages of services to individuals; tackle so-called 'wicked issues'; reduce the impact of organisational fragmentation (and minimise the impact of any perverse incentives that result from it); bid for or gain access to new resources; align services provided by all partners with the needs of users; make better use of resources; stimulate more creative approaches to problems; and influence the behaviour of the partners or of third parties in ways that none of the partners acting alone could achieve. Similarly, Payne's (2000) work on multidisciplinary teamwork holds out the hope that effective teams can, in theory: help to bring together key skills; share information; achieve continuity of care; apportion and ensure responsibility and accountability; coordinate the planning of resources; and coordinate in delivering the resources for professionals to apply for the benefit of service users. These are powerful claims, but possibly ones that must be treated with a degree of scepticism – while these proposed benefits seem common sense, achieving them may be more complex than the literature often suggests.

In spite of this, the English Department of Health provides a very strong but very helpful critique of agencies that fail to work in partnership, setting out a clear rationale why services must work together more effectively (DH 1998: 3):

> All too often when people have complex needs spanning both health and social care good quality services are sacrificed for sterile arguments about boundaries. When this happens people, often the most vulnerable in our society . . . and those who care for them find themselves in the no man's land between health and social services. This is not what people want or need. It places the needs of the organisation above the needs of the people they are there to serve. It is poor organisation, poor practice, poor use of taxpayers' money – it is unacceptable.

Behind this official pronouncement and behind much of the literature is a working hypothesis that effective partnerships should lead to better services and better outcomes for service users and their families (see Figure 17.1).

Unfortunately, many of these links currently remain unproven, and

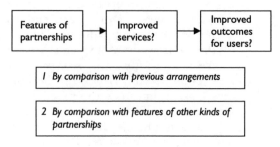

Figure 17.1   Effective partnership working (in theory)

further research is required to understand this model in more detail. For example, which approaches to partnership work best for whom in what circumstances? Until such questions receive more definitive answers, however, the Department of Health summary above remains one of the most powerful arguments for working together, even if it is stronger on its critique of the current situation than it is on possible ways forward.

The policy context

In a UK context, the post-war welfare state that was developed in the late 1940s is based on the assumption that it is possible to distinguish between people who are *sick* (who have 'health' needs and receive care free at the point of delivery) and those who are merely *frail* or *disabled* (who receive 'social care' services that are often means tested and subject to charges). In addition to this, many wider services (for example, education, policing, social security, etc.) have tended to be organised on hierarchical lines, with resources and policy flowing from the centre downwards. More recently, there has been increasing recognition of the need to create links between these different central government functions at a regional and, in particular, at a local level, with more effective inter-agency working for people who have range of needs. Thus, a disabled person who lives in local-authority housing may need adaptations making to their house, have particular transport needs, have particular health and social care support needs, and be keen to access training opportunities in order to gain employment. Similarly, a child at risk of abuse may be living in poor housing in a rundown inner-city area with few social amenities, be in trouble at school, at risk of crime (either as a victim of crime or as a perpetrator), and may self-harm or have substance misuse problems (or both). In both these hypothetical scenarios, the person concerned will need a wide range of agencies to work together in a coordinated way to meet their needs.

In response to this need to coordinate local services more effectively, there have been a number of key policy initiatives. For example, in 1973 the NHS Reorganisataion Act placed a statutory duty on health and local authorities to collaborate with each other through joint consultative committees. Advisory rather than executive, these bodies were soon seen to be inadequate for the task in hand (Wistow and Fuller 1982), prompting calls for further reform. In 1976, these arrangements were strengthened by the creation of joint care planning teams of senior officers and by a joint finance programme to provide short-term funding for social services projects deemed to be beneficial to the health services. Despite growing criticisms of these mechanisms for joint working, formal arrangements for collaboration remained substantially unchanged until the community care reforms of the 1990s (Hudson et al. 1997). Here, there was an attempt to create a more market-based approach to the delivery of public services, with a purchaser–provider split in healthcare and the stimulation of a much more mixed economy of provision in adult social care. Since 1997, the emphasis has arguably been more on creating local networks or partnerships between local agencies. Key policies include:

- The Health Act 1999: three new legal powers (or 'flexibilities') enabled health and social care to create pooled budgets, to develop lead commissioning arrangements or to create integrated providers (see Glendinning et al. 2002b).
- The creation of Care Trusts (NHS bodies with social care responsibilities delegated to them). With nine such organisations currently in existence, this is the closest model to a full merger of health and social care (see Glasby and Peck 2003).
- The creation of Children's Trusts: more virtual in nature than adult Care Trusts, these typically bring together a wider range of partners than just health and social care, and are local authority based. Alongside these new organisational arrangements, there is also an emphasis on a common assessment framework for children, greater information sharing, a lead professional to coordinate care and greater co-location of different professions working with children and young people (HM Treasury 2003).

In recent years, political devolution has allowed a series of new approaches to develop in the different countries of the UK. While England is formally integrating some services via the Care Trust and Children's Trust model, Scotland is developing a joint performance information and assessment framework to explore the outcomes (rather than just process issues) that whole systems working is achieving (see, for example, Hudson 2005). In addition, rather than distinguish between free healthcare and means-tested social care, Scotland is also seeking to provide all personal care free of charge, developing a new way of conceptualising needs that moves beyond the traditional health and social care divide. In Wales, use has been made of the Health Act flexibilities (Young et al. 2003), but further changes will also undoubtedly follow after an influential review of health and social in Wales by Derek Wanless (2003). In contrast, Northern Ireland has long had integrated health and social care structures, although some commentators debate the extent to which this system is truly integrated and delivers different outcomes to other parts of the UK (see, for example, Hudson 2004; Hudson and Henwood 2002). More recently, greater local flexibility in England has also enabled new models to emerge in individual health and social care communities, with, for example, proposals to integrate primary, secondary and social care on the Isle of Wight. Throughout all these changes, however, it is important to remember that partnership working is not a panacea and should never be an automatic response to a policy problem. Instead, policymakers and health and social care managers need to think through the outcomes they are trying to achieve, and choose the most appropriate organisational structures and processes to deliver these goals.

Useful theoretical frameworks

Against this background, there are a number of theoretical frameworks and models available that may help local managers and systems to think through their aspirations for local people and the different ways in which they might need to engage partner organisations. These are tools that my own organisation – the Health Services Management Centre (HSMC) – uses regularly in its consultancy and development work, and so we have considerable experience of applying them in practice.

Theories of change

When working with health and social systems around the country, HSMC often draws on an approach adapted from the 'theories of change' literature (utilised, for example, in the national evaluation of Health Action Zones; see Figure 17.2). In particular, this asks systems to explore:

- the outcomes which different stakeholders wish to achieve for service users
- the current context (including both strengths and weaknesses)
- possible ways forward and issues to be resolved.

In particular, HSMC uses this approach to prevent controversial discussion about issues of process and structure from dominating initial inter-agency debate. Instead, this model encourages services to ask themselves the following questions:

- Where do we want to be/what do we want to achieve? (outcomes)
- Where are we now? (context)
- What do we need to do to achieve our desired outcomes? (process)

In our experience, this allows greater time to surface and potentially reconcile different interpretations about desired outcomes and the current context before moving on to more practical discussions about next steps at a later stage. In particular, it allows managers and practitioners to see partnership working (and any structural changes that may ensue) as a means to an end (of better services and hence better outcomes for users and carers). While partnership working should never be an end in itself, it is easy to see how this happens when an already busy manager is tasked with setting up a new partnership. However well intentioned, it is all too

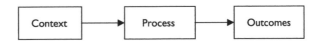

Figure 17.2   Theories of change
Source: Adapted from Judge (2000).

easy to lose sight of why the partnership was so important in the first place and the outcomes it was meant to deliver. Instead, having the partnership becomes the main aim. In contrast, 'theories of change' encourages a difficult but helpful focus on outcomes.

Depth v breadth of partnership

Having clarified desired outcomes and the strengths and limitations of the current context, there is scope for individual organisations to reflect in more detail on the partners they need to engage and the way in which they might need to work with different partners. Depending on desired outcomes, there may need to be very different organisations involved, and a range of options exist with regard to the depth and breadth of partnership that may be appropriate. This is set out in Figure 17.3 and it may be helpful for local services to map existing partnerships onto this graph in order to reflect on current relationships and their fitness for purpose.

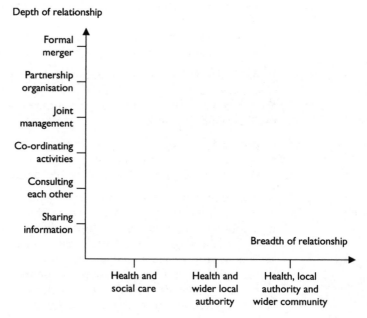

Figure 17.3   Depth v breadth
Source: Adapted from Peck (2002).

Different levels of partnership working

In addition, Glasby's (2003) research into delayed hospital discharges identifies three different levels of activity which health and social care agencies need to address in order to develop effective partnerships (see Figure 17.4): individual (I), organisational (O) and structural (S). While there is much more that can be done to encourage joint working between individual practitioners and local health and social care organisations (the I and O levels), Glasby argues that more action is required at a central government level to tackle some of the legal, administrative and bureaucratic barriers to partnership working. These are deeply ingrained in our current service structures and, ultimately, derive from the fact that the current health and social care system is based on an underlying division between two very different organisations with different priorities, values and ways of working. The framework is presented in terms of a series of interlocking circles, as each level of activity has the capacity to influence or be reinforced by the others. Thus, the way in which individuals behave is based in part on the norms, values and policies of their organisations, which in turn are shaped by a series of structural barriers to partnership working at a central government level. Similarly, these structural barriers depend in part on the characteristics of particular types of health and social care organisation, which depend ultimately on the people working in these organisations. As a result, any policy designed to achieve true partnership working will need to operate at all three levels of activity at the same time if it is to be successful.

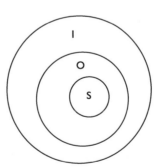

I: Individual level

O: Organisational level

S: Structural level

Figure 17.4   Different levels of partnership working
Source: Glasby (2003).

Key factors that may help or hinder partnership working

Although focusing on outcomes can be difficult, there is a large and growing body of evidence with regard to process. Over time, a series of consistent messages has emerged from various studies about the underlying factors and local conditions that may assist or hamper attempts to work together across organisational boundaries. Two of the most prominent frameworks are set out in Boxes 17.1 and 17.2 There is scope to use these in conjunction with external facilitation to explore shared understandings of progress to date, outstanding barriers, mutual perceptions of current partnerships and the 'readiness' of local services for new ways of joint working.

Box 17.1   Partnership working: what helps and what hinders?

Barriers

- *Structural* (the fragmentation of service responsibilities across and within agency boundaries)
- *Procedural* (differences in planning and budget cycles)
- *Financial* (differences in funding mechanisms and resource flows)
- *Professional* (differences in ideologies, values and professional interests)
- *Perceived threats to status, autonomy and legitimacy*

Principles for strengthening strategic approaches to collaboration

- *Shared vision*: Specifying what is to be achieved in terms of user-centred goals, clarifying the purpose of collaboration as a mechanism for achieving such goals, and mobilising commitment around goals, outcomes and mechanisms.
- *Clarity of roles and responsibilities*: Specifying and agreeing who does what and designing organisational arrangements by which roles and responsibilities are to be fulfilled.
- *Appropriate incentives and rewards*: Promoting organisational behaviour consistent with agreed goals and responsibilities, and harnessing organisational self-interest to collective goals.
- *Accountability for joint working*: Monitoring achievements in relation to the stated vision, holding individuals and agencies to account for the fulfilment of predetermined roles and responsibilities, and providing feedback and review of vision, responsibilities, incentives, and their interrelationship.

These factors have also been summarised in a Partnership Assessment Tool to help local systems evaluate the 'health' of their inter-agency relationships (available via www.odpm.gov.uk).

Source: Hudson et al. (1997).

> **Box 17.2   The partnership readiness framework**
>
> 1 Building shared values and principles.
> 2 Agreeing specific policy shifts.
> 3 Being prepared to explore new service options.
> 4 Determining agreed boundaries.
> 5 Agreeing respective roles with regard to commissioning, purchasing and providing.
> 6 Identifying agreed resource pools.
> 7 Ensuring effective leadership.
> 8 Providing sufficient development capacity.
> 9 Developing and sustaining good personal relationships.
> 10 Paying specific attention to mutual trust and attitude.
>
> *Source*: Poxton (2003)

The limits of structural change

In addition to factors that help the development of partnerships, there is a growing literature on what does not help and, in particular, on the limits of structural change. This material is summarised in detail elsewhere (see, for example, Social Services Inspectorate/Audit Commission 2004; Peck and Freeman 2005). However, messages from research and from practice seem to suggest that:

• structural change by itself rarely achieves stated objectives
• mergers typically do not save money – the economic benefits are often modest at best and are more than offset by unintended negative consequences such as a potential reduction in productivity and morale
• mergers are potentially very disruptive for managers, staff and service users and can give a false impression of change
• mergers can stall positive service development for at least 18 months.

Instead, research suggests (Peck and Freeman 2005) that successful mergers may depend upon the following:

• clarifying the real (as opposed to the stated) reasons behind the merger
• resourcing adequate organisational development support
• matching activities closely to intentions to reduce cynicism among key staff groups whose support will be crucial in realising the intended benefits.

A more detailed discussion of partnership working and organisational culture is available from the Integrated Care Network website (Peck and Crawford 2004).

Conclusion

While the key points raised in this chapter are set out in the Summary Box below, the current partnership agenda raises significant issues about the management styles and behaviours that will be required in the future. For example, what knowledge do current and future NHS managers have of social care, wider services and the voluntary and private sectors? Is there scope for interprofessional education and training to help NHS managers learn more about the roles and responsibilities of other agencies? Could the current NHS Management Training Scheme be reformed to become more of a generic public sector management scheme, with a common foundation and then greater specialism later in the course? What sorts of skills and values will future managers need to empathise with other agencies, lead by example, model effective collaboration and influence across boundaries? Whatever the detailed answers to these questions, it seems likely that NHS management in the future will not be the same as it is now, and that a new generation of managers with new skills, new horizons and new worldviews may have a very different role to play in future inter-agency collaborations.

Summary box

- People do not live their lives according to the categories we create in our welfare services.
- Meeting healthcare needs in a joined up and holistic way means working with other agencies.
- Partnership is a current government priority and a range of different models is developing in services for particular user groups and in different parts of the UK.
- Against this background, there is a range of theoretical models available to help managers think through the outcomes they are trying to achieve, the partners they need to engage and common factors that help or hinder partnership working.
- In the future, healthcare managers may need very different skills, values and experiences in order to be able to work effectively across agency boundaries.

Self-test exercises

1 What are service users and their families telling you about the experience of using your service and about the outcomes they are seeking from local health and social care? What opportunities are there for involving users in evaluating current partnerships and planning new services?

2 What knowledge do you have of social care and of other services in

your area? What fora exist to meet relevant people from different agencies, and is there scope to shadow a manager from a different organisational background to yourself?

3 What interpersonal and management skills do you possess, and are these the right ones to work in partnership with other agencies?

4 How can you support more junior staff to work effectively with other agencies?

5 How can you influence upwards in order to encourage senior commitment to partnership working?

6 With a mixed group of staff (for example, social workers and district nurses) ask each professional group to list the attributes of their profession/organisation they admire and those that frustrate them. Ask them also to list things that they admire about the other profession/organisation and those that they find frustrating. Bring the groups back together to share these perceptions, and facilitate a discussion about the extent to which these perceptions of each other are true, why each organisation/profession is like that, and what can be done locally to build on commonalities and tackle potential barriers to more effective joint working.

References and further reading

Audit Commission (1998) *A Fruitful Partnership: Effective Partnership Working.* London: Audit Commission.

Balloch, S. and Taylor, M. (2001) *Partnership Working: Policy and Practice.* Bristol: The Policy Press.

Banks, P. (2004) *Policy Framework for Integrated Care for Older People.* London: King's Fund/CARMEN Network.

Department of Health (DH, 1998) *Partnership in Action: New Opportunities for Joint Working between Health and Social Services – A Discussion Document.* London: DH.

Dowling, B., Powell, M. and Glendinning, C. (2004) Conceptualising successful partnerships. *Health and Social Care in the Community,* 12(4): 309–17.

Glasby, J. (2003) *Hospital Discharge: Integrating Health and Social Care.* Abingdon: Radcliffe.

Glasby, J. (2004) *Integrated Care for Older People.* Leeds: Integrated Care Network.

Glasby, J. and Littlechild, R. (2004) *The Health and Social Care Divide: The Experiences of Older People,* 2nd edn Bristol: The Policy Press.

Glasby, J. and Peck, E. (eds) (2003) *Care Trusts: Partnership Working in Action.* Abingdon: Radcliffe Medical Press.

Glendinning, C., Powell, M. and Rummery, K. (2002a) *Partnerships, New Labour and the Governance of Welfare.* Bristol: The Policy Press.

Glendinning, C., Hudson, B., Hardy, B. and Young, R. (2002b) *National Evaluation of Notifications for the Use of the Section 31 Partnership Flexibilities in the Health Act 1999: Final Project Report.* Leeds/Manchester: Nuffield Institute for Health/National Primary Care Research and Development Centre.

HM Treasury (2003) *Every Child Matters.* London: The Stationery Office.

Hudson, B. (2000) Inter-agency collaboration: A sceptical view. In A. Brechin, H.

Brown and M.A. Eby (eds) *Critical Practice in Health and Social Care*. Maidenhead: Open University Press.

Hudson, B. (2004) Care Trusts: A sceptical view. In J. Glasby and E. Peck (eds) *Care Trusts: Partnership Working in Action*. Abingdon: Radcliffe Medical Press.

Hudson, B. (2005) Pick up the pieces. *Community Care*, 22 September. Available at www.communitycare.co.uk (accessed 11 October 2005).

Hudson, B. and Henwood, M. (2002) The NHS and social care: The final countdown? *Policy and Politics*, 30(2): 153–66.

Hudson, B., Hardy, B., Henwood, M. and Wistow, G. (1997) *Inter-Agency Collaboration: Final Report*. Leeds: Nuffield Institute for Health.

Judge, K. (2000) Testing evaluation to the limits: The case of English Health Action Zones. *Journal of Health Services Research and Policy*, 5(1): 3–5.

Kodner, D. and Kay Kyriacou, C. (2000) Fully integrated care for frail elderly: Two American models. *International Journal of Integrated Care*, 1. Available at http://www.ijic.org/ (accessed 25 February 2004).

Leichsenring, K. and Alaszewski, A. (eds) (2004) *Providing Integrated Health and Social Care for Older Persons: A European Overview of Issues at Stake*. Ashgate: Aldershot.

Means, R. and Smith, R. (1998) *From Poor Law to Community Care*. Basingstoke: Macmillan.

Nies, H. and Berman, P.C. (2005) *Integrating Services for Older People: A Resource Book for Managers*. Dublin: European Health Management Association (available to download free online).

Payne, M. (2000) *Teamwork in Multiprofessional Care*. Basingstoke: Macmillan.

Peck, E. (2002) Integrating health and social care, *Managing Community Care*, 10(3): 16–19.

Peck, E. and Crawford, A. (2004) *'Culture' in Partnerships: What Do We Mean by It and What Can We Do About It?* Leeds: Integrated Care Network.

Peck, E. and Freeman, T. (2005) *Reconfiguring PCTs: Influences and Options*. Briefing paper prepared for the NHS Alliance. Birmingham: HSMC, University of Birmingham.

Poxton, R. (2003) What makes effective partnerships between health and social care? In J. Glasby and E. Peck (eds) *Care Trusts: Partnership Working in Action*. Abingdon: Radcliffe Medical Press.

Rummery, K. and Glendinning, C. (2000) *Primary Care and Social Services: Developing New Partnerships for Older People*. Oxford: Radcliffe Medical Press.

Social Services Inspectorate/Audit Commission (2004) *Old Virtues, New Virtues: An Overview of the Changes in Social Care Services over the Seven Years of Joint Reviews in England, 1996–2003*. London: SSI/Audit Commission.

Sullivan, H. and Skelcher, C. (2002) *Working Across Boundaries: Collaboration in Public Services*. Basingstoke: Macmillan Palgrave.

Wanless, D. (2003) *The Review of Health and Social Care in Wales*. Cardiff: Welsh Assembly.

Wistow, G. and Fuller, S. (1982) *Joint Planning in Perspective*. Birmingham: Centre for Research in Social Policy and National Association of Health Authorities.

Young, R., Hardy, B., Waddington, E. and Jones, N. (2003) *Partnership Working: A Study of NHS and Local Authority Services in Wales*. Manchester/Leeds: Centre for Healthcare Management/Nuffield Institute for Health.

Websites and resources

CARMEN. Network of organisations and countries focusing on the care and management of services for older people across the European Union. Supported by the European Health Management Association, the CARMEN website contains links to a range of reports, good practice guides and resources for managers: www.ehma.org/projects/carmen.asp

Centre for the Advancement of Interprofessional Education (CAIPE). National body dedicated to supporting education and training that helps workers from different backgrounds to come together to learn from and with each other: www.caipe.org.uk

Change Agent Team. Department of Health, part of the Care Services Improvement Partnership working to support frontline services working across agency boundaries in older people's services: www.csip.org.uk

Every Child Matters. Department for Education and Skills website dedicated to this agenda and the integration of children's services: www.everychildmatters.gov.uk

Integrated Care Network. Key UK resource for anyone interested in partnership working, with an online bulletin board, news of forthcoming events and series of practical publications on topics such as culture, governance and human resources: www.integratedcarenetwrok.gov.uk

International Journal of Integrated Care. Free online journal with articles from a range of different countries and continents: www.ijic.org

International Network for Integrated Care (INIC). Runs a series of international conferences and study tours on the subject of integrated care: www.integratedcarenetwork.org

Joint Future Unit. Responsible for promoting collaboration between local government, the NHS and other partners: www.scotland.gov.uk

Journal of Integrated Care. Practice-focused UK publication devoted to exploring inter-agency working. With contributions from managers, practitioners and academics, it contains a range of very accessible discussion pieces, summaries and new research studies with regard to partnership working: *www.pavpub.com*

Social Care Institute for Excellence (SCIE). Independent body funded by government to identify and disseminate good practice in social care. SCIE also hosts Social Care Online, a free database that enables users to search key social care databases and documents. SCIE currently covers England, Wales and Northern Ireland and has a series of practice guides, discussion papers and toolkits available to download free of charge: www.scie.org.uk

Welsh Assembly. Guidance on the health, social care and well-being agenda in Wales. (See, for example: www.wales.gov.uk/subihealth/content/keypubs/pdf/policy-guide-e.pdf).

18 Performance measurement and improvement

Tim Freeman

Too much policing will not create a culture of quality. Rather it is likely to distort practice and prioritise the conventional and the measurable. (Smith 1995c: 308)

Introduction

This chapter avoids the limitations of rapid obsolescence and inability to explain change associated with simple 'lists' of contemporary regulatory practice by providing a conceptual overview. Drawing on cultural theory, regulation is considered within the context of international trends in governance, and regulatory approaches such as accreditation, inspection, performance management and peer review are situated within a conceptual framework consisting of two independent dimensions: control location (internal/external); and nature of resultant action (formative/summative). The axes combine to produce quadrants: internal control, formative action (Q1); external control, formative action (Q2); internal control, summative action (Q3); and external control, summative action (Q4). The focus is firmly on Q4, with a consideration of the interplay of the summative and formative within real-world regulatory and inspection systems.

Recent UK NHS regulatory experience is considered, together with an overview of the generic empirical and theoretical literature on use of performance indicators in performance management. Conceptual and technical issues are explored, including the potential displacement of informal modes of quality assurance; the status of indicators as 'conceptual technologies'; difficulties associated with availability, reliability, validity and confounding; the importance of sensitivity and specificity; and the potential for unintended negative consequences. The chapter concludes with a cautious assessment of the potential value of performance measurement in governance systems.

The rise of regulatory and inspection systems

The role of external regulation is perhaps best understood in the context of governance, where governance is defined as a form of social coordination (Mayntz 1993), of which multiple patterns or modes are available. Cultural theory (Hood 1998; Hood et al. 1999) identifies four 'ideal types': oversight (bureaucracy); mutuality (professional or 'clan'); competition (market); and contrived randomness (fatalism). Each has its strengths and weaknesses, so that while markets provide flexibility and dynamism, the competitive environment makes collaboration on joint ventures difficult. Cultural theory's assertion that the pursuit of each 'ideal type' in isolation leads to negative feedback that undermines its ability to function provides a rationale for drawing on each of the four ideal types, continually readjusting the blend of hybrid governance forms operating in any system, to maintain a dynamic tension between the elements – a complex dance, in which the music never stops (Figure 18.1).

While it is important not to overemphasise the degree of homogeneity in emergent public sector management practices, during the 1980s public services in western Europe increasingly became managed rather than administrated, governance practices tending to emphasise market provision and indirect regulatory systems rather than hierarchical control (Hoggett 1996; Jacobs and Manzi 2000; McLaughlin et al. 2001). Marrying central control with local responsibility, New Public Management (NPM) sought to verify the compliance of semi-autonomous provider agencies by auditing performance against targets (Carter et al. 1992; Power 1997). While strongly associated with New Right political theory and the entrepreneurial governance thesis (Osborne and Gaebeler 1992), in which clients are conceptualised as customers and service provision decentralised to competing autonomous providers in regulated markets, the demands of political accountability required close management of the market leading to a rapid expansion in systems of inspection, accounting, regulation and review (Clarke et al. 2000). Indeed, the simultaneous use of both centralisation and decentralisation is a defining paradox of the approach (Clarke and Newman 1997), regulatory mechanisms providing

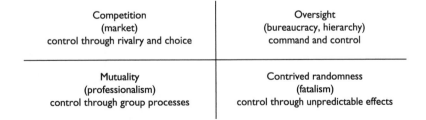

Competition (market) control through rivalry and choice	Oversight (bureaucracy, hierarchy) command and control
Mutuality (professionalism) control through group processes	Contrived randomness (fatalism) control through unpredictable effects

Figure 18.1   Modes of governance
Source: Adapted from Hood (2000)

the means to 'steer' the behaviour of semi-autonomous organisations at a distance.

While the UK Labour Party vehemently opposed the use of internal markets in healthcare provision while in opposition during the early 1990s, when elected to government in 1997 the new administration retained and extended the emphasis on decentralisation and performance management, with additional elements of central direction and new regulatory bodies to set and monitor standards. Thus, care standards were to be set nationally via a new National Institute for Clinical Excellence (NICE) and new National Service Frameworks (NSFs). National standards were monitored through performance management and external regulation via a rolling programme of visits from a new Commission for Health Improvement (CHI) and a series of high-level performance indicators under a Performance Assessment Framework (PAF). While commentators satirised the continuities with the earlier NPM by coining the term Modern Public Management ('MPM'; Newman 2000), the new regulatory bodies signalled a significant step away from market modes of governance associated with competition and contracting towards new forms of regulatory oversight associated with guidance and monitoring. They constituted a strong system of performance improvement, with an underlying emphasis on the increased accountability of professionals to government, drawing on a comprehensive set of high-level performance indicators and central targets (McLaughlin et al. 2001). At the time of writing, more recent policy innovations such as Payment by Results (PbR), Patient Choice and use of Independent Sector Treatment Centres (ISTCs) for clinical and diagnostic procedures may be seen as reintroducing a number of market-based incentives into governance systems. (See Box 18.1.)

From the perspective of cultural theory the above shifts in emphasis over time are less new 'post-bureaucratic' forms than a dynamic blend of different forms of social coordination drawing on market, hierarchy, clan and fatalist modes of governance to address emerging negative feedback over time. The increased centralism of NICE and CHI could be seen as an attempt to increase collaboration and standardisation in the face of competitive pressures; and the introduction of PbR, patient choice and ISTCs as an attempt to increase competitive incentives in the light of concern over 'management by targets'. While the number of ideal types of governance mode is limited, the relative balance between these

---

Box 18.1   Cultural theory

- Suggests that all governance systems require blends of competition, oversight, mutuality and contrived randomness.
- Blends are only ever in unstable, dynamic balance: all governance systems require continual renewal to offset emerging negative unintended consequences.

approaches and their hybrids is almost without limit and there is much scope for new forms of regulatory practices within these emergent governance hybrids. For example, publication of *Creating a Patient-led NHS: Delivering the NHS Improvement Plan* (DH 2005) raised the prospect of contestable provision from multiple providers in primary as well as secondary care within the UK NHS, necessitating the development of market regulation mechanisms for entry, exit and consumer protection. At the time of writing, it is unclear which agency or agencies will be charged with these functions, or how they will be organised.

Conceptual framework: control location and resultant action matrix

Given the fluidity of governance hybrids considered above, there is a wide and potentially bewildering array of measurement indices for assessing the quality of healthcare provision at the level of local health economy, organisation, clinical directorate or service team. Options include accreditation, quality management frameworks, performance management systems, benchmarking and statistical process control, among many others. The emphasis placed on the various elements has continued to evolve necessitating periodic 'shuffles' of structural and institutional arrangements, such as the expansion of CHAI's responsibilities to include performance indicators and the reconfiguration of the Modernisation Agency into the NHS Institute for Innovation and Improvement (NIII).

In the context of such dynamic complexity, Boland and Fowler (2000) provide a useful conceptual framework of performance measurement, indicators and improvement initiatives (Figure 18.2). Their model is expressed as a simple matrix with two axes: the source of control (internal or external); and the nature of resultant action – positive (supportive and formative) or negative (punitive or summative).

The vertical axis identifies the source of authority for control, either

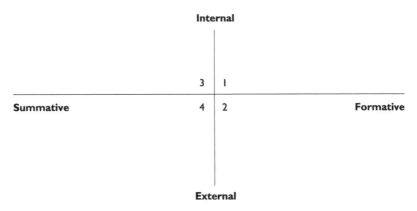

Figure 18.2   Control locations and resultant action matrix
Source: Adapted from Boland and Fowler (2000)

from within the organisation (internal) or from outside (external). While the former implies using indicators for internal purposes, the latter implies the existence of an outside body holding the organisation to account for its actions – regulation. The horizontal axis concerns perceptions of the nature of resultant controlling actions: supportive and formative (positive) or punitive and summative (negative). Negative action implies an assumption that underperformance is due to inefficiency, leading to actions such as a reduction in resource allocation. In contrast, positive action implies that in the same situation an investigation would be undertaken to explore why the situation had arisen, leading to redeployment of resources or organisational development activities such as staff development. Considered as two independent dimensions of control location and resultant action, the axes combine to produce four potential options (Box 18.2):

Box 18.2   Control location and resulting action quadrants

- Q1: controlled by the organisation and used formatively for development
- Q2: controlled by an external agency and used formatively for development
- Q3: controlled by the organisation and used for sanction and blame
- Q4: controlled by an external agency and used for sanction and blame

---

1 *Quadrant 1: Internal control, positive action.* These typically include internal quality improvement procedures such as total quality management (TQM), benchmarking and statistical process control – measurements are taken in order to support internal quality improvement.
2 *Quadrant 2: External control, positive action.* This quadrant includes external bodies charged with auditing the performance measurement and quality improvement systems of organisations, i.e. audit of systems at one step removed, in order to offer advice on how the whole organisation can develop component parts to ensure continued improvements. It is positive in nature given its supportive, largely nurturing role.
3 *Quadrant 3: Internal control, negative action.* This concerns measurement of internal subunits as in Quadrant 1, but here negative actions may arise. Although data may be gathered internally, in practice information is often required by an external agency. Thus in the UK the collection and reporting of waiting time data in hospitals is an internal concern, but also required by a central agency. Such local collection of data used externally to monitor performance is a defining feature of New Public Management (NPM) approaches.
4 *Quadrant 4: External control, negative action.* As in Quadrant 3, organisations may expect to be judged on their activities with punitive consequences for poor performers. However, in this quadrant authority is imposed through lines of accountability to an external regulatory agency.

The remainder of this chapter concentrates largely on the regulatory options available in Quadrant 4, as internal quality improvement approaches such as statistical process control (SPC) and benchmarking are considered elsewhere in this book. It is important to note at this point that the potential of internal formative approaches such as TQM in influencing behaviour should not be underestimated. Indeed, when considered in Foucaultian terms as a series of techniques and practices that encourage clinicians in their own self-surveillance, TQM may be characterised as a particularly subtle internal regulatory practice, in which the behaviours accepted internally by clinicians as the hallmark of professionalism become increasingly aligned with those expected by the external 'gaze' of the performance manager (Flynn 2004).

Regulation

The external quadrants Q2 and Q4 are in essence regulatory, the key feature being placement of responsibility for overseeing performance with an external body, i.e. the regulator. Walshe (2002) identifies two paradigms of regulation – deterrence and compliance – each with a distinctive perspective on the nature of those regulated and the behaviour required of the regulator. The former assumes that regulatees need to be coerced to behave well through strict enforcement of demanding standards, lest they pursue their own interests to the detriment of others. They require searching judgement and it is the duty of the regulator to bring them to account. In contrast, the compliance model assumes that those regulated are well meaning and seeking to comply, requiring support and advice from their external assessors. Given the above, it is clear that Walshe's deterrence and compliance models equate respectively to Q4 (external summative) and Q2 (external formative) in Boland and Fowler's model (Box 18.3).

While the above distinctions are helpful in conceptualising the options available within external regulatory systems, Walshe (2002) is careful to emphasise their heuristic status. In practice, regulators may seek to differentiate their behaviour, drawing on deterrence or compliance approaches according to the demands of the situation, the degree of discretion

---

Box 18.3   Regulation

- *Deterrence-based approaches* assume actors are self-interested and will seek to avoid regulation unless coerced.
- *Compliance-based approaches* assume well-intentioned actors who are seeking to comply.
- *Real-world regulatory systems* seek latitude to balance these two approaches as appropriate

available to them and political exigencies. Thus an organisation in which management is open and honest about shortcomings and has been working towards solutions may well receive rather more sympathetic treatment than one where management have hidden their difficulties and attempted to 'hoodwink' the regulators, if such differentiation is within the gift of the regulator and will not cause political disquiet when exercised. The following section considers recent healthcare examples of four major regulatory forms: accreditation; inspection; performance management; and external peer review.

Accreditation: a healthcare organisation perspective

Organisational accreditation originated in the USA with the Joint Commission on the Accreditation of Healthcare Organisations, and was exported to Canada via Australia and then to Europe in the 1980s (Shaw 2000). Usually voluntary in nature, accreditation is typically undertaken by a multidisciplinary team of healthcare professionals against published standards, and those organisations which are able to show their conformance to standards receive accreditation from the award-making body. Examples that have been used internationally within the context of healthcare provision include the Malcolm Baldrige and European Foundation for Quality Management approaches to organisational excellence, as well as the International Organisation for Standardisation (ISO 9000) approach to quality management. In the UK, accreditation became increasingly widespread (see Box 18.4), evinced by a wide range of programmes such as the Hospital Accreditation Programme (HAP), the King's Fund Organisational Audit (now HQS), Investors In People (IIP) for training and development of staff, and Clinical Pathology Accreditation (CPA) (Heaton 2000).

Box 18.4   Accreditation – the US experience

The US accreditation model for external evaluation of healthcare organisation quality, initiated by the American College of Surgeons (ACS) in 1917, evolved into the Joint Commission in 1951. This was entirely professionally driven (standards set, results used exclusively by health professionals for quality improvement and graduate education) until 1964. The subsequent pervasive influence of the Joint Commission is the result of government, purchaser and public use of accreditation. Establishment of the Medicare programme for older Americans in 1965 created 'deemed status' for provider eligibility for funding – thus accreditation became a mechanism for public accountability and control of costs, involving government, purchasers and the public. The primary reasons for seeking accreditation under this arrangement are thus rather different than those under the earlier professionally controlled ACS external evaluation.

Inspection: Commission for Health Improvement (CHI)

CHI was created in the UK under the Health Act (1999) as an independent body charged with monitoring performance and facilitating improvements in clinical care quality, through routine reviews and special investigations. This constitutes a potential double paradox: that of supportive and developmental in the context of reviews and the hard-edged investigator charged with naming and shaming; and the extent of its independence from government, given that Secretary of State may request investigations. The dual identity has been discussed by classical allusion to Janus, the Roman god of beginnings with two faces (Rowland 2003).

From its inception, senior CHI personnel consistently sought to place the emphasis firmly on facilitating improvement. While generally well received within the service, Day and Klein (2002) raised a number of important tensions within the clinical governance reviews undertaken by CHI. These included the combination of summative and formative dimensions of the reviews; the balance between checking for the implementation of mechanisms and assessing their impact; and queries over data quality and the extent of critical evaluation of data in context. The NHS Reform and Healthcare Professions Act 2002 and *Delivering the NHS Plan* (DH 2002) outlined new powers and responsibilities for CHI, along with a change of name to Commission for Healthcare Audit and Inspection (CHAI), and latterly Healthcare Commission. Its expanded portfolio included performance management, waiting lists and value for money. These included the creation of an Office for Information on Health Care Performance, licensing private healthcare provision, conducting value for money audits, validating published performance statistics, publishing star ratings and an ability to recommend special measures. (See Box 18.5.)

Box 18.5   Inspection – the Dutch experience of 'Visitatie'

Originating in the Netherlands, 'visitatie' (to visit) was introduced in the late 1980s by the specialist medical community to assure patient quality and reconfirming the trust of the public, financiers and government in professional self-regulatory mechanisms. The collegial peer-review system was doctor-led, and aimed to assess the quality of practice of hospital-based specialist groups. On completion of a visit, findings are documented in a confidential report, listing recommendations for improvement, and implementation is left to the specialists who were reviewed. While there are no formal sanctions for failure to comply with recommendations, the specialist societies expect members to act on the recommendations; governance is collegiate rather than hierarchical.

Performance management

The NHS Performance Assessment Framework (PAF)

Central influence over policy implementation in England increased dramatically under reforms instituted by New Labour, principally via Public Service Agreements (PSAs) between Whitehall departments and the Treasury, and service delivery agreements explaining how the high-level targets contained in the PSAs are to be reached (Lee and Woodward 2002). Agreements were implemented through the Performance Assessment Framework (PAF), the routine quantitative instrument for monitoring the progress of healthcare organisations under the 1997 reforms (NHSE 1999). Six areas of the PAF were agreed in 1999: health improvement; deaths from all causes; fair access; effective delivery of appropriate healthcare; efficiency; patient/carer experience of the NHS; health outcomes. Under the Health and Social Care (Community Health and Standards) Act 2003, the performance assessment framework for 2005–8 ('Standards for Better Health') promised fewer national targets and a renewed focus on outcomes and patient experience, in order to stimulate local flexibility and innovation. Seven domains are identified: safety; clinical and cost effectiveness; governance; patient focus; accessible and responsive care; care environment and amenities; public health. However, while the new system offered the prospect of greater autonomy for trusts within the national framework given the system of 'core' and 'developmental' standards within the seven domains, they are still based on Treasury Public Service Agreements.

Box 18.6   Performance management: New Zealand PHOs

Similar to the UK Quality Outcomes Framework, primary healthcare organisations (PHOs) in New Zealand receive financial incentives for improvements in performance against a range of nationally agreed indicators under the PHO performance management programme. The indicators were developed by a PHO clinical governance advisory group and government representatives, and include clinical, process/capacity and financial indicators. PHOs become eligible for payments as they improve their performance on the indicators against targets as laid out in an agreed development plan with the district health board (DHB). Additionally, DHBs agree with PHOs on how the performance payments will be used.

Performance ratings ('stars')

Under the 'star' rating system of NHS trusts in England, three sets of information were combined to produce a summary measure of performance from 'excellent' (three stars) to 'poor' (zero stars). The first area comprised performance under key targets in the PAF such as waiting times; the second a battery of additional indicators under headings of patient, clinical and capacity focus; and the third CHI review information, used (where available) for adjustment. Star ratings had important effects as only three-star trusts were allowed to spend improvement fund monies at their discretion, or to apply for foundation status. Crucially, trusts failing badly on the key targets received no stars, no matter how good the CHI report or how well it performed under the other measures. Given the possibility of reward or sanction, the potential for perverse incentives leading to misrepresentation was high.

National Service Frameworks (NSFs)

NSFs are developed with the intention of setting national standards and defining service models for specific services or care groups including mental health (DH 1999), coronary heart disease (DH 2000), diabetes (DH 2003) and older people (DH 2001); and establishing implementation programmes and performance measures against which progress may be measured. Each NSF includes national standards of care which patients may expect, a definition of the evidence base associated with interventions and their associated costs, as well as work commissioned to support implementation such as research, appraisal, benchmarks and outcome indicators, and supporting programmes including workforce planning, education and information management.

Local authority Overview and Scrutiny Committees (OSCs)

Introduced from 2002, OSCs have the ability to require local NHS representatives to answer questions concerning local health service matters, and provides an opportunity for lay elected representatives to influence the development of local health services on behalf of the community. Guidance from the Audit Commission (2002) emphasises the need for inclusive local processes in drawing up its scrutiny programme; careful organisation around a series of subpanels; extensive and robust evidence gathering and review cycles; and extensive 'informal' lines of communication. (See Box 18.6.)

External peer review

A review of the scope, mechanisms and use of external peer review techniques (ExPeRT) operative in western European healthcare systems (Shaw 2000) identified four assessment mechanisms: accreditation, ISO 9000, EFQM and visitatie, each of which are used in the UK (Heaton 2000). Klazinga (2000) embeds these assessment mechanisms within broader perspectives of external review: organisational (accreditation); process control (ISO 9000); quality management (European Foundation for Quality Monitoring Excellence Model EFQM EM); and professional (visitatie). Traditionally, the focus of the standards in each model reflected their original purpose: professional standards (visitatie), health service delivery (accreditation); management systems (EFQM); and quality assurance systems (ISO). Models are typically complementary rather than mutually exclusive, the differences in uptake in any healthcare system being a function of the attributes of the models and the interests of different professional groupings (Heaton 2000). Thus, debates over models and methods are ultimately concerned with professional control, and the perceived value of approaches is dependent upon judgements concerning the appropriate balance between professional self-regulation and external accountability.

At the level of healthcare organisations, clinical professionals tend to be supportive of visitatie and accreditation. Their enthusiasm is, however, dependent on who is going to use the model and to what aims, and they will seek to limit accreditation programmes to areas of professional performance that they deem appropriate. Similarly, managers may either promote or oppose visitatie depending on their perspective on the value of self-regulation, and those managers intent on increasing managerial control will tend to pursue accreditation and ISO. At the government level, debate among policymakers ultimately concerns the ability of the mix of models to achieve a balance of power between stakeholders congruent with government policy towards accountability (Klazinga 2000). Figure 18.3 identifies a range of contemporary regulatory practices within Boland and Fowler's framework.

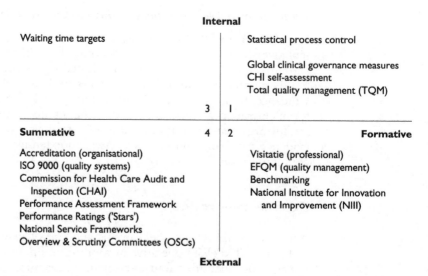

Figure 18.3   Populated control locations and resultant action matrix

Using performance indicators in performance management

While the previous section considered a number of contemporary regulatory mechanisms, there is an extensive literature on the generic issues associated with use of performance indicators in any performance management system (Freeman 2002), and a careful reading reveals two broad traditions. The first is practice oriented, prescriptive and optimistic of the value and use of performance indicators, while in contrast the second is more critically engaged and sceptical. Much of the practice-oriented literature focuses on matters internal to healthcare organisations and links conceptually to total quality management (TQM) and continuous quality improvement (CQI) approaches. In contrast, the academic literature is more consistently negative, and forms a discourse defined in terms of conceptual difficulties and statistical proof. In the UK, the use of performance indicators in assurance and performance management systems has heavily influenced debate over their value. Indeed, many of the conceptual and technical problems considered below arise due to problems over validity, reliability and perverse incentives that tend to characterise such systems.

Conceptual difficulties

In common with all assurance approaches, the primary goal of assurance-focused performance indicator systems is the verification of improvements – quality must not only improve but be seen to do so. Yet faith in measurement may be misplaced. In the context of external assurance, the existence of indicators does not remove the need for trust but relocates it from the internal control systems of professionals to audit systems (Power 1997). Under such circumstances performance indicator frameworks may simply displace existing informal modes of quality assurance. The irony is that new structures may displace these informal strategies, and in seeking to verify the accountability of agents may generate suspicion and fear, undermining the conditions of trust required for quality improvement (Sitkin and Roth 1993).

Indicators provide information on a potentially limitless number of dimensions. As indicator systems are unable to capture more than a fragment of what is important about the human experience of healthcare, some selection is required. A delicate balance needs to be struck between coverage and practicality: too few indicators and important aspects will be missed; too many indicators and the instrument will be impractical to use and costly to maintain. By making some aspects visible, indicators marginalise other aspects and perspectives (Van Peursem et al. 1995). They are thus conceptual technologies (Barnetson and Cutright 2000), shaping which issues are thought about and how people think about them. (See Box 18.7.)

> **Box 18.7   Conceptual difficulties with performance indicators**
>
> • They risk displacing formal quality assurance approaches and undermine the conditions of trust and openness required for quality improvement.
> • Given the limited number of indicators that may be incorporated into any system, they inevitably marginalise other aspects and perspectives which are not included.

Technical difficulties

One of the main attractions of indicators is that they promise visible and concrete proof of performance. The claim to objectivity is essential to the use of indicators in performance league tables, yet poses many difficulties. Much of the debate is conducted in terms of statistical proof, but includes indicator selection, meaningfulness, and robustness in the light of adjustments for confounding factors, as well as difficulties that arise when using them to inform service change. Indicators based on a limited range of items available in pre-existing information systems may additionally have significant problems with their validity, reliability and comparability.

Imprecision

The structured reporting of indicators further obscures the layered meanings involved in interpretation, and subtle variations in definitions of indicators such as 'readmission' at different centres may lead to the failure to compare like with like (Gross et al. 2000; McColl et al. 2000; Jackson 2001). Further difficulties in operationalising indicators arise specifically in the public sector because of the existence of multiple conflicting objectives and overriding importance of political objectives (Hepworth 1988). There are no technical solutions to these problems and value judgements are required given the existence of legitimate political debates surrounding the definition of 'appropriate' measures (Stewart and Walsh 1994).

Data: availability and reliability

There are often problems with the availability of data, resulting in a tendency to focus on measuring what there is data for, rather than items that correlate with the system's goals and objectives (Lowry 1988; McKee and James 1997; Lorence et al. 2002). Data accuracy is also important, the issue being whether between-group differences reflect quality of data rather than quality of care (Kazandjian et al. 1996), a particular problem in the context of summative assurance. All data collection relies on the goodwill of clinicians and is thus susceptible to manipulation, particularly when reward and censure depend on results (Audit Commission 2000).

Data: validity and confounding

Even where data is available and reliable, it may be potentially misleading and easily misinterpreted (Smith 1995b; McColl et al. 1998). Measurement validity reflects the extent to which indicators truly represent a more abstract variable. In order to be valid measures of healthcare quality, indicators need to reflect attributes of the healthcare system, rather than attributes of the patient or of other non-healthcare characteristics. For example, readmission rates are a valid indicator of care quality to the extent that readmission is due solely to deficiencies in the quality of the previous care. The point at issue here is that indicators should only relate to factors that are under the control of those under scrutiny (Parry et al. 1998; Hauck et al. 2003).

To avoid confounding, all other exogenous and endogenous factors affecting the indicators must be controlled (Barnsley et al. 1996; Davenport et al. 1996). Potential confounding factors include configuration of the local health economy (Carter 1989; Brown et al. 1995), socioeconomic variations (Giuffrida et al. 1999), case mix, comorbidity and severity (Mant and Hicks 1996; Rigby et al. 2001). Without adjustment, it is not clear to what extent indicators identify the contribution of health services to healthcare (Mulligan et al. 2000). There are particular problems associated with outcome measures, as they may occur over long time scales and suffer from problems of attribution, especially in measures of chronic illness (Smith 1995c).

Dealing with confounding

Risk adjustment models such as standardisation, cluster analysis, multiple regression and data envelope analysis (DEA) may be used (Blumberg 1986; Giuffrida et al. 2000; Giuffrida and Gravelle 2001). Perhaps the greatest difficulty with such methods is that they are not transparent to the end user so that attempts to increase the validity of the data may simply undermine its credibility. The tendency of different adjustment methods to yield different results brings the robustness of the process further into question (Nutley and Smith 1998).

Indicators: robustness, sensitivity and specificity

Indicators may falsely convey an impression of objectivity to what is often weak and ambiguous evidence (Davies and Lampel 1998). Small numbers of cases mean low significance (McGlynn 1998; Sheldon 1998), the data requirements for precision are excessive (Mant 1995), and random variation in measures may be misinterpreted (Smith 1995c). In short, comparisons become difficult and potentially deceptive. It is important that indicators are able to identify all poorly performing units (sensitivity) and that all units identified by indicators as performing poorly really are performing poorly (specificity); poor sensitivity and specificity results in false assurance or denigration, where indicators incorrectly identify individuals/organisations as poor, or fail to identify

the poorly performing (Goldstein and Spiegelhalter 1996; Davies 1998).
(See Box 18.8.)

Box 18.8   Technical difficulties with performance indicator systems

- Imprecision and lack of technical solutions to political objectives.
- Limited availability and reliability.
- Poor validity due to difficulties in attribution of outcomes to processes, a
  result of extraneous confounding factors.
- Techniques for dealing with confounding may be subject to legitimate challenge.

Perverse incentives

Performance management systems may give rise to perverse incentives
and unintended consequences (Smith 1990, 1995a; Goddard et al. 2000),
arising from the fact that people anticipate the reactions of those charged
with controlling them (Thompson and Lally 2000). Smith (1995c) outlines the potential distortions induced by performance indicators by
drawing attention to the implicit management incentives of such
schemes (Table 18.1). Drawing on a wealth of literature, he concludes
that the almost universal finding is that performance indicators distort
behaviour in unintended ways.

Table 18.1   Unintended consequences of public sector performance indicator systems

Emphasis on phenomena quantified in the measurement scheme
Pursuit of narrow local objectives, rather than those of the organisation
Pursuit of short-term targets
Pursuit of strategies enhancing the measure rather than the associated objective
Deliberate manipulation of data
Drawing misleading inferences from raw performance data
Deliberate manipulation of behaviour to secure strategic advantage
Organisational paralysis due to rigid performance evaluation

Source: Adapted from Smith (1995c)

Conclusion

The recent exponential growth in external regulatory mechanisms
throughout western Europe has been occasioned by increased decentralisation and use of regulated markets in healthcare service delivery, with
greater emphasis on oversight methods of accountability (Power 1997;
Hood et al. 1998). Consistent with the growing influence of managerialism, since the early 1990s the European Union experience is of convergence between external peer review models, each moving towards
comprehensive standards for organisation, management and clinical

performance. Thus, accreditation systems are embracing ISO 9000 standards (Heaton 2000) and EFQM is being used as a framework within which the other models are incorporated (Moullin 2002). Notwithstanding such pressures of convergence, the shifting balance of formative and summative elements within these various approaches to external review remains. Indeed the recent UK experience suggests that the general international picture of convergence of techniques around the New Public Management agenda may be deceptive, as new variant approaches are continuously added to the mix in an attempt to avoid the unintended negative effects of the previous regimes.

In the context of performance indicators, the weight of evidence considered in this chapter suggests that their use in a summative way without adequate recourse to countervailing governance strategies is almost inevitably corrosive and corrupting. Such accounting systems place trust in systems rather than individuals, potentially undermining the conditions of trust required for quality improvement. A range of technical problems arise due to the precision of data required to make summative comparisons, and further negative unintended consequences follow due to the pressures on clinicians and managers to 'get good results'. Performance measurement may thus be considered a complex art rather than a science, requiring considerable sensitivity and sophistication.

Summary box

- Regulatory practices are dynamic over time and best considered within the context of shifting modes of governance. Cultural theory suggests that all governance systems will require additions to offset emerging negative unintended consequences in the previous 'blend'.
- The rise of external inspection from the 1980s onwards across western Europe is linked to the requirement for mechanisms capable of 'steering' the behaviour of semi-autonomous organisations from a distance. While New Labour's 'modernisation' project initially increased regulatory oversight, later reforms such as Payment by Results (PbR) and patient choice may be seen as a reaction against the excesses of oversight and 'target culture' and reintroduction of quasi-market incentives.
- Regulatory frameworks may be conceptualised in a simple matrix with two axes: the source of control (internal or external); and the nature of resultant action (summative or formative).
- While regulation can be either 'deterrence' or 'compliance' focused, real-world external regulatory systems typically contain elements of each in order to differentiate their response to regulate behaviour.
- The major approaches are: accreditation; inspection; performance management; external peer review.
- Use of performance indicators in performance management systems poses serious technical and conceptual difficulties. The former include aspects of availability and reliability; validity and confounding; and robustness, sensitivity and specificity. More fundamentally, they may displace informal assurance mechanisms.

Self-test exercises

1 Identify an indicator that others use to judge your work performance. In what ways has the existence of this indicator changed the way that you both *think* about and *do* your work? Identify the positive and negative consequences of these changes for you, your organisation and your professional group.
2 Think about the regulatory mechanisms (accreditation, inspection, performance management, peer review) to which you are subject. What is the relative balance between them and how has this changed over time?

References and further reading

Audit Commission (2000) *On Target: The Practice of Performance Indicators.* London: Audit Commission.

Audit Commission (2002) *A Healthy Outlook: Local Authority Overview and Scrutiny of Health.* London: Audit Commission.

Barnetson, B. and Cutright, M. (2000) Performance indicators as conceptual technologies. *Higher Education,* 40: 277–92.

Barnsley, J., Lemieux-Charles, L. and Baker, G.R. (1996) Selecting clinical outcome indicators for monitoring quality of care. *Healthcare Management Forum,* 9(1): 5–12.

Blumberg, M. (1986) Risk adjusting health care outcomes: A methodologic review. *Medical Care Review,* 43(2): 351–93.

Boland, T. and Fowler, A. (2000) A systems perspective of performance management in public sector organisations. *International Journal of Public Sector Management,* 13(5): 417–46.

Brown, R.B., McCartney, S. and Bell, L. (1995) Why the NHS should abandon the search for the universal outcome measure. *Health Care Analysis,* 3: 191–5.

Carter, N. (1989) Performance indicators: Backseat driving or hands off control? *Policy and Politics,* 17(2): 131–8.

Carter, N., Klein, R. and Day, P. (1992) *How Organizations Measure Success: The Use of Performance Indicators in Government.* London: Routledge.

Clarke, J. and Newman, J. (1997) *The Managerial State.* London: Sage.

Clarke, J., Gewirtz, S. and McLaughlin, E. (eds) (2000) *New Managerialism, New Welfare?* London: Sage.

Davenport, R.J., Dennis, M.S. and Warlow, C.P. (1996) Effect of correcting outcome data for case mix: An example from stroke medicine. *British Medical Journal,* 312: 1503–1505.

Davies, H.T.O. (1998) Performance management using health outcomes: In search of instrumentality. *Journal of Evaluation in Clinical Practice,* 4(4): 359–62.

Davies, H.T.O. and Lampel, J. (1998) Trust in performance indicators? *Quality in Health Care,* 7: 159–62.

Day, P. and Klein, R. (2002) Who nose best? *Health Services Journal,* 112(5799): 26–9.

Department of Health (DH, 1999) *National Service Framework for Mental Health Services: Modern Standards and Service Models.* London: The Stationery Office.

Department of Health (DH, 2000) *National Service Framework for Coronary Heart Disease: Modern Standards and Service Models.* London: The Stationery Office.

Department of Health (DH, 2001) *National Service Framework for Older People: Modern Standards and Service Models.* London: The Stationery Office.

Department of Health (DH, 2002) *Delivering the NHS Plan.* London: The Stationery Office.

Department of Health (DH, 2003) *National Service Framework for Diabetes: Modern Standards and Service Models.* London: The Stationery Office.

Department of Health (DH, 2005) *Creating a Patient-led NHS: Delivering the NHS Improvement Plan.* London: The Stationery Office.

Flynn, R. (2004) 'Soft bureaucracy', governmentality and clinical governance: Theoretical approaches to emerging policy. In A. Gray and S. Harrison (eds) *Governing Medicine: Theory and Practice.* Maidenhead: Open University Press.

Freeman, T. (2002) Using performance indicators to improve health care quality in the public sector: A review of the literature, *Health Services Management Research*, 15: 126–37.

Giuffrida, A. and Gravelle, H. (2001) Measuring performance in primary care: Econometric analysis and DEA. *Applied Economics*, 33(2): 163–75.

Giuffrida, A., Gravelle, H. and Roland, M. (1999) Measuring quality of care with routine data: Avoiding confusion between performance indicators and health outcomes, *British Medical Journal*, 319: 94–8.

Giuffrida, A., Gravelle, H. and Roland, M. (2000) Performance indicators for managing primary care: The confounding problem. In P. Smith (ed.) *Reforming Markets in Health Care: An Economic Perspective.* Buckingham: Open University Press.

Goddard, M., Mannion, R. and Smith, P. (2000) The performance framework: Taking account of economic behaviour. In P. Smith (ed.) *Reforming Markets in Health Care: An Economic Perspective.* Buckingham: Open University Pres.

Goldstein, H. and Spiegelhalter, D.J. (1996) League tables and their limitations: Statistical issues in comparisons of institutional performance. *Journal of the Royal Statistical Society*, A159: 385–443.

Gross, P.A., Braun, B., Kritchevsky, S.B. and Simmons, B.P. (2000) Comparison of clinical indicators for performance measurement of health care quality: A cautionary note. *British Journal of Clinical Governance.* 5(4): 202–11.

Hauck, K., Rice, N. and Smith, P. (2003) The influence of health care organisations on health system performance. *Journal of Health Services Research and Policy*, 8(2): 68–74.

Heaton, C. (2000) External peer review in Europe: An overview from the EXPeRT project. *International Journal for Quality in Health Care*, 12(3): 177–82.

Hepworth, N.P. (1988) Measuring performance in non-market organizations. *International Journal of Public Sector Management*, 1(1): 16–26.

Hoggett, P. (1996) New modes of control in the public service. *Public Administration*, 74: 9–32.

Hood, C. (1998) *The Art of the State: Culture, Rhetoric and Public Management.* Oxford: Clarendon Press.

Hood, C., James, O., Jones, G., Scott, C. and Travers, T. (1998) Regulation inside government: Where the new public management meets the audit explosion. *Public Money and Management*, 18(2): 61–8.

Hood, C., Scott, C., James, O., Jones, G. and Travers, T. (eds) (1999) *Regulation Inside Government: Waste Watchers, Quality Police and Sleaze Busters.* Oxford: Oxford University Press.

Jackson, A. (2001) An evaluation of evaluation: problems with performance measurement in small business loan and grant schemes. *Progress in Planning*, 55: 1–64.

Jacobs, K. and Manzi, T. (2000) Performance indicators and social constructivism: Conflict and control in housing management. *Critical Social Policy*, 20(1): 85–103.

Kazandjian, V.A., Thomson, R.G., Law, W.R. and Waldron, K. (1996) Do performance indicators make a difference? *Joint Commission Journal of Quality Improvement*, 22(7): 482–91.

Klazinga, N. (2000) Re-engineering trust: The adoption and adaption of four models for external quality assurance of health care services in western European health care systems. *International Journal for Quality in Health Care*, 12(3): 183–9.

Lee, S. and Woodward, R. (2002) Implementing the third way: The delivery of public services under the Blair government. *Public Money and Management*, 22(4): 49–56.

Lorence, D.P., Spink, A. and Jameson, R. (2002) Information in medical decision-making: How consistent is our management? *Medical Decision-Making*, 22(6): 514–21.

Lowry, S. (1988) Focus on performance indicators. *British Medical Journal*, 296: 992–4.

McColl, A., Gabbay, J. and Roderick, P. (1998) Improving health outcomes – a review of case studies from English health authorities. *Journal of Public Health Medicine*, 20(3): 302–11.

McColl, A., Roderick, P., Smith, H., Wilkinson, E., Moore, M., Exworthy, M. and Gabbay, J. (2000) Clinical governance in primary care groups: The feasibility of deriving evidence-based performance indicators. *Quality in Health Care*, 9: 90–97.

McGlynn, E.A. (1998) Choosing and evaluating clinical performance measures. *Joint Commission Journal on Quality Improvement*, 24(9): 470–479.

McKee, M. and James, P. (1997) Using routine data to evaluate quality of care in British hospitals. *Medical Care*, 35(10): OS102–OS111.

McLaughlin, V., Leatherman, S., Fletcher, M. and Wyn-Owen, J. (2001) Improving performance using indicators: Recent experiences in the Unites States, the United Kingdom, and Australia. *International Journal for Quality in Health Care*, 13(6): 455–62.

Mant, J. (1995) Detecting differences in quality of care: the sensitivity of measures of process and outcome in treating acute myocardial infarction. *British Medical Journal*, 311: 793–6.

Mant, J. and Hicks, N. (1996) Health status measurement and the assessment of medical care. *International Journal for Quality in Health Care*, 8(2): 107–109.

Mayntz, R. (1993) Governing failures and the problems of governability: Some comments on a theoretical paradigm. In J. Kooiman (ed.) *Modern Governance*. London: Sage.

Moullin, M. (2002) *Delivering Excellence in Health and Social Care*. Maidenhead: Open University Press.

Mulligan, J., Appleby, J. and Harrison, A. (2000) Measuring the performance of health systems: Indicators still fail to take socio-economic factors into account. *British Medical Journal*, 321: 191–2.

Newman, J. (2000) Beyond the new public management? Modernising public services. In J. Clarke, S. Gerwitz and E. McLaughlin (eds) *New Managerialism, New Welfare?* London: Sage.

NHS Executive (NHSE, 1999) *The NHS Performance Assessment Framework*. Wetherby: Department of Health.

Nutley, S. and Smith, P.C. (1998) League tables for performance improvement in health care. *Journal of Health Services Research and Policy*, 3(1): 50–57.

Osborne, D. and Gaebler, T. (1992) *Reinventing Government: How the Entrepreneurial Spirit is Transforming the Public Sector*. Reading, MA: Addison-Wesley.

Parry, G.J., Gould, C.R., McCabe, C.J. and Tarnow-Mordi, W.O. (1998) Annual league tables of mortality in neonatal intensive care units: Longitudinal study. *British Medical Journal*, 316: 1932–5.

Power, M. (1997) *The Audit Society: Rituals of Verification*. Oxford: Oxford University Press.

Rigby, K.A., Palfreyman, S. and Michaels, J.A. (2001) Performance indicators from routine hospital data: Death following aortic surgery as a potential measure of quality of care. *British Journal of Surgery*, 88: 964–8.

Rowland, H. (2003) Janus: The two faces of the Commission for Health Improvement. *Clinical Governance: An International Journal*, 8(1): 33–8.

Shaw, C.D. (2000) External quality mechanisms for health care: Summary of the ExPeRT Project on visitatie, accreditation, EFQM and ISO assessment in European Union countries. *International Journal for Quality in Health Care*, 12: 169–75.

Sheldon, T. (1998) Promoting health care quality: What role performance indicators? *Quality in Health Care*, 7: S45–S50.

Sitkin, S.B. and Roth, N.L. (1993) Explaining the limited effectiveness of legalistic 'remedies' for trust / distrust. *Organizational Science*, 4(3): 367–92.

Smith, P. (1990) The use of performance indicators in the public sector. *Journal of the Royal Statistical Society* A153(1): 53–72.

Smith, P. (1995a) Outcomes related performance indicators and organisational control in the public sector. In J. Holloway and G. Mallory (eds) *Performance Measurement and Evaluation*. London: Sage.

Smith, P. (1995b) Performance indicators and outcome in the public sector. *Public Money and Management*, 15(4): 13–16.

Smith, P. (1995c) The unintended consequences of publishing performance data in the public sector. *International Journal of Public Administration*, 18(2): 277–310.

Stewart, J. and Walsh, K. (1994) Performance measurement: When performance can never be finally defined. *Public Money and Management*, 14: 45–9.

Thompson, R.G. and Lally, J. (2000) Performance management at the crossroads in the NHS: Don't go into the red. *Quality in Health Care*, 9(1): 201–202.

Van Peursem, K.A., Pratt, M.J. and Lawrence, S.R. (1995) Health management performance: A review of measures and indicators, *Accounting, Auditing and Accountability Journal*, 8(5): 34–70.

Walshe, K. (2002) The rise of regulation in the NHS. *British Medical Journal*, 324: 967–70.

Websites and resources

Healthcare Commission. Provides an overview of the Commission's regulatory and external inspection programmes, as well as its annual report and forward plan. Also includes detail on performance ratings and 'star' rating systems: *http://www.healthcarecommission.org.uk/Homepage/fs/en*

International Organisation for Standardisation (ISO). Overview of the ISO approach, its systems and products, together with news and workshops: *http://www.iso.org/iso/en/ISOOnline.frontpage*

Investors In People. Provides an introduction to the IIP approach to accreditation in human resource development: *http://inverstorsinpeople.co.uk/IIP/Web/default.htm*

Joint Commission on Accreditation of Hospital Organisations (JCAHO). Provides access to detail on US hospital accreditation programmes: *http://www.jcaho.org*

Monitor. Provides access to annual reports, regulatory activity, and discussion documents concerning the role of a regulator in a quasi-market: *http://www.monitor-nhsft.gov.uk/index.php*

National Institute of Clinical Excellence (NICE). Provides an overview of the work of the institute: *http://www.nice.org.uk/page.aspx?o=*home

NHS Institute for Innovation and Improvement (NIII). Resources for learning and leadership, together with forward plan: *http://www.institute.nhs.uk*

Overview and Scrutiny Committees (OSCs). Overview of responsibilities, together with series of case studies: *http://www.dh.gov.uk/PolicyAndGuidance/HealthAndSocialCareTopics/BuildingQualityInSocialCare/fs/en*

Total Quality Management (TQM). Outline of the historical evolution of the approach, together with information on tools such as Statistical Process Control (SPC) and force-field analysis: *http://www.dti.gov.uk/quality/6i.htm*

Visitatie. Provides a comparative overview of expert peer review systems in the UK and Netherlands: *http://caspe.co.uk/expert/nl-uk.htm*

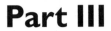

Part III
Management theories, models and techniques

19 Leadership and its development in healthcare

Edward Peck

Introduction

This chapter explores four themes around leadership:

- the main theories of leadership that have emerged over the last 50 years, drawing out the ongoing influence of each
- the ways in which these theories are reflected in specific policy documents on leadership in UK healthcare
- the components of one typical model for leadership development
- the evidence – such as it is – of the impact of leadership development in healthcare, both on individuals and on the system.

The chapter finishes with a summary of the key points. Before embarking on these more detailed discussions, however, I want to set the context by making four broader points about leadership.

First, the current interest in leadership in UK healthcare is relatively recent. Up until the late 1990s the word 'leadership' appeared infrequently in policy pronouncements in healthcare. In contrast, the concept now occupies a prominent position in most major documents issued, for example, by the English Department of Health. In this respect, the UK NHS is merely following a broader trend in the public sector, both nationally and internationally. Storey (2004a) charts the explosion in papers, programmes and projects dedicated to leadership in public services over the preceding ten years. Both Storey and myself (Davidson and Peck 2005) have mapped out the reasons why leadership has risen to such prominence. However, the very variety of challenges discussed in this book suggest why some form of organisational alchemy has been seen to be necessary (and leadership is often discussed in such florid language – see Rooke and Torbert 2005 for a discussion of leaders as alchemists). Nevertheless, fashions in management theory – and thus practice – ebb and flow (Abrahamson 1991, 1996) and the current focus on leadership may yet prove ephemeral. Already much of the discussion is turning to followership (for example, Daft 1999), and even non-followership (for instance, Prince 1998), and the connected notion of authenticity (for example, Alvolio et al. 2004; Illes et al. 2005). Furthermore, there is a whole school of writers who have always argued for the importance of fundamental organisational assumptions and arrangements (e.g. forms of accountability) rather than the impact of individuals (for instance, Giddens 1993). In response, some champions of leadership acknowledge that leaders may indeed experience constraints – but no more – on their influence (for example, Dubrin 2004). I have explored this debate elsewhere (Peck 2005b) and limitations of space prohibit further examination of this significant issue. There are also critiques of leadership texts that challenge their predominantly Anglo-American assumptions (e.g. Prince 2005); again, space precludes more investigation here.

Second, Storey also identifies some of the major problems with this enthusiasm for leadership: 'precise meanings are . . . usually under-specified . . . its value is simply asserted and its nature assumed . . . there is a tendency to assume and assert that leadership is the answer to a whole array of intractable problems' (2004a: 5). Collins (2001: 21) goes further: 'the "Leadership is the answer to everything" perspective is the modern equivalent of the "God is the answer to everything" perspective . . . in the Dark Ages'. We shall return to these problems of definition and attribution when we consider below the evidence on impact. This is not to suggest that there are no commentators who venture apparently helpful definitions of leadership. Based on his review of previous formulations, Bass (1990: 19) suggests:

> Leadership is an interaction between two or more members of a group that often involves a structuring or restructuring of the situation, perceptions and expectations of the members. Leaders are agents of change – persons whose acts affect other people more than other people's affect them. Leadership occurs when one group member modifies the motivation or competencies of others in the group . . . any member of the group can exhibit some amount of leadership and the members will vary in the extent to which they do so.

This definition draws out three themes that are important later in this chapter: leadership is enacted through relationships with others (who might be termed 'followers'); leadership – or at least the potential for leadership – is widely distributed throughout an organisation; and much writing on leadership has developed out of the authors' in-depth work with small groups rather than with large organisations.

Third, it is worth pondering for a moment the distinction between leadership and management, especially given that many of you reading this volume will have titles that refer to you as managers. Much of the literature seems to assume that leaders are butterflies whilst managers are caterpillars. It is proclaimed regularly that leaders are transformational and managers are transactional (Zaleznik 1992; Dubrin 2004); the former do the right thing whilst the latter merely do the thing right (Bennis 1994). The contrast between transformational and transactional approaches is summarised by one contemporary guru of public sector leadership – Alimo-Metcalfe – as follows:

> Leadership has experienced a major reinterpretation from represent-ing an authority relationship (now referred to as management or Transactional Leadership which may or may not involve some form of pushing or coercion) to a process of influencing followers or staff for whom one is responsible, by inspiring them, or pulling them towards the vision of some future state . . . this new model of leader-ship is referred to as Transformational Leadership because such individuals transform followers. (Alimo-Metcalfe 1998: 7)

Presented as a simple dichotomy, this distinction seems to me misguided (not to mention potentially intimidating to those of us who are being expected to make the alleged move from one to the other (see Fullan 2001). At the outset, therefore, I want to establish an alternative meta-phor: if artistic creation is 90% perspiration (for example, the under-standing of your materials) and 10% inspiration (Harrison 1979), then leadership in healthcare may be a similar mix of transaction (for example, the putting in place of performance review procedures) and transform-ation (for example, the creating of new meanings for colleagues). Fortu-nately, there are other commentators who share this more balanced view (e.g. Fullan 2001; Alvolio and Bass 2002).

The quotation from Alimo-Metcalfe takes me to my fourth and final broader point. Much as the theme is underplayed in many – especially contemporary – accounts, leadership has a lot to do with power (see Lukes 1974 for a seminal debate on three forms of power). When the concept of power appears at all in the recent literature, it is often viewed pejoratively (for example, in the reference to 'coercion' in the previous quotation). Ignoring the reality of power in discussions of leadership has at least two major dangers. On the one hand, it can render some analyses of leadership rather fanciful, not to say naive, apparently regarding the exercise of any hierarchical or professional authority as almost illegitim-ate. On the other hand, it can overlook the 'shadow side' of leadership, the abuses of authority that can take place under its banner (DeCelles and Pfarrer 2004). With these four points in mind, it is time to turn to a short history of leadership.

The evolution of leadership theory

The history of leadership has been told chronologically many times, perhaps most magisterially by Bass (1990), but also by the present author (Davidson and Peck 2005, and this chapter draws on that source), as well as thematically by Storey (2004b). I shall therefore compress this history, giving copious references for further reading, and focusing on those aspects of the various theories that still seem influential.

Great man and trait theories

Much of the early literature initially focused on the leadership of 'great men' (for instance, Woods 1913; Wiggam 1931). Examples tended to be military or political leaders and the predominant organisational forms were large, apparently requiring command and control. There was interest in establishing the inherent traits that might make these great men such great leaders (for example, Bernard 1926; Tead 1929). However, as the context for leadership research changed from these settings to other human systems (for instance, education) the prevalent leadership traits seemed to change. As a consequence, simple trait theory fell out of favour; for example, Stogdill (1948) concluded that both the person and the situation (see next paragraph) had to be considered in the emergence of leadership. Nonetheless, the residue of this theory – or maybe just the everyday perception that some individuals prominent in public life seem to exhibit extraordinary self-confidence or intelligence or whatever – still shape our view of leadership (and, therefore, it is still necessary, for contemporary writers to assert that 'leaders are made, not born' – see Rooke and Torbert 2005: 67). Thus, the search for the personality types of successful leaders still continues (e.g. Antonikas et al. 2004, who identifies emotional maturity, integrity, various forms of intelligence and task-relevant knowledge). Certainly in healthcare settings the great man approach seems alive and kicking, particularly amongst politicians (presumably because they see one regularly in the mirror); for example, it is evident in the New Labour proposal for management 'franchising' in healthcare, where a chief executive apparently successful in one organisation would be given responsibility for another that is perceived to be failing.

Personal-situational theories I

In contrast to trait theorists, the situational approach suggested that leadership styles have to be adopted as a response to the demands of a given situation; contextual factors thus determine who emerges as a leader. Initially these theorists argued that 'great men' were a product of the particular situation that required them to step forward (see Schneider 1937; Murphy 1941). At this stage it was still thought that some personality factors made a difference to who could emerge and, therefore, trait theory could not be completely dismissed. In time, this led to the evolution of personal-situational theories. These maintain that, in any given case of leadership, some aspects are due to the situation, some result from the person and yet others are consequent on the combination of the two (Bass 1960). This way of thinking established that there was a crucial relationship between context and leadership which was to prove increasingly influential and, indeed, still shapes many leadership development programmes delivered today.

Humanistic theories

After the 1939–1945 war, psychologists and social scientists brought a renewed energy to the search for an understanding of the causes of such events, including the ways in which they affected – and were affected by – leadership behaviours. These writers concluded that leadership was based on a number of factors which again put the individual centre stage: the interrelations between individuals (Likert 1961); individual motivation (Maslow 1954); the interdependence between individuals and organisations (Blake and Moulton 1965); and the fit between individual and organisational needs (McGregor 1966). These writers established the importance of the individual's psychological profile to leadership, and also the potential benefits of their examination. Perhaps the best known psychological inventory – the Myers Briggs Type Inventory – was initially put together by psychologists in the 1940s (Briggs Myers 2000); it is still widely used in leadership development programmes.

These writers also set the stage for the entrance of concepts which are also now commonplace in such programmes. For example, 'emotional intelligence' (EI; Salovey and Mayer 1990; Goleman 1996). George (2000) stresses the importance of four aspects of EI to leadership (the appraisal and expression of emotion, the use of emotion to enhance decision making, knowledge about emotions and the management of emotions). These theorists – with their stress on the importance of the personal resources of the individual – found their ideas very much back in favour when the solution to the problems of late twentieth century corporations was seen as lying in the capabilities of chief executives (Storey 2004a).

Personal-situational theorists II

During the same period, a number of accounts took forward the idea that the interaction between the person and the situation was of paramount importance. *Path–goal theory* (House 1971) suggested that successful leaders show their follower the rewards that are available and the paths (that is, the behaviours) through which these rewards may be obtained (and this seems to have resonance with the approach adopted by the Department of Health in England three decades later in the notion of 'earned autonomy' – see below). *Contingency theory* (Fiedler 1967) argued, rather simplistically, that leaders have a tendency towards either task-orientation or relation-oriented leadership. Later, Vroom and colleagues (Vroom and Yetton 1973; Vroom and Jago 1988) elaborated this theory. They postulated that three factors influence the choice of leadership style: the degree of structuring of the problem; the amount of information available; and the quality of decision required. Hersey and Blanchard (1988) added as an additional variable the readiness of followers to accept leadership. Whilst sharing the limitations of other theories in this tradition – for example, paying no regard to the constraints imposed on leaders by the pre-existing assumptions and arrangements of organisations (Giddens 1993) – the suggestion that leaders can identify certain factors which might shape their selection of leadership style has become important in leadership development.

Charismatic and transformational leadership

Before transformational leadership made its entrance onto the theoretical stage, it was preceded by charismatic leadership. In many respects, this signalled a return to the certainties of the great man era. Perhaps best seen as one, and only one, characteristic of transformational leaders – a necessary but not a sufficient condition – the charisma of chief executives was a cause for celebration in the 1980s (e.g. Peters and Waterman 1985) and a cause for concern 20 years later (Mangham 2004). Perhaps the most considered overview of this theory is provided by Bryman (1992). Although many writers (e.g. Bass 1990) have given sober accounts of the attributes of transformational leaders towards their followers – individualised consideration, intellectual stimulation, inspirational motivation and idealised influence (that is, providing a role model) – and these undoubtedly contain some wisdom, the concept has become tainted by the corporate scandals, primarily Enron, that Mangham (2004) discusses.

Nonetheless, this account can draw attention to two often overlooked aspects of leadership, both of which are highlighted by Grint (2005). First, the identity of a leader – charismatic or otherwise – is relational rather than individual: 'leadership is a function of a community not a result derived from an individual deemed to be objectively superhuman' (p.2). Second, leadership has to be embodied: 'leadership is essentially hybrid in nature – it comprises humans, clothes, adornments, technologies, cultures, rules and so on' (p.2). This dimension of leadership is central to the approach to leadership development that is introduced below.

Post-transformational leadership

Despite losing some of its currency in the private sector (and also being challenged by studies in the public sector, see Currie et al. 2005), transformational leadership continues to exercise significant influence in the NHS (for example, Bevan 2005). Nonetheless, there are also signs of some new trends emerging. These seem to suggest a number of directions that have not yet coalesced into a 'school' (which is presumably why Storey 2004b gives them the name 'post-transformational'). The extent to which these will catch the imagination of politicians and policymakers is still unclear, so I will restrict myself to two examples.

The first is servant leadership (e.g. Greenleaf 1977; Boje and Dennehey 1999). At first sight, this seems at the opposite end of the spectrum to charismatic leadership, about as far as the pendulum could realistically swing. Boje and Dennehey (1999) make 'servant' an acronym where the letters stand for: Servant, Empowers, Recounter of stories, Visionary, Androgynous (that is, being able to speak in the voices of both genders), Networker and Team Builder. However, as Clegg et al. (2005) point out, rather than representing a radical departure, this account has much in common with its forebears. For instance, the Transformational Leadership Questionnaire – another example of a feedback instrument for putative leaders which may enable them to learn from their followers – was developed following an investigation into leadership styles across the public and private sectors in the UK (Alimo-Metcalfe 1998). The framework contains 3 dimensions with 14 scales and is shown in Figure 19.1. The points of overlap with the acronym of Boje and Dennehey (1999) are clear. However, it could be argued that this checklist starts to appear overly aspirational, not to say fanciful, in its description of the characteristics that we would like to see in our perfect leader (and perhaps in ourselves). This tendency is no doubt influenced by its origins in a survey – albeit very extensive – of employees. Perhaps we are also seeing here the development of a 'great woman' theory of leadership (see Alimo-Metcalfe and Alban Metcalfe 2003).

The second is leadership as sense-making (Fullan 2001), building on the earlier work of writers such as Brown and Duguid (2000) on organisational learning, Stacey (2000) on chaos and complexity theory and Goleman (1996) on emotional intelligence. He identifies five independent but mutually reinforcing components of effective leadership: moral purpose; understanding the change process; relationship building; knowledge creation and sharing; and coherence making (and there are obvious links here to the seminal work of Weick 1995 on sense-making in organisations; see also Peck 2005a; Pye 2005, who explores in depth the idea of leading as sense-making).

Given all of these sources to draw upon, how have policymakers conceptualised leadership? In the next section, I want to look at a few of the leadership frameworks developed for use in UK healthcare in the early twenty-first century.

Leading and developing others
- Showing genuine concern
- Enabling
- Being accessible
- Encouraging change

Personal qualities
- Being honest and consistent
- Acting with integrity
- Being decisive
- Inspiring others
- Resolving complex problems

Leading the organisation
- Networking and achieving
- Focusing effort
- Building shared vision
- Supporting a developmental culture
- Facilitating change sensitively

Figure 19.1   Transformational leadership questionnaire.

Conceptual frameworks for leadership in healthcare

In the early years of the twenty-first century, there has been a flurry of frameworks for leadership in UK healthcare (e.g. DH 2001, Scottish

Executive 2004). For reasons of space, I want to focus here on the first: the NHS Leadership Qualities Framework (DH 2001). This is reproduced in Figure 19.2. Initially aimed at NHS chief executives and subsequently adapted to cover other roles, it consisted of three dimensions and 15 scales; its influence can be clearly seen in its successors. Its own origins lay in a comparison of existing frameworks used in the UK and US health sectors and also from existing models in commerce and industry. It can thus be seen as being both timeless and very much of its time.

What do I mean by this apparent paradox? The timeless aspect can be seen in the importance given to personal qualities; arguably, this is trait theory reinvented for the twenty-first century. A later derivative of the framework argued: 'the scale and complexity of the change agenda and the level of accountability mean that NHS leaders need to draw deeply on their personal qualities' (Modernisation Agency 2003: 4). These personal qualities seem largely to derive from notions articulated by advocates of *emotional intelligence* (e.g. Goleman 1998). Furthermore, the emphasis on delivery seems to echo *path–goal theory* (House 1971) whilst its aspirational language appears to draw upon ideas from *transformational leadership* (e.g. Alimo–Metcalfe 1998). In many respects, therefore, this framework – and its successors – is a bold attempt to apply 50 years of leadership theory to the challenges of contemporary healthcare reform. Possession of this portfolio of characteristics would undoubtedly assist good managers to be more effective leaders.

So why, then, is it very much of its time? For me, the foreword to a later document from the Scottish Executive (2005) captures the moment: 'Leadership is not a peripheral issue; it is central to improving performance, redesigning services and securing better delivery' (p.1). Investment in leadership is thus an intervention in healthcare that will support the reform agenda of government. In these circumstances, as I have argued at greater length elsewhere (Peck and 6 2006), good leadership starts to look suspiciously like smart followership. This trend is perhaps particularly apparent in the notion of 'earned autonomy' (which has been extensively critiqued, by, for example, Wall 2004). Furthermore, this emphasis on followership seems to be manifest in the apparent aspiration of the Modernisation Agency (2005) for so-called Improvement Leaders to become more adept at encouraging peers to adopt innovations initiated in other organisations. Finally, Grint (2005: 31) suggests that if leadership is too

Setting direction	Personal qualities	Delivering the service
• Seizing the future	• Self-belief	• Leading change through people
• Intellectual flexibility	• Self-awareness	
• Broad scanning	• Self-management	• Holding to account
• Political astuteness	• Drive for improvement	• Empowering others
• Drive for results	• Personal integrity	• Effective and strategic influencing
		• Collaborative working

Figure 19.2   The NHS leadership qualities framework
Source: Department of Health (2001)

focused on achieving targets then 'we should not be surprised to find hospitals . . . manipulating their activities to generate the requisite results even if the overall performance . . . plummets'.

A model of leadership development

I want briefly to describe the model that Deborah Davidson and I have developed over recent years (and one programme based on this approach is described in Davidson et al. 2002). The 'repertoire' model is based on the idea that the key characteristic of good leaders is their ability to adjust their behaviours to the context in which they are operating in order to deliver an effective outcome (see also Davidson and Peck 2005).

At first sight, this notion of 'repertoire' might seem like little more than a resurrection of *situational leadership* (Bass 1960), suggesting that divergent situations demand different styles of leadership. This should not be a surprise; any leadership development programme ought to have its roots firmly planted in established theory. At the same time, this concept of 'repertoire' leadership has a more extensive range of 'dimensions'. These can be summarised under three headings:

* *Intellectual* – the range of theories and concepts available to the leader.
* *Psychological* – the depth of understanding that the leader has of her or his responses and relationships with others.
* *Performative* – the breadth of behaviours that the leader can call upon to enact leadership in the system.

In addition to these three 'dimensions' of repertoire, there are three related 'mechanisms' through which repertoire can be exercised:

* Use of *multiple aspects of the self* which are brought to the fore by different demands and situations (and where the challenge of leadership is to select the aspect of self that will have the most impact) in contrast to the reliance on the so-called essential self.
* Use of *emotional intelligence*, of being sensitive to the needs and responses of oneself and others as a way of linking performance to integrity and credibility.
* Use of the *physical enactment* of the performance, that is, body language, dress, speech, text, symbols, etc.

As with many other leadership programmes (see below), these dimensions and mechanisms are nurtured through a combination of: seminars and directed reading around theories and frameworks or organisational development (see Chapter 20); action learning, coaching and mentoring (see Chapter 21); work-based projects; and explorations of personal and presentational styles.

To date I have focused on the prescriptive parts of the literature; that is, the broad theories, the specific frameworks and one development programme. These tell us what leadership in healthcare ought to be like, albeit that these prescriptions are not all mutually consistent. However, they do not reveal the impact of attempts to develop leadership in UK healthcare that follow from these prescriptions. For such insight, we have to turn to the research evidence.

Evidence on leadership development in healthcare

A literature search looking for papers published since 1997 deploying the words 'leadership', 'healthcare', 'UK' and 'development' produced reports of six separate studies published in peer-review or professional journals. The key characteristics of these leadership development programmes and the central findings arising from their evaluation are summarised in Table 19.1. Broadly speaking, the nature and length of the interventions are similar both with each other and also with the programme described in the previous section, with two clear outliers in approaches lasting only 3 days and 75 minutes. Further, the evaluative approaches are generally consistent, focusing on pre- and post-programme questionnaires from participants and their colleagues. It would appear that a consensus has emerged, therefore, over the past decade about the most appropriate methods for developing leadership and for assessing the impact of such development. Let us reflect for a moment on the design and delivery issues that arise from these studies.

A number of important assumptions seem to underpin most of these programmes. The obvious one is that leadership can be developed through structured interventions. Indeed, a review (Williams 2004) commissioned by the erstwhile NHS Leadership Centre of literature derived from a number of sectors concluded that: 'leadership development for professional groups can be effective in driving organisations forward . . . [it] does however need to be the appropriate kind, to be both work-based and programme-based, and to take into account organisational culture' (p. 4). The second is that leadership is best seen as distributed throughout organisations. As Cooper (2003) notes: 'the government . . . hopes to create visionary leaders at all levels' (p. 33) and programme participants range from junior nurses to board members. The third is that developing leadership is a small-group activity to be undertaken at a distance from the system in which it will be exercised, albeit linked to some form of work-connected project. Both of these last two assumptions seem to reflect the influence of Bass (1990) that was noted earlier. A fourth is that clinicians and managers can make a significant – indeed a transformational – difference to organisations based on the enhancement of their individual knowledge and skills alone. As has been suggested above, this may be an overly optimistic view and a study by Stordeur et al. (2000) provides evidence from healthcare that 'structure and culture are major determinants of leadership styles' (p. 40). Fifth – and finally – these programmes (as well as the review by Williams) seem to assume that the notion of leadership is unproblematic. Interestingly, this is not the view of the more senior participants involved in the studies by Edmonstone and Western (2002) or that emerges from the review of leadership development in UK companies undertaken by Alimo-Metcalfe and Lawler (2001).

There are methodological problems shared by all of these studies. Leaving to one side concerns about programme facilitators in some cases also being programme evaluators and the small size of many of the samples, there are three major weaknesses: the absence of comparison (i.e. the lack of any studies that compare programmes with contrasting process and content leading to the suspicion that any competent intervention focused on the personal development of a small group of selected individuals would be viewed positively by participants); the typically short length of the follow-up regarding perceived individual and organisational impact; and the routine lack of any quantitative data derived from measures of organisational performance that supports any claims about benefits for organisations. Morgan (2005) is the most marked exception here in linking the programme to reduced staff turnover amongst the target group albeit without any discussion of the problem of attribution identified by Edmonstone and Western (2003). Nonetheless, we do seem to be a little further on than Goodwin's (2000) reflection that 'evaluations of current NHS leadership programmes are at best, anecdotal;' (p. 399). best, anecdotal' (p. 399).

Conclusion

It would seem churlish to conclude other than that the programmes discussed in Table 19.1 supported the personal development of their participants. Whether they contributed to the creation of a cadre of distributed leaders who can transform the NHS through the power of their enhanced ideas is much more debateable. In this respect, the NHS may be consistent with the UK private sector. Alimo-Metcalfe and Lawler (2001) conclude that 'although leadership development may assist individuals in their self-development, their impact on organisations is, at best, inconclusive' (p. 402).

Overall, then, the recent focus on leadership in healthcare may be producing managers and clinicians who are much more adept at handling the everyday transactions of organisational life. The positive impact of this focus should not, therefore, be underestimated, even if it often falls short of the transformational aspirations of many contemporary leadership games

Table 19.1 Summary of studies of leadership development in the NHS since 1997

Programme name (reference) Role of evaluator in programme	Interventions	Intensity/duration	Sample site of participants and length of follow-up	Methodology	Impact
1) Leading an empowered organisation (Cooper 2003) None	• Teaching sessions and group work	3 days	15 6 months	• Pre- and post-programme leadership skills questionnaire completed by participants • Interviews with and pre- and post-programme questionnaires from members of participants' teams	• Statistically significant improvement reported by participants in: – articulating goals – maintaining organisational objectives – exhibiting trust – getting outside support • 'No overall improvement in team members' ratings of their leader' (p.35) although improvement perceived in: – maintaining organisational objectives – presenting them with challenging opportunities
2) Advanced Life Support Programme Leadership Module (Cooper 2001) Author was trainer	• Lectures, videos and discussion groups	75 minutes	68 Immediate	• Randomised control trial • Observation of participants' facilitation of group scenario before and after leadership training session for experimental group • Pre- and post-programme questionnaires for participants and staff	• 'There was a generalised improvement in leadership performance for both control and experimental groups' (p.37), although 'more work is required to evaluate the degree to which this improvement is transferred to practice' (p.38). • 'In summary, 76% of leaders rated themselves as more effective overall; 63% of the followers rated their leaders as being more effective overall' (p.36).
3) RCN Clinical Leadership Development Programme (Cunningham and Kitson 2000a, 2000b) Lead author was 'expert' facilitator on programme	• Personal Development Plan • Action Learning • Teaching Sessions • Mentorship • Observation of participants' work environments • Use of patient narratives	18 months	27 Immediate		• Five themes emerged: – learning how to manage self – building, developing and managing team relationships – patient focus – networking – political awareness • 'Results show a significant improvement in the organisation of care in eight out of 24 wards as judged by ward leaders, and ten wards as judged by ward staff' (p.39).

Table 19.1 continued

Programme name (reference) Role of evaluator in programme	Interventions	Intensity/duration	Sample site of participants and length of follow-up	Methodology	Impact
4) Trent Leadership Development Programme (Edmonstone and Western 2002) None	• Action learning • Mentoring • Learning network	2 years	Just under 200 who underwent programme Immediate	All participants received questionnaire following programme (but no information on response rate) and range of interviews with participants and 'sponsors' (i.e. line managers) over three cohorts	• Seven themes emerged: – need for a common vision of leadership – design issues – making programme bespoke – promoting leadership development (i.e. ensuring participation of all professions) – creating more coherence between a number of leadership programmes – achieving a balance between tight client specification and provider flexibility to respond to participants – challenges arising from geographical dispersal of participants – differences in individual and organisational benefit' (p.46).
5) Northern and Yorkshire Board-level Development Programme (Edmonstone and Western 2002) None	• Development Centre • Personal Development Plan • Teaching Sessions • Action Learning	As above	As above	As above	As above
6) 'Grow its own' future leaders (Morgan 2005) Design and Delivery	• Teaching sessions • Personal Development Plan • Action Learning	One day a month for six months	Unclear Three months	Unclear but based around six-point pragmatic approach derived from Pawson and Tilley (1997)	• Met original objectives based around trust competency framework and: – increased participants' confidence – increased professional voice – increased organisational understanding – reduced turnover of junior sisters from 19.3% to 10%

Summary box

- Theories of leadership have a long and in some respects contested history.
- Despite this history, the importance of leadership has only come to prominence in healthcare relatively recently and has resulted in the UK in frameworks which draw selectively on those theories.
- In common with much of the recent literature, these frameworks tend to focus on the potential benefits of transformational leadership at the expense of consideration of the positive impact of transactional leadership where it is the combination of the two that may be most efficacious.
- At the same time, at least in England, effective leadership by local managers has, for some politicians and policymakers, come to be seen as identical with smart followership.
- Effective leadership development programmes may have to address simultaneously the intellectual, psychological and performative aspects of leadership.
- The evidence suggests that the programmes designed to enhance leadership do contribute to the personal development of their participants, but it is less certain whether they are creating a cadre of leaders who can transform the NHS through the power of their enhanced ideas.
- Many accounts of leadership can be accused of being too Anglo-American in their assumptions, too narrow in their focus on the influence of individuals on change rather than considering the impact of organisational assumptions (culture) and arrangements (structure) and too naive in their consideration of power (especially when leadership pursues goals that for much of society may be morally reprehensible).
- Finally, 'it may well be that one of the secrets of leadership is not a list of innate skills and competences, or how much charisma you have . . . but whether you have a capacity to learn from your followers' (Grint 2005: 105).

Self-test exercises

1 Identify three leaders who you admire, one who is a national figure (for example, a politician or sportsperson), another who is an important figure in your profession and a third who is a manager in your organisation. Then think about the intellectual, psychological and performative characteristics that they bring to their leadership and which prompt your admiration. How much do you already or could you in future adapt these characteristics into your own approach to leadership?

2 Reflect on a recent work experience where you can see that you possessed some followers (and were thus a leader). On a scale of 1 (I did not do this) to 10 (I could not have done more of this) analyse your approach to leadership on this occasion against the characteristics in Figure 19.2 (NHS Leadership Qualities Framework). For those items

where you rate yourself as 6 or below, think through what you could have done to have rated yourself 7 or above.

References and further reading

Abrahamson, E. (1991) Managerial fads and fashions: The diffusion and rejection of innovations. *Academy of Management Review*, 16(3): 586–612.

Abrahamson, E. (1996) Management fashion. *Academy of Management Review*, 21(1): 254–85.

Alimo-Metcalfe, B. (1998) *Effective Leadership*. London, Local Government Management Board.

Alimo-Metcalfe, B. and Alban Metcalfe, J. (2003) Gender and leadership – a masculine past, but a feminine future? *Proceedings of the BPS Annual Occupational Psychology Conference*, Brighton, 8–10 January, 67–70.

Alimo-Metcalfe, B. and Lawler, J. (2001) Leadership development in UK companies at the beginning of the twenty-first century: Lessons for the NHS? *Journal of Management in Medicine*, 15(5): 387–404.

Alvolio, B. and Bass, B. (eds) (2002) *Developing Potential across a Full Range of Leadership Styles: Cases on Transactional and Transformational Leadership*. Mahwah, NJ: Lawrence Erlbaum Associates.

Alvolio, B., Gardner, W., Walumbwa, F. and May, D. (2004) Unlocking the mask: A look at the process by which authentic leaders impact upon follower attitudes and behaviour. *Leadership Quarterly*, 15: 801–15.

Antonakis, J., Cianicolo, A.T. and Sternberg, R.J. (eds) (2004) *The Nature of Leadership*. London: Sage.

Bass, B. (1960) *Leadership, Psychology, and Organizational Behaviour*. New York: Harper.

Bass, B. (1990) *Bass and Stogdill's Handbook of Leadership Theory, Research and Managerial Applications*, 3rd edn. New York: Free Press.

Bennis, W. (1994) *On Becoming a Leader*. Reading, MA: Addison-Wesley.

Bernard, L. (1926) *An Introduction to Social Psychology*. New York: Holt.

Bevan, H. (2005) On reform from within. *Health Service Journal*, 1 September: 19.

Blake, R. and Moulton, J. (1965) A 9,9 approach for increasing organizational productivity. In M. Sherif (ed.) *Intergroup Relations and Leadership*. New York: Wiley.

Boje, D. and Dennehey, R. (1999) *Managing in a Post-modern World*. Dubuque, IA: Kendall-Hunt.

Briggs Myers, I. (2000) *Introduction to Type*, 6th edn. Oxford: Oxford Psychologists Press.

Brown, J. and Duguid, P. (2000) *The Social Life of Information*. Boston: Harvard Business School Press.

Bryman, A. (1992) *Charisma and Leadership in Organizations*. London: Sage.

Clegg, S., Kornberger, M. and Pitsis, T. (2005) *Managing and Organisations: An Introduction to Theory and Practice*. London: Sage.

Collins, J. (2001) *Good to Great: Why Some Companies Make the Leap and Others Don't*. London: Random House.

Cooper, S. (2001) Developing leaders for advanced life support: Evaluation of a training programme. *Resuscitation*, 49: 33–8.

Cooper, S. (2003) An evaluation of the Leading an Empowered Organisation Programme. *Nursing Standard*, 17(24): 33–9.

Cunningham, G. and Kitson, A. (2000a) An evaluation of the RCN Clinical Leadership Programme: Part 1. *Nursing Standard*, 15(12): 34–7.

Cunningham, G. and Kitson, A. (2000b) An evaluation of the RCN Clinical Leadership Programme: Part 2. *Nursing Standard*, 15(13): 34–40.

Currie, G., Boyett, I. and Suhomlinova, T. (2005) Transformational leadership in secondary schools in England: A panacea for organizational ills? *Public Administration*, 83(2): 265–96.

Daft, R. (1999) *Leadership: Theory and Practice*. Fort Worth, TX: Dryden Press.

Davidson, D. and Peck, E. (2005) Organisational development and the 'repertoire' of healthcare leaders. In E. Peck (ed.) *Organisational Development in Healthcare: Approaches, Innovations, Achievements*. Oxford: Radcliffe.

Davidson, D., Newbigging, K. and Peck, E. (2002) Leadership development: Reflections and learning on a two-year programme. *Mental Health Review*, 7(4): 10–14.

DeCelles, K. and Pfarrer, M. (2004) Heroes or villains?: Corruption and the charismatic leader. *Journal of Leadership and Organizational Studies*, 11(1): 67–77.

Department of Health (DH, 2001) *NHS Leadership Qualities Framework*. http:// www.nhsleadershipqualities.nhs.uk/

Dubrin, A. (2004) *Leadership: Research Findings, Practice and Skills*. New York: Houghton Mifflin.

Edmonstone, J. and Western, J. (2002) Leadership development in health care: What do we know? *Journal of Management in Medicine*, 16(1): 34–47.

Fiedler, F. (1967) *A Theory of Leadership Effectiveness*. New York: McGraw-Hill.

Fullan, M. (2001) *Leading in a Culture of Change*. San Francisco: Jossey-Bass.

George, J. (2000) Emotions and leadership: The role of emotional intelligence. *Human Relations*, 53(8): 1027–55.

Giddens, A. (1993) Structuration theory: Past, present and future. In C. Bryant and D. Jary (eds) *Giddens' Theory of Structuration*. London: Routledge.

Goleman, D. (1996) *Emotional Intelligence: Why It Can Matter More Than IQ*. London: Bloomsbury.

Goleman, D. (1998) *Working with Emotional Intelligence*. London: Bloomsbury.

Goodwin, N. (2000) The National Leadership Centre and the NHS Plan. *British Journal of Healthcare Management*, 6(9): 399–401.

Greenleaf, R. (1977) *Servant Leadership*. New York: Paulist Press.

Grint, K. (2005) *Leadership: Limits and Possibilities*. Basingstoke: Palgrave Macmillan.

Harrison, A. (1979) *Making and Thinking*. Brighton: Wheatsheaf.

Hersey, P. and Blanchard, K. (1988) *Management of Organisational Behaviour: Utilizing Human Resources*. Englewood Cliffs, NJ: Prentice-Hall.

House, R. (1971) A path–goal theory of leader effectiveness. *Administrative Science Quarterly*, 16: 321–38.

Illes, R., Morgeson, F. and Nahrgang, J. (2005) Authentic leadership and eudaemonic well-being: Understanding leader–follower outcomes. *Leadership Quarterly*, 16: 373–94.

Kotter, J. (1990) *A Force for Change: How Leadership Differs from Management*. New York: Free Press.

Likert, R. (1961) An emerging theory of organizations, leadership and management. In L. Petrullo and E. Bass (eds) *Leadership and Interpersonal Behaviour*. New York: Holt, Rinehart and Winston.

Lukes, S. (1974) *Power: A Radical View*. London: Macmillan.

McGregor, D. (1966) *Leadership and Motivation*. Cambridge, MA: MIT Press.

Mangham, I. (2004) Leadership and integrity. In J. Storey (ed.) *Leadership in Organisations: Key Issues and Trends*. Oxford: Routledge.

Maslow, A. (1954) *Motivation and Personality*. New York: Harper.

Modernisation Agency (2003) *NHS Leadership Qualities Framework*. London: Modernisation Agency.

Modernisation Agency (2005) *Improvement Leaders' Guides*. London: Modernisation Agency.

Morgan, C. (2005) Growing our own: A model for encouraging and nurturing aspiring leaders. *Nursing Management*, 11(9): 27–30.

Murphy, A. (1941) Social factors in child development. In T. Newcomb and E. Hartley (eds) *Readings in Social Psychology*. New York: Holt.

Pawson, R. and Tilley, N. (1997) *Realistic Evaluation*. London: Sage.

Peck, E. (2005a) Introduction. In E. Peck (ed.) *Organisational Development in Healthcare: Approaches, Innovations, Achievements*. Oxford: Radcliffe.

Peck, E. (2005b) Conclusion. In E. Peck (ed.) *Organisational Development in Healthcare: Approaches, Innovations, Achievements*. Oxford: Radcliffe.

Peck, E. and 6, P. (2006) *Beyond Delivery: Policy Implementation as Settlement and Sense-Making*. London: Palgrave Macmillan.

Peters, T. and Waterman, R. (1985) *In Search of Excellence*. New York: Harper and Row.

Prince, L. (1998) The neglected rules: On leadership and dissent. In A. Coulson (ed.) *Trust and Contracts: Relationships in Local Government, Health and Public Services*. Bristol: The Policy Press.

Prince, L. (2005) Eating the menu rather then the dinner: Tao and leadership. *Leadership*, 1(1): 105–26.

Pye, A. (2005) Leadership and organizing: Sensemaking in action. *Leadership*, 1(1): 31–50.

Rooke, D. and Torbert, W. (2005) Transformations of leadership. *Harvard Business Review*, April: 67–76.

Salovey, P. and Mayer, J. (1990) Emotional intelligence. *Imagination, Cognition and Personality*, 9(3): 185–211.

Schneider, J. (1937) The cultural situation as a condition for the achievement of fame. *American Sociology Review*, 2: 480–91.

Scottish Executive (2004) *Leadership Development Framework: For Discussion*. Edinburgh: Scottish Executive.

Scottish Executive (2005) *Delivery Through Leadership*. Edinburgh: Scottish Executive.

Senge, P. (1990) The leader's new work: Building learning organisations. *Sloan Management Review*, Fall: 7–23.

Stacey, R. (2000) *Strategic Management and Organizational Dynamics*, 3rd edn. London: Prentice-Hall.

Stogdill, R. (1948) Personal factors associated with leadership: A survey of the literature. *Journal of Psychology*, 25: 35–71.

Stordeur, S., Vandenberghe, C. and D'hoore, W. (2000) Leadership styles in hierarchical levels in nursing departments. *Nursing Research*, 49(1): 37–43.

Storey, J. (ed.) (2004) *Leadership in Organisations: Key Issues and Trends*, Oxford: Routledge.

Storey, J. (2004a) Signs of change: Damned rascals and beyond. In J. Storey (ed.) *Leadership in Organisations: Key issues and Trends*. Oxford: Routledge.

Storey, J. (2004b) Changing theories of leadership and leadership development. In J. Storey (ed.) *Leadership in Organisations: Key Issues and Trends*. Oxford: Routledge.

Tead, O. (1929) *Human Nature and Management*. New York: McGraw-Hill.

Vroom, V. and Jago, A. (1988) *The New Leadership: Managing Participation in Organisations*. Englewood Cliffs, NJ: Prentice-Hall.

Vroom, V. and Yetton, P. (1973) *Leadership and Decision-Making*. Pittsburgh, PA: University of Pittsburgh Press.

Wall, A. (2004) Is health service management a profession? In S. Pattison and R. Pill (eds) *Values in Professional Practice: Lessons for Health, Social Care and Other Professionals*. Oxford: Radcliffe.

Weick, K. (1995) *Sensemaking in Organizations*. London: Sage.

Wiggam, A. (1931) The biology of leadership. In H. Metcalf (ed.) *Business Leadership*. New York: Pitman.

Williams, S. (2004) *Evidence of the Contribution Leadership Development for Professional Groups Makes in Driving Organisations Forward*. Henley: Henley Management College.

Woods, F. (1913) *The Influence of Monarchs*. New York: Macmillan.

Zalzenik, A. (1992) Managers and leaders: Are they different? *Harvard Business Review*, March–April: 126–35.

Websites and resources

Art and Science of Leadership. Offers articles and links exploring numerous aspects of leadership: *www.nwlink.com/~donclark/leader/leader.html*

Businessballs. Free management and training templates, resources and tools: *www.businessballs.com/freeonlineresources.htm*

Cabinet Office Leadership Programme. CMPS courses, programmes and tailored training provided by the Cabinet Office's Corporate Development Group (CDG) cover the skills and knowledge that public servants need to meet the challenges of improving delivery in the twenty-first century: *www.cmps.gov.uk/*

Center for Health Leadership and Practice (CHLP). Provides health leadership development consultation and training: *www.cfhl.org/*

Council for Excellence in Management and Leadership. Appointed by Secretary of State for Education and Skills and the Secretary of State for Trade and Industry to develop a strategy to ensure that the UK has the managers and leaders of the future to match the best in the world: *http://www.managementandleadershipcouncil.org/*

Health Services Management Centre Quarterly Leadership and Management Bulletin. Latest news on issues and publications around leadership and links to other useful sites: *www.bham.ac.uk/hsmc*

Leadership through effective HR management. Good people management in the NHS is everybody's business – chief executives, board members and non executives, HR professionals and staff, general managers, doctors, nurses, allied health professionals, line managers and frontline staff: *www.hrmdev.com/*

Leadership Trust. Established in 1975 to enhance and develop managers' and directors' leadership skills: *www.leadership.co.uk*

Leader Values. Provides resources focused on leadership and value systems, innovation, complexity, and organizational change: *www.leader-values.com*

Managing and Organizations: An Introduction to Theory and Practice by Stewart Clegg, Martin Kornberger and Tyrone Pitsis. A portal from where you can connect the literature on management and organizations to that of leadership. The goal is to provide readers with information, resources, and interactive features that allow them to get what they want, just in time, updated, wherever they are: *www.ckmanagement.net*

National Leadership and Innovation Agency for Healthcare in Wales. Provides strategic support to NHS Wales in building leadership capacity and capability to secure continuous service improvement underpinned by technology, innovation, leading-edge thinking and best practice to deliver the service change agenda: *www.nliah.wales.nhs.uk*

NHS Institute for Innovation and Improvement. Focus on expertise in service transformation, technology and product innovation, leadership development and learning on a small number of big priorities at any one time: *www.institute.nhs.uk*

NHS leadership qualities framework. The framework is evidence based being grounded in research with 150 NHS chief executives and directors of all disciplines. The framework sets the standard for outstanding leadership in the NHS: *www.nhsleadershipqualities.nhs.uk/*

NHS Leaders. The NHS Leaders team at the NHS Institute for Innovation and Improvement provides supported personal development for leaders in the NHS: *www.nhsleaders.nhs.uk/brochure/brochurewareRUN.asp?url*=NHS%20 Leaders

Northern Ireland Office. Home page of the Department of Health and Social Services in Northern Ireland: *www.dhsspsni.gov.uk*

Scottish Executive. A range of resources linked to leadership in healthcare and public services more generally are accessible through this site: *www.scotland.gov.uk*

20 Organisational development and organisational design

Deborah Davidson and Edward Peck

Introduction

Across the world, governments are devoting increasing amounts of time and energy to the design and development of healthcare services – and the organisations that deliver them – so as to meet the demand of the public for improvements in access, choice and quality (Dixon and Mossialoss 2002). In the UK, where healthcare systems seem to be in a state of permanent 'structural revolution', New Labour's Performance and Innovation Unit has analysed these pressures (see Box 20.1); taken together they represent a challenging agenda which is broadly familiar across the developed world.

Box 20.1   Demands and new expectations on public services in the UK

- The increase in the size and complexity of service organisations.
- The demand for joined up inter-sectoral provision.
- The delivery of individualised services.
- The need to rapidly and continuously improve, innovate and learn.
- The need to be more outward looking, strategic and business focused.

Source: Adapted from performance and Innovation Unit (PIU, 2001: 3).

In the context of this heightened interest in organisational design and development, this chapter addresses three key questions:

1. How does the dominant model of organisations influence the ways in which they are designed and developed?
2. How can alternative understandings of organisations help to establish a richer palette from which to draw structures and processes for change?
3. What are the approaches in the literature on organisational design and development that might enable these understandings to be influential?

In so doing, the text summarises a number of arguments that are dealt with in much more depth in Peck (2005a).

The dominant model of organisations

From the early eighteenth century to the mid-twentieth century, most frameworks for understanding the world of work shared an increasingly strong belief in the power of reason, from the outset placing accounts of organisations in the broader context of social, political and scientific thought (in this case, broadly aligning with the so-called 'Enlightenment' – see Porter 2000). As Parker (2000) notes, within this school of thought 'the world is seen as a system, one that comes increasingly under human control as our knowledge increases . . . a rationalism that is unchallengeable and a faith that it is ultimately possible to communicate the results of enquiry to other rational beings' (p. 3). This dominant model – which might be seen as one aspect of modernism – gave life to the notion of the organisation as machine reflecting its origins in such social institutions as the church and the military. Subsequently, the model was refined by the routinisation of work following the Industrial Revolution, where it started to attract the attention of the initial generation of commentators specifically interested in organisational design. Two important points should be noted here: first, the trend towards descriptions of organisations that rely on metaphors derived from other areas of human intellectual endeavour was there from the start (and we return to the importance of metaphors below); second, to a large extent, the organisation in our mind remains rooted in this rational model such that other perspectives are frequently squeezed out.

The first famous contribution to the literature on organisations came from the German sociologist Max Weber (e.g. 1947) at the turn of the twentieth century, who developed the idea of the 'bureaucracy' as the ideal type of organisation (at least, it has been argued, for that particular time). He suggested that bureaucracies are goal-oriented organisations designed according to rational principles in order to achieve them efficiently (Coser 1977). This understanding of organisation emphasised precision, regularity and reliability. These characteristics were to be achieved through a specialised division of task, hierarchy of authority and impersonally applied explicit rules that stated duties, responsibilities and standard procedures.

Two more authors are very important to the growth of the dominant model. Scientific management theory is associated most with an American engineer, Frederick Taylor (e.g. 1967/1911), who believed that enormous gains would result from the substituting of 'rule-of-thumb' methods with more 'scientific' methods. He set about codifying the most efficient methods of working for specific tasks: 'the development of each man [could deliver] . . . his state of maximum efficiency, so that he may be able to do . . . the highest grade of work for which his natural abilities fit him' (1967/1911: 8). Apparently, productivity dramatically increased using such methods and the introduction of mass production lines into large-scale industries were significantly influenced by Taylor's ideas. Advocates of such techniques live on – suitably updated – in the writings of the gurus, for example, of business process *re-engineering*, where the idea of the organisation as a machine could scarcely be more prominent (e.g. Hammer and Champy 1995).

At about the same time, a French engineer – Henri Fayol (e.g. 1949) – began identifying the elements that seemed to make organisations successful. He became particularly interested in the exercise of authority and developed his famous five functions of management: plan, organise, command, coordinate and control (that is, inspect the output). He then went on to develop a set of 14 principles of management – classical management theory – that he argued were common to all effective organisations. These included: specialisation of input; unity of command; clear line of authority; coordination by managers. The links to Weber's and Taylor's ideas of command and control through hierarchy are obvious (and the key characteristics of a machine bureaucracy are summarised in Box 20.2). Fayol's principles live on in the popular texts of writers like Peter Drucker (e.g. 1954) and Charles Handy (e.g.1985).

Box 20.2   Summary characteristics of a machine bureaucracy

- Designed according to rational principles in order to attain goals efficiently.
- Emphasises precision, regularity and reliability.
- Specialised division of tasks.
- Hierarchy of authority with chain of command.
- Impersonally applied explicit rules that state duties, responsibilities and standard procedures.

It is hardly surprising that this dominant model is readily apparent in the design and development of healthcare (most branches of nursing, after all, have their origins in the convent and the army). To support this interpretation we can call on writers on the UK healthcare system in recent years who have highlighted:

- a highly developed focus on hierarchy, structure and rules (Attwood 1994)
- a command and control approach (Green 1995)
- a centralised unitary system (Laing 1994)
- a tiered, specialised approach to management tasks (Ham 1999).

The extent to which the organisation in our minds is a machine bureaucracy is illustrated by the report into neonatal surgery at the Bristol Royal Infirmary in the 1990s (Kennedy 2001). First, the features summarised in Box 20.2 are vividly represented in the all too familiar depiction of the management structure of the Bristol and Weston District Health Authority reproduced in the report (see Figure 20.1). Second, the apparent influence of the machine bureaucracy is discussed, albeit implicitly, in the report:

The fundamental political driving forces of the 1980s and 1990s

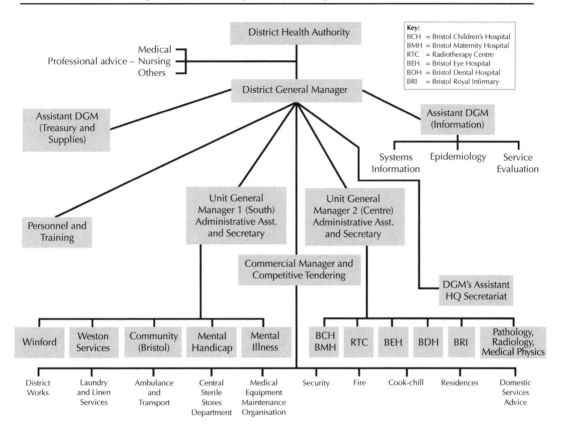

Figure 20.1   Example of NHS organisational design – management structure of the Bristol & Weston District Health Authority, May 1985
Source: Reproduced from the *Royal Bristol Infirmary Inquiry* (Kennedy 2001: 63).

were the desire to transform the economy to make it more efficient and competitive and to control (and if possible reduce) public spending . . . The NHS, as part of the public sector, attracted attention . . . because it was part of the public sector . . . The changes introduced, therefore, were the application to the NHS of a more general set of ideas . . . those of commerce, of output and throughput, of cost control and cost-efficiencies, of managerial rather than professional direction. (Kennedy 2001: 50–51)

Other writers have looked at the influence of machine bureaucracy on the way hospitals are managed more directly:

The 'machine bureaucracy' model often influences current thinking in hospitals. This assumes that all knowledge, responsibility, authority, and power is [sic] vested at the top of the organisation, from where it is delegated to lower levels. Leading therefore means controlling all processes and decisions. (Koeck 1998: 1268)

The argument suggests that there was a concerted attempt in the NHS in the late twentieth century to extend the prevalent notions of hierarchical command and control – already very familiar to nursing – to the medical profession (that is, to make the neat contours of the organisational chart in Figure 20.1 encompass the accountabilities of consultants). That this trend may have been sufficiently successful to contribute in some way to the tragic events in Bristol should give us pause for thought. It certainly contrasts with the view in much of the academic literature that senior doctors were largely able to resist the assertion of hierarchical control by NHS managers earlier in this period (e.g. Harrison et al. 1992). Indeed, there is a case for saying that, in the initial years of the twenty-first century, the approach has changed, at least in England, from one based on the assertion of national hierarchy – which broadly failed to bring these senior doctors into the chain of command – to the empowerment of local hierarchy equipped with the real or imagined incentives and threats of market pressures which may be able to succeed in so doing (on the basis that private hospitals have no problem in getting their doctors to conform to organisational norms and rules).

This is not to say that the dominant model went unchallenged on its own terms. Parallel strands of work arose which focused on cooperation between management and workers in order to achieve improved productivity and to provide better working conditions (Follett 1918) as well as on the relationship of individual motivations to the formal structures of organisations (Mayo 1922). Overall, these approaches combined the needs and interests of individuals working in organisations with the earlier concerns around productivity. Perhaps the best known example from the period are the Hawthorne Studies. These found that informal social relationships between workers in a group and between workers and their bosses were key factors in productivity gains: 'For responsibilities to be discharged, sentiments had to be engaged; the rationality of functions alone could not be relied on. Authority, similarly was insufficient in itself; it had to be buttressed by moral leadership that could produce cooperation and collaboration within organizations' (Clegg et al. 2005: 33).

Moving beyond the dominant model

More profoundly, however, from the mid–twentieth century onward, the ideas available for understanding the world of work broadened to embrace other fields of study such as, for example, philosophy, sociology and the so-called 'new science'. At their core, these ideas challenged the Enlightenment faith in the explanatory power of *rationality* and *reason*. We shall return to the link between this 'new science' and theories of organisational design and development later in this chapter.

Postmodernism

A slippery concept, originating in architecture and literary criticism, for present purposes postmodernism can be defined as the death of the grand narrative of society. For example, Lyotard (e.g. 1979) suggested that the dominant narrative of the modern era was that of Newtonian science which subordinated all other narratives. In contrast, postmodernism offers the idea that there are multiple and often competing narratives and accounts of reality. As a consequence, it rejects the search for one definitive truth which is central to modernism. Postmodernism also asserts that the world is both more complex and less controllable than modernism would have us believe. In the world of healthcare, the promotion of the importance of the voice of patients – through schemes in England such as the expert patient programme and patient choice – can be interpreted as a manifestation of postmodernism in action as the previously prevailing narrative of the medical profession is increasingly brought into question.

Social constructionism

This asserts that the world is constantly formed and reformed by our interactions with it. Given the wide variety of our emotions, experience and expertise, the world within which each of us lives is therefore unique. Thus, social constructionism argues (e.g. Berger and Luckman 1967) that all of our social institutions – including our organisations – are phenomena that come about as a consequence of the local conversations (in talk or in text) that take place between participants in these institutions. The meanings that we attribute to organisations are thus multiple (because each of us has our own), negotiated (because we seek to find common ground with others), contested (because finding such common ground can be difficult) and transient (because we are frequently discovering new meanings in these conversations and discarding old ones). Social constructionism holds that such conversations have the power to shape the culture of the organisation and thus the attitudes of its members to change.

Applying postmodernism and social constructionism

Clearly, these two ideas are mutually reinforcing, but how do they relate to understanding the design and development of organisations? Box 20.3 sets out the implications for ways in which management practice would change as a result of a rigorous application of such thinking. Two central tenets of current organisational theory – the acknowledgement of multiple accounts of reality and the recognition of the power of organisational narratives – derived from these two schools of thought feature strongly in the remainder of this chapter. They are each represented by a major contribution to the literature: the first by Gareth Morgan's *Images*

Box 20.3 Implications of postmodern and social constructionist thinking for management practice

Postmodern and social constructionist principles	Implications
Multiple and often competing narratives and accounts of reality	Recognise the legitimacy and influence of a number of disparate voices
Paradox and ambiguity are core elements of organisational culture	Respect the divergent interests and perspectives represented in organisations as valid
World is both more complex and less controllable	Acknowledge the uncertainty and unpredictability of the environment within which multiple perspectives interact
Narratives that emerge are constructed as a collective regulated system of statements. These statements are iterations of ideas, formed and reformed, as new conversations influence new ideas and produce new social practices. They both inform and are informed by the institutions within which they take place.	The problem of understanding organisations could be formulated as that of understanding which narratives constitute and come to constitute organisations, what effects they have, for what reasons and what resistances they incur.

of Organisations (1997), which looks at the metaphorical analysis of organisations, and the second by Karl Weick's *Sensemaking in Organizations* (1995), which explores the ways in which organisational members construct their understanding of the organisations in which they work. In the following two sections, we examine these two different – albeit interconnected – approaches to understanding organisational design and development.

Understanding organisational design and development through metaphors

In his seminal text, Morgan suggests that there is a danger in focusing on a certain way of thinking about organisations – for example, the 'machine bureaucracy' – as 'it tends to force others into the background' (1997: 4). He asserts that we need to read situations 'with *various* scenarios in mind' (1997: 3) until a more comprehensive view is formed. Morgan advocates we develop this more rounded understanding of organisations through using different metaphorical lenses. Morgan argues that all theories of organisation are based on implicit images or metaphors that lead us to see and understand organisations in distinctive yet partial ways. By using different metaphors to understand the complex and paradoxical character of organisational life, he suggests that we will be able to understand organisations in new ways. The importance of this argument is the insight that drawing on new or unfamiliar ways of understanding organisations can help us design and develop them differently from the ways that they have been designed and developed previously; that is, the use of metaphors can guide action and not just analysis.

In addition to understanding organisations as *machines*, Morgan offers readers seven other 'images' by which to understand organisations (and in so doing largely summarises the twentieth-century canon on the subject):

- *as organisms living in ecosystems* – focuses our attention on the interface between the human and technological aspects of the organisation, the importance of the environment and subsystems, adapting to the environment, different 'species' of organisation and their ability to 'evolve' and survive (Burns and Stalker 1961; Lawrence and Lorsch 1967).
- *as brains engaging in learning and self-organisation* – focuses our attention on the importance of information processing, cybernetics and learning to learn, learning organisations, holographic design and self-managed teams (e.g. Simon 1947).
- *as cultures creating social realities* – focuses our attention on culture and organisation, corporate and subcultures, creating shared organisational reality (see below).
- *as political systems reflecting interests, conflicts and power* – focuses our attention on systems of government, modes of political rule, systems of political activity, power and control (decision making, knowledge, information and technology, boundaries, coping with uncertainty, interpersonal alliances, gender relations), symbolism and the management of meaning (e.g. Pfeffer 1981).
- *as psychic prisons containing constraints of our own creation* – focuses our attention on the trap of favoured ways of thinking, the unconscious, repression, anxiety, transitional objects, shadows and archetypes (e.g. Obholzer and Roberts 1994)
- *as flux and transformation dealing with the unfolding logics of change* – focuses our attention on the nature of the relationship between organisations and their environments, chaos and complexity, mutual causality, dialectical change (how opposing forces can drive change; see below).
- *as instruments of domination possessing negative aspects* – focuses our attention on charismatic, traditional and rational-legal domination, the use and exploitation of employees, work hazards, occupational disease and industrial accidents, social and psychological stress, politics and the radicalised organisation (Weber 1978).

In essence, Morgan is providing an alternative method of approaching the tradition of organisational theory, presenting the key ideas as a series of lenses through which to consider the design and development of organisations. However, for Morgan there is no one grand narrative which contains the 'truth'; to a certain extent, therefore, he is an arche-typal postmodernist author (Box 20.4). Morgan has his critics (see Peck 2005b, for instance), but he has made the theories he considers accessible as well as practical.

Box 20.4   Summary of metaphorical analysis

- All theories of organisation are based on implicit images or metaphors that lead us to see and understand organisations in distinctive yet partial ways.
- Because metaphors can create powerful insights that can also become distortions, we can appreciate no single metaphor will ever give us a perfect all-purpose viewpoint.
- We need to read situations with various scenarios in mind until a more comprehensive view of the situation emerges.
- By using different metaphors to understand the complex and paradoxical character of organisational life, we are able to understand organisations in ways that we may not have thought possible before.
- Drawing on new or unfamiliar ways of understanding organisations can help us design organisations differently from the ways that they have been designed before.

Indeed, Elkind (1998) applied two of Morgan's metaphors and two of her own devising to the National Health Service and concluded that each illustrates different characteristics of the enterprise:

- 'the machine metaphor allows us to understand . . . the "single right answer" view of problem solving, which in turn underpins the structural approach repeatedly taken to organisational change' (p. 1723)
- 'the value of the idea of the NHS as an organism is its emphasis on need for the organisation to be responsive and adaptive to its environment' (p. 1724)
- 'the value of the image of religion is that it identifies the high aspir-ations, ideals and mission of the NHS and its positive role *contributing* to social cohesion' (p. 1723)
- 'the value of the metaphor of the market is that it emphasises the efficient use of NHS resources and acknowledges the role of *incentives* in developing innovative and quality services . . . it gives prominence to the role and needs of the consumer' (p. 1724).

Elkind agrees that every one of these metaphors inevitably has its limita-tions, but argues that by deploying them 'we have arrived at a reading that . . . captures the complex uniqueness of the NHS' (p. 1725). Almost ten years on, a reform agenda that still seeks to achieve a satisfactory compromise between centrally imposed structures, market mechanisms and professional commitments seems to demonstrate the longevity of these insights.

Understanding organisational design and development through sensemaking

If Morgan is our representative of postmodernism, Weick is our standard bearer for social constructionism. He provides an accessible introduction to the notion of sensemaking: 'Active agents construct sensible, sensable . . . events. They "structure the unknown" . . . How they construct what they construct, why, and with what effects are the central questions for people interested in sensemaking' (1995: 4). For Weick, 'sensemaking is about authoring as well as reading' (p.7); for him, it involves creation as much as discovery. Unlike Morgan's and his metaphors, however, Weick means us to accept sensemaking non-figuratively: 'sensemaking . . . may have an informal poetic flavor, that should not disguise the fact that is literally just what it says it is' (p.8). Box 20.5 summarises the seven distinguishing features of sensemaking discussed by Weick (1995). He describes the expression 'how can I know what I think until I see what I

Box 20.5   Weick's seven properties of sensemaking

1   It is grounded in the importance of sensemaking in the construction of the identity of the self (and of the organisation): 'Who I am as indicated by discovery of how and what I think.'

2   It is retrospective in its focus on sensemaking as rendering meaningful lived experience: 'To learn what I think, I look back over what I said earlier.'

3   It recognises that people produce at least part of the environment (e.g. the constraints and opportunities) within which they are sensemaking: 'I create the object to be seen and inspected when I say or do something.'

4   It stresses that sensemaking is a social process undertaken with others: 'What I say and single out and conclude are determined by who socialised me and how I was socialised, as well as by the audience I anticipate will audit the conclusions I reach.'

5   It argues that sensemaking is always ongoing in that it never starts and it never stops (even though events may be chopped out of this flow in order to be presented to others): 'My talking is spread across time, competes for attention with other ongoing projects, and is reflected on after it is finished, which means my interests may already have changed.'

6   It acknowledges that sensemaking is typically based on cues, where one simple and familiar item can initiate a process that encompasses a much broader range of meanings and implications: 'The "what" that I single out and embellish as the content of the thought is only a small proportion of the utterance that becomes salient because of context and personal dispositions.'

7   It is driven by plausibility rather than accuracy: 'I need to know enough about what I think to get on with my projects but no more, which means that sufficiency and plausibility take precedence over accuracy.'

Source: Derived from Weick (1995: 61–2), from Peck, E. (ed.), *Organisational Development in Healthcare: Approaches, Innovations, Achievements.* Oxford: Radcliffe Publishing, 2005. Reproduced with kind permission of the copyright holder.

say' as a 'recipe' through which each of these seven properties can be parsed (and the seven statements that result are in the quotation marks in the box). The importance of Weick's work to organisational design and development is that it emphasises the potential for changing the way in which organisational pasts, presents and futures are constructed by organisational members. In particular, he argues that 'occasions for sensemaking are themselves constructed' (p. 85) and may be particularly common where people reach a threshold of dissatisfaction that previous patterns of sensemaking are unable to reduce.

In the following two sections, we look in a little more details at two metaphors – lenses as we term them – through which sensemaking in and about organisations may be filtered. The first sees organisations as complex adaptive systems, often also informed by ideas from chaos theory. The second sees them as cultures. We are focusing on these two approaches both because they are becoming increasingly commonplace in the literature on management and the language of managers in healthcare (e.g. Plsek and Wilson 2001 on complexity; Peck et al. 2001 on culture) and also as they are typically presented as being in stark contrast to ideas based in the notion of the machine bureaucracy (see Sweeney 2005 for an example of this approach).

Understanding the design and development of organisations through the lens of complex adaptive systems and chaos theory

Included in Morgan's metaphor of flux and transformation – arguably rather unhelpfully – are ideas derived from scientific notions of complex adaptive systems and chaos theory. In most accounts (e.g. Sweeney 2005, on which this section draws), there are a number of important concepts adapted from these ideas that are then applied to organisations. Non-linearity is central and related to the key processes of sensitivity to initial conditions (often called receptive contexts) and self-organisation. Unpacking the title of this section, this framework suggests: a *system* – that is, the coming together of parts and their interaction – which is *complex* – that is, functions with a large number of elements interacting richly – and which can *adapt* – that is, the elements can co-evolve as a result of their interaction.

A non-linear effect occurs when the output is disproportionate to the input. Put another way, in a linear world a direct relationship between cause and effect is accepted and therefore a given action is assumed to have only one outcome. However, in non-linear relationships, it is assumed that any action can have many different outcomes and that more than one outcome is possible. Perhaps the most frequently referred to example is the butterfly effect where 'a butterfly flapping its wings over the Amazon leads to a hurricane on the other side of the world'. A receptive context is a prerequisite for organisations as complex adaptive systems if they are to self-organise. It assumes the ability of the agents in the system to interact through a set of shared values in order to sustain coherent behaviour. Self-organising behaviour refers to the tendency within complex systems for patterns of coherent behaviour to emerge from what initially appear to be random interactions.

In human systems, interactions predominantly occur through the conversations which the participants conduct with each other. Stacey (2001) has described the nature and importance of these interactions in human complex systems. In organisational terms, he argues, the ways in which participants in a system communicate, interact and co-evolve is crucial to the development of the system. One of the tasks of managers, therefore, is to create opportunities for organisational members to interact in novel and creative ways. In so doing, they will 'craft' strategy (and the links to Weick and his arguments around sensemaking are clear). This approach contrasts with the rational approach to strategy dominant in the machine paradigm. It has been characterised as distinction between the 'deliberate' approach to strategy and the 'emergent' approach (Mintzberg and van der Heyden 1999). Mintzberg, in common with many other commentators, has come to the view that the key skill of strategists is pattern recognition, their most important attributes are intuition and their most important contribution is the ability to recognise and respond to unexpected changes as they occur. On this account, managers cannot command and control and to think they ever could – as the machine bureaucracy suggests – is unrealistic.

Plsek (2000) has incorporated the principles of complex adaptive systems into what he calls a set of simple rules for healthcare systems. Plsek's rules are summarised in Box 20.6 and contrasted with the approaches that would be favoured by more linear, machine-orientated theorists. These rules make the connections between ideas derived from complex adaptive systems and the priorities of healthcare management very tangible indeed (they do so in a manner perhaps which could itself be criticised for being overly linear).

Understanding organisational design and development through the lens of culture

Culture constantly recurs in both theoretical and managerial discussions of organisational design and development. It is one of Morgan's metaphors and regularly appears in counterpoint to the structural focus of the 'machine bureaucracy'. Nonetheless, there is a distinct lack of consensus regarding the term 'culture' in the field of organisational studies. As Scott et al. (2003) point out, several scholars have contributed to the literature on organisational culture that has appeared since the late 1970s and many have introduced new frameworks. As they go on to comment: 'there has been little agreement between scholars over the years as to what the terms "organisation" and "culture" mean, how each can be observed and measured or in particular how different methodologies can

---

Box 20.6   Plsek's simple rules for the twenty-first century US healthcare system

Former linear approach	New complexity approach
• Healthcare based on episodic office visits	• Care based on continuous healing relationships
• Variability driven by professional autonomy	• Care customised according to patient needs and values
• Professional-centred care	• Patient-centred care
• Information located in medical record	• Knowledge is freely available and shared
• Decision making based predominantly on experience	• Evidence-based decision making
• Do no harm seen as individual's responsibility	• Safety an inherent feature of the system
• Secrecy is necessary	• Transparency is necessary
• System reacts to needs	• System anticipates needs
• Cost reduction is sought	• Waste is continuously diminished
• Preference given to professionals' roles over the system	• Co-operation and collaboration among professionals a priority for the system

Source: Adapted from Plsek (2000) by Sweeney (2005), by Peck, E. (ed.), *Organisational Development in Healthcare: Approaches, Innovations, Achievements*. Oxford: Radcliffe Publishing, 2005. Reproduced with kind permission of the copyright holder.

---

be used to inform both practical administration and organisational change' (p. 1).

Whilst a wide variety of conceptions of culture exist, Smircich (1983) suggests that two main perspectives have emerged. The first treats culture as a critical variable of organisation, in short a component part of a tangible entity. The second treats culture as a 'root' metaphor for organising, a lens through which to view organisational life (this is the Morgan approach). It is to a consideration of these two conceptions that we turn next.

The critical variable approach proposes a direct correlation between organisational culture and organisational performance. It suggested that by analysing and actively manipulating this critical variable improvements in quality and competitiveness can be achieved (Wilkins and Ouchi 1983). However, from their exhaustive study of the literature in healthcare, Scott et al. (2003) conclude that 'empirical studies . . . do not provide clear answers' (p.129) as to whether there is a link between organisational culture and organisational performance, whilst noting that the available research is small in quantity, mixed in quality and variable in methodology (thus making comparisons between studies difficult).

The most commonly cited writer in this tradition is, however, Schein (for example, 1985). Schein's theory specifies three layers: *cultural artefacts*;

espoused values; *basic assumptions*. Artefacts are the outermost layer and the most visible manifestations of culture, such as its rituals and rewards. The second layer, espoused values, refers to those values used to justify behaviour and constitute the grounds on which alternative courses of action are justified. At the core lie assumptions, that is, the unspoken and often unconscious beliefs and expectations shared by individuals.

Can we see these three layers within healthcare settings? A recent briefing from the Department of Health's Integrated Care Network (Peck and Crawford 2004: 5) suggests:

> The fundamental cultural divide between health and social care is frequently claimed to be exemplified in the contrast between the 'medical model' and the 'social model' . . . One cultural artefact of the 'medical model' is its emphasis on the rituals of diagnosis of the specific part of the individual patient that is perceived to be mal-functioning. This is underpinned by the espoused value of the pre-dominance of the clinician's opinion over that of patient. The underlying assumption is of the dependent nature of the patient in relation to the clinician. . . . This is often contrasted with the 'social model' prevalent in social care where one cultural artefact is an emphasis on an assessment of the individual client within their wider social environment. This is underpinned by the espoused value of the importance of a dialogue between practitioner and client. The underlying assumption is of the independent nature of the client in active negotiation with the practitioner.

This may appear to be something of a parody, but its importance lies in it being a recognisable parody. The popularity of Schein's framework may lie in its ability to represent aspects of organisational experience that managers and clinicians recognise.

Meyerson and Martin (1987) argue that Schein's account represents the 'integration' view of culture, where it is an influence which promotes cohesion within organisations. Cultural artefacts, including management styles, are seen as powerful symbolic means of communication which can be used to 'build organisational commitment, convey a philosophy of management, rationalize and legitimate activity, motivate personnel and facilitate socialisation' (Smircich 1983: 345).

Meyerson and Martin (1987; see also Peck et al. 2001; Peck and Crawford 2004) suggest two other views of culture – culture as differ-ence and culture as ambiguity – which to some extent undermine this integrative account. Parker (2000) reflects these contrasting dimensions in his two conclusions about the potential for managers to 'shape' cul-ture. The first is that 'cultural management in the sense of creating an enduring set of shared beliefs is impossible' (p. 228). On the other hand, he suggests that 'it seems perverse to argue that the "climate", "atmos-phere", "personality", or culture of an organisation cannot be con-sciously altered' (p. 229). So, a considered position might be that some manipulation of culture is possible, but the impact may be limited and/ or unpredictable.

Intervening in organisational design and development: the role of organisational development

So, finally, we arrive at organisational development (OD) as a structured intervention in the design and development or organisations. There are numerous lengthy texts on this subject (see Peck 2005a for an account of the history of OD). Unsurprisingly, definitions of OD vary from the very rational-scientific:

> 'A system-wide application of behavioural science knowledge to the planned development and reinforcement of organisational strategies, structures and processes for improving an organisation's effectiveness' (Cummings and Worley 2001: 1)

to those more sympathetic to ideas of culture and complexity:

> The overall goal of organisation development is not just enhanced organisational effectiveness and organisational health but, in addition, it aims for an organisation's culture and processes to change in order that it is continually reflexive and self-examining. (French et al. 2000)

Whichever definition is preferred, either the 'scientific knowledge' or the models for reflection, will be derived from the theories – or metaphors – that the organisation (or more likely its leaders) favour. At present, much OD is based around the three metaphors explored above, although others are also common (in particular, organisation as psychic prison). Perhaps, unsurprisingly, healthcare systems frequently utilise linear techniques to oversee the delivery of projects, especially where they are required to deliver against very tight deadlines. While Iles and Sutherland (2001) point out that traditional project management is useful in 'situations in which there is a defined beginning and end, and in which a discrete and identifiable set of sub-tasks must be completed' (p. 70), we can see from the section above on complexity that such linear processes may not be the most effective way in which to intervene in complex organisations. Instead, we need to look to a more iterative and sophisticated approach to plan development and change, all the time knowing that we cannot predict how it will turn out.

The 'OD cycle' is just such an iterative tool and acts as a 'map' to guide participants through a process of change whilst neither specifying the exact theories or interventions that should be used nor suggesting that the process will unfold in exactly the way that it is envisaged at the beginning. Underlying this tool is a belief in the fundamental importance of engaging organisational stakeholders' active participation so as to build ownership of and support for the innovations in practice that emerge. This cycle is summarised in Figure 20.2 which shows there are six phases to the OD cycle. While these phases are depicted as discrete stages, and the cycle as a whole process appears linear, experience of using it with complex and emergent processes of change prove that it is as applicable in

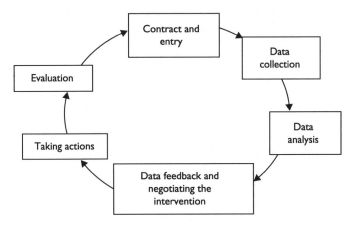

Figure 20.2   The OD cycle
Source: Adapted from Kolb and Frohmann (1970)

those situations as it is with more simple and predictable processes of change. They are described in more detail in Davidson and Peck (2005).

Conclusion

In tying the ideas of this chapter together, one device is to link the temporal component of this cycle to the notions of planned and emergent change. The cycle implies three stages of a strategic process: prospective (looking forward); real time; and reflection (looking back). Iles (2004) has conceptualised the contribution of emergence to organisational strategy in these three stages. As Sweeney (2005: 160) summarises her argument:

> Running a large organisation obliges managers to have a plan, that is, to identify a set of critical issues the organisation must address and to implement a programme to address those issues. There simply must be a prospective element to strategy and this is where a classic rational approach is best suited. But in real time, those managers need to be able to expect the unexpected, to adapt and evolve with circumstances as they emerge in sometimes unforeseen ways and to be sufficiently agile to respond to changes in circumstances.

In other words, one message from this chapter is: 'talk rationally about the future, think emergently about the present!' Looking back, of course, the only way to make sense of what happened in the process of the design and development of a change programme may be to compare the initial ambitions with the unpredicted (and perhaps unpredictable) elements and events that ultimately influenced the outcome.

Summary box

- The dominant model in the design and development of organisations – the organisation in our minds – is based on scientific rationalism and the metaphor of the machine.
- However, ideas derived from postmodernism and social constructionism are creating an environment where the dominance of any one model is unsustainable.
- As a consequence, there are number of other ways of looking at organisations which are increasingly seen as metaphors which illuminate distinct aspects of organisations.
- These metaphors can help the process of sensemaking through which organisational members both understand and shape their organisations.
- There are two other frameworks – organisations as complex adaptive systems and organisations as cultures – that are becoming common in discussions of organisational design and development.
- It is these ideas that inform – either overtly or covertly – the organisational development cycle which informs structured interventions in design and development.

Self-test exercises

1 *Understanding the organisation using metaphorical lenses.* Ask members of your team to pair up with another person and read one of the following chapters from Gareth Morgan's book *Images of Organizations* (1997):

- Organisations as Machines
- Organisations as Organisms
- Organisations as Brains
- Organisations as Cultures
- Organisations as Psychic Prisons
- Organisations as Political Systems.

Each pair will need to read and understand the chapter. At a team meeting ask the pairs to provide:

- an overview explanation of three of the core concepts that is provided by that image/metaphor (10 minutes)
- an example of the way in which they have seen this image exemplified in their service or organisation (5 minutes)
- the leadership style best suited to leading an organisation/service viewed in this way.

After each pair has presented their understanding, provide some time for the team to ask questions and discuss this understanding further. At the end of the explanations, get the team as a whole to discuss the strengths and limitations of the metaphors used in making sense of your service or organisation.

2 *Multiple accounts of reality.* Using a recent organisational event that involved staff, service delivery issue that involved staff and patients, or process of change that was announced, each person to write down (on their own):

- their account of that event – what happened – or of how they see the change needing to take place
- how they made sense of other people's behaviours and intents or of other people's responses to the announced change
- how they thought and felt about what happened
- the way in which this influences their approach to a similar situation.

Place three chairs in the middle of the room and the remaining chairs in the room in a circle around the three in the middle (goldfish bowl). Invite three team members to sit on the three chairs and have a dialogue about their different accounts of what happened. Ask the remaining team members (sitting on the outside to remain quiet but actively listen).

Taking opportunities to pause the conversation from time to time, ask the three members to remain quiet, and draw out the observations and thoughts of the other members of staff. Allow them to contribute without direction. You can run this exercise for as long as seems useful. It might be useful at the end to bring the whole team together to observe:

- the different ways in which people made sense of the same situation (without attributing a right or a wrong way)
- the rationale behind the sensemaking of each individual
- whether once the different accounts were contributed, a more integrated account emerged.

3 *Defining your context.* With other members of your team or service, take 30 minutes to explore the wider context within which your services are situated. Discuss whether any of the following factors affect your organisation now or will they in the future:

- active 'choice' of different clinical services by patients
- hospital or community services competing to attract patients to use their services
- use of the web to advertise and market services to patients, e.g. in relation to clinical outcomes
- focus on services where costs enable you to generate a surplus
- new public service business models, for example, hospitals taking over neighbouring providers (public or private), reducing hospital-based care and moving services into the community, shopfront networks developing in local retail sites

- other changes in response to political, social, economic or technological influences.

4 *Predicting the future.* How certain are you about what exists and what is
to come in two years, five years or 10 years:

- Can you predict how your organisation/you will change and adapt
  in relation to these future challenges?
- What methods and processes are/will be used to respond to change?

References and further reading

Attwood, M. (1994) *Developing Organisations Across Boundaries.* Briefing Paper 3.
Bristol: NHS Training Directorate.

Berger, P. and Luckman, T. (1967) *The Social Construction of Reality.* Harmondsworth: Penguin.

Burns, T. and Stalker, G. (1961) *The Management of Innovation.* London: Tavistock.

Clegg, S., Kornberger, M. and Pitsis, T. (2005) *Managing and Organizations: An
Introduction to Theory and Practice.* London: Sage.

Coser, L. A. (1977) *Masters of Sociological Thought: Ideas in Historical and Social
Context,* 2nd edn. New York: Harcourt Brace Jovanovich.

Cummings, T. and Worley, C. (2001) *Organization Development and Change.*
Cincinatti, OH: South-Western College Publishing.

Davidson, D. and Peck, E. (2005) The organisational cycle: Putting the
approaches into a cycle. In E. Peck (ed.) (2005) *Organisational Development in
Healthcare: Approaches, innovations, achievements.* Oxford, Radcliffe.

Dixon, A. and Mossialos, E. (eds) (2002) *Health Care Systems in Eight Countries:
Trends and Challenges.* The London School of Economics and Political Science:
European Observatory on Health Care Systems.

Drucker, P. (1954) *The Practice of Management.* New York: Harper and Row.

DuGay, P. (2000) *In Praise of Bureaucracy.* London: Sage

Elkind, A. (1998) Using metaphor to read the organisation of the NHS. *Social
Science and Medicine,* 47(11): 1715–27.

Fayol, H. (1949) *Industrial and General Administration.* London: Pitman.

Follett, M.P. (1918) *The New State: Group Organization, The Solution for Popular
Government.* New York: Longman, Green.

French, W., Bell, C. and Zawacki, R. (2000) *Organization Development and
Transformation.* Singapore: McGraw-Hill.

Green, D.G. (1995) *A Note of Dissent in UK Health and Healthcare Services:
Challenges and Policy Options.* London: Healthcare.

Ham, C. (1999) *Health Policy in Britain,* 4th edn. Basingstoke: Macmillan.

Hammer, M. and Champy, J. (1995) *Reengineering the Corporation: A Manifesto for
a Business Revolution.* London: Nicholas Brealey.

Handy, C. (1985) *Understanding Organizations,* 3rd edn. Harmondsworth: Penguin.

Hardacre, J. and Peck, E. (2005) What is organisational development? In E. Peck
(ed.) *Organisational Development in Healthcare: Approaches, Innovations, Achievements.* Oxford: Radcliffe.

Harrison, S., Hunter, D., Marnoch, G. and Pollitt, C. (1992) *Just Managing: Power
and culture in the National Health Service.* London: Macmillan.

Iles, V. (2004) *Developing Strategy in Complex Organisations*. London: NHS Confederation.

Iles, V. and Sutherland, K. (2001) *Organisational Change: A Review for Health Care Managers, Professionals and Researchers*. London: National Co-ordinating Centre for NHS Service Delivery and Organisation R&D.

Kennedy, I. (2001) *Learning from Bristol: The Report of the Public Inquiry into Children's Heart Surgery at the Bristol Royal Infirmary 1984–1995*. London: Public Record Office.

Kolb, D. and Frohmann, A. (1970) An organization development approach to consulting, *Sloan Management Review*, 12(1): 51–65.

Koeck, C. (1998) Time for organisational development in healthcare organisations: Improving quality for patients means changing the organisation. *British Medical Journal*, 317: 1267–8.

Laing, W. (1994) *Managing the NHS: Past, Present and Agenda for the Future*. London: Office of Health Economics.

Lawrence, P. and Lorsch, J. (1967) *Organization and Environment*. Cambridge, MA: Harvard Graduate School of Business Administration.

Lyotard, J.-F. (1979) *The Post Modern Condition: A Report on Knowledge*. Minneapolis: University of Minnesota Press.

Mayo, E. (1922) Industrial unrest and 'nervous breakdowns', *Industrial Australian and Mining Standard*, 63–4.

Meyerson, D. and Martin, J. (1987) Cultural change: An integration of three different views. *Journal of Management Studies*, 24(6): 623–43.

Mintzberg, H. and van der Heyden, L. (1999) Drawing how companies really work. *Harvard Business Review*, September–October.

Morgan, G. (1997) *Images of Organizations*. London: Sage.

Obholzer, A. and Roberts, V.Z. (eds) (1994) *The Unconscious At Work: Individual and Organisational Stress in the Human Services*. London: Routledge.

Parker, M. (1992) Post-modern organizations or post-modern organization theory? *Organization Studies*, 13(1): 1–17.

Parker, M. (2000) *Organisational Culture and Identity*. London: Sage.

Peck, (ed.) (2005a) *Organisational Development in Healthcare: Approaches, Innovations, Achievements*. Oxford: Radcliffe.

Peck (2005b) Conclusion. In E. Peck (ed.) *Organisational Development in Healthcare: Approaches, Innovations, Achievements*. Oxford: Radcliffe.

Peck, E. and Crawford, A. (2004) *Culture in Partnerships: What Do We Mean By It and What Can We Do About It?* London: Integrated Care Network.

Peck, E., Towell, D. and Gulliver, P. (2001) The meanings of culture in health and social care: A study of the combined trust in Somerset. *Journal of Interprofessional Care*, 15(4): 319–27.

Performance and Innovation Unit (PIU, 2001) *Strengthening Leadership in the Public Sector*. London: The Cabinet Office.

Pfeffer, J. (1981) *Power in Organizations*. Marshfield, MA: Pitman.

Plsek, P. (2000) *Crossing the Quality Chasm: A New Health System for the 21st Century*. Washington, DC: National Academy Press.

Plsek, P. and Wilson, T. (2001) Complexity, leadership and management in healthcare organisations. *British Medical Journal*, 323: 746–9.

Porter, R. (2000) *Enlightenment: Britain and the Creation of the Modern World*. London: Allen Lane.

Schein, E. (1985) *Organizational Culture and Leadership*. San Francisco: Bass.

Scott, T., Mannion, R., Davies, H. and Marshall, M. (2003) *Healthcare Performance and Organisational Culture*. Oxford: Radcliffe.

Simon, H. (1947) *Administrative Behaviour*. New York: Macmillan.

Smircich, L. (1983) Concepts of culture and organizational analysis. *Administrative Science Quarterly*, 28: 339–58.

Stacey, R. (2001) *Complex Responsive Processes in Organisations*. London: Routledge.

Sweeney, K. (2005) Emergence, complexity and organisation development. In E. Peck (ed.) *Organisational Development in Healthcare: Approaches, Innovations, Achievements*. Oxford: Radcliffe.

Taylor, F. (1967/1911) *The Principles of Scientific Management*. New York: Harper Brothers.

Weber, M. (1947) *The Theory of Social and Economic Organisation*. Oxford: Oxford University Press.

Weber, M. (1978) *Economy and Society: An Outline of Interpretative Sociology*. Berkeley: University of California Press.

Weick, K.E. (1995) *Sensemaking in Organizations*. London: Sage.

Weick, K.E. (2001) *Making Sense of the Organization*. Oxford: Blackwell

Weick, K.E. and Sutcliffe, K.M. (2001) *Managing the Unexpected: Assuring High Performance in an Age of Complexity*. San Francisco, CA: Jossey-Bass.

Wilkins, L. and Ouchi, W. (1983) Efficient cultures: Exploring the relationship between culture and organisational performance. *Administrative Science Quarterly*, 28: 468–81.

Websites and resources

Bureaucracy. Paul du Gay, Professor of Sociology and Organization Studies and Co-Director of the Centre for Citizenship, Identities and Governance and the Open University is one of the few academics that continues to support the notion of bureaucracy: (*http://www.open.ac.uk/socialsciences/staff/pdugay/info.html*)

Change and Innovation. Helps staff in Scotland develop new solutions by providing information about best practice in healthcare and encouraging innovative, flexible working to improve patient care: *http://www.cci.scot.nhs.uk/*

Complexity and Management Centre. Set up to create links between academic work and organisational practice using a complexity perspective, in which the inevitable paradoxes and ambiguities of organisational life are not finally resolved but held in creative tension. This perspective draws on insights into evolutionary theory emerging in the natural sciences, strands of social constructionist thought in the social sciences and various psychological understandings of the dynamics at work in networks of human relationship. The Complexity and Management Centre seeks new ways of working with these ideas, emphasising the self-organising potential of ordinary conversation in which people reflect together on their personal experiences. There are a number of useful working papers available on request from: *http://www.herts.ac.uk/business/centres/cmc/*

Directed Creativity Involves using specific techniques to perceive things freshly, break free of the current patterns stored in memory, make novel associations among concepts stored in memory, and use judgement to develop rather than reject new ideas: *http://www.directedcreativity.com/pages/CycleFrameset.html*

Improvement Leaders Guides. These improvement guides provide a summary of current thinking and practical advice and tips for improving patient care and experience: *http://www.institute.nhs.uk/improvementguides/default.htm*

Institute for Healthcare Improvement (IHI). US not-for-profit organisation, driving the improvement of health by advancing the quality and value of healthcare: *http://www.ihi.org/ihi*

Karl Weick and sense making. See Michigan Ross School of Business. There are series of papers on leadership and change, including one Karl Weick called 'Leadership When Events Don't Play by the Rules': *http://www.bus.umich.edu/FacultyResearch/Research/TryingTimes/Rules.htm*

NHS Institute for Innovation and Improvement. Focuses expertise in service transformation, technology and product innovation, leadership development and learning: *www.institute.nhs.uk*. One of its key publications is *10 High Impact Changes for Service Improvement and Delivery*, accessible at: *http://www.wise.nhs.uk/NR/rdonlyres/6E0D282A-4896-46DF-B8C7-068AA5EA1121/654/HIC_for_web.pdf*

NHS Service Delivery and Organisation R&D Programme. Produces and promotes the use of research evidence about how the organisation and delivery of services can be improved to increase the quality of patient care, ensure better strategic outcomes and contribute to improved public health: *http://www.sdo.lshtm.ac.uk/*

Social constructionism. For further information go to: *http://en.wikipedia.org/wiki/Social_constructionism*

21 Personal effectiveness

Kim Jelphs

Introduction

Mastery and an appreciation of the importance of personal effectiveness are both fundamental to being a successful manager and leader working in and across complex ever-changing environments, where situations are often far from clear and there is no right answer to the problems and dilemmas that are posed. Leaders and managers do not work in isolation, and how you behave and react in given situations can be essential to the outcome and to the relationships with others at all levels of and across organisations. Equally important is the sense of personal well-being when individuals are working effectively and both they and others recognise and value their unique skills.

This chapter aims to give an overview of personal effectiveness and has chosen to focus upon self-awareness, self-management, working successfully with others and becoming a reflective practitioner as complementary themes in this essential development arena. In recognition that leaders need to develop real skills, together with an appreciation of why they need that skill base, this chapter aims to draw upon literature that is academic and evidence based, together with hints and tips for practical application in the real world.

Some of the areas covered in this chapter may perhaps be perceived as 'soft skills' but that belies their importance, and such an attitude is perhaps rooted in somewhat dated thinking about learning that tends to appreciate and reward more traditional and didactic methods of teaching over experiential techniques, where people discover for themselves – a theme to which this chapter will return.

Learning about ourselves is not always comfortable, for in fact the most powerful learning experiences are often very uncomfortable because they challenge individuals to think and sometimes act outside their comfort zones. Looking at oneself encourages an individual to be honest, sometimes about areas they do not like and may find hard to acknowledge and face up to. Fundamental to being honest with ourselves is the need to develop an enhanced understanding and appreciation of who we are, how we work and why we do the things we do (or do not do), and a key component of this is to develop self-awareness.

Self-awareness

Knowing oneself and having an appreciation of the perceptions of how others see us is key to being an effective leader. But how often do we take the time to try and see ourselves and reflect upon our behaviour and personality as others see it? The Johari window (Figure 21.1) was developed by two researchers at the University of California in the 1950s (Rogers 2004), and the model provides a framework for identifying what you and others see (or not) by looking at yourself as if through a window which has four distinct panes:

1 *Open free area* – known by individual and also known by others.
2 *Blind area* – unknown by individual but known to others.
3 *Hidden area* – known by individual and not known by others.
4 *Unknown area* – unknown to individual and unknown to others.

360-degree review

Another valuable tool is the 360-degree process where people who work with you are invited to provide feedback and comment upon your performance as a leader. A variety of people (chosen by the leader undergoing the review, typically including peers, managers, service users, carers and people who report directly) are invited to comment upon a range of attributes and skills and the effect they perceive these characteristics to have upon the organisation and individual relationships. The real value is in receiving the comments and perceptions of a number of people across a whole range of relationships and associations (Rogers 2004),

1 Open/free area	2 Blind area
3 Hidden area	4 Unknown area

Figure 21.1   Johari window
Source: Adapted from Chapman (1995, 2005, *www.businessballs.com*)
Origin: Luft (1970)

recognising that perception can vary amongst peers, supervisors and sub-ordinates (Latham et al. 2005). There are many different 360-degree review systems available but it is essential to consider the following:

1 *Confidentiality of the process.* How is the information to be used and by whom?
2 *Feedback mechanisms.* Who is going to feed back to you and how?
3 *Anonymity of the contributors.* This is important for their honesty.
4 *Cost and funding of the exercise.* This is time consuming and most processes will have a cost.
5 *Coordination and planning.* How will the process work?
6 *Evaluation.* How will the value of the exercise and subsequent actions be determined? (Adapted from Modernisation Agency 2005.)

We all see the world in different ways but the insights of others can be invaluable to developing as a leader because those insights often challenge presumptions and importantly are not always negative insights but an appreciation of positive traits that are valued and respected by others. The real challenge lies in using learning and insights in a positive way to develop further.

Learning and learning styles

Many of us recognise that we enjoy learning in certain ways or situations, but do we consciously know how we learn best and how to make the most of learning opportunities? Often we will have been in learning situations as part of a group of people and yet the reactions to the experience will be fundamentally different, with some people being really positive about the experience and others being totally bemused by this reaction because for them the experience was not helpful or enjoyable (See Self-test Exercise 1.)

Conscious learning is an essential skill that can improve performance (Honey and Mumford 1992) and is especially valuable when sharing learning with others. It is not only important to understand how we learn as individuals, but to consider the learning needs and styles of individuals, teams and groups if we are to maximise understanding, sharing and learning together (Honey and Mumford 1992); for example, when learning about an incident that has taken place in one part of an organisation that impacts across the whole.

Cameron and Green (2004: 11) argue that 'learning is not just an acquisition of knowledge, but the application of it through doing something different'. David Kolb (1984) developed a model of learning which demonstrates that people go through a cycle of both doing and thinking in order to learn (Cameron and Green 2004). This work has been further enhanced by Honey and Mumford (1992) who have developed a tool (Honey and Mumford 2000) that helps individuals assess and understand their preference for one of the four distinct stages on this learning cycle. Rogers (2001: 23) describes the stages:

- *Activity* – doing something or undergoing an experience.
- *Reflection* – thinking about the experience.
- *Theory* – seeing where it fits in with theoretical ideas.
- *Pragmatism* – applying the learning to real situations.

To be effective, adult learning has to have some special characteristics that: recognise and value experiential learning; are challenging, learner centred and interactive; are relevant (directly related to daily work); and provide feedback (adapted from Jones 1992). Additionally, it can be helpful to think about how you learn to make associations and links (Buzan 2003) and to learn to respect intuition (Figure 21.2). Claxton (2001: 37) argues that 'when people are learning to manage a complex environment, their intuitive grasp, their "know-how", develops much faster than their ability to describe what they are doing'. Expertise precedes explanation, meaning that often people underestimate their performance if they are unable to articulate what they are doing and why. They need to learn to trust their intuition which will be rooted in prior learning and experiences. Self-discovery and reflection are critical to this process and perhaps enhanced by the use of psychometric tests.

The role of psychometrics

The English dictionary suggests that psychometrics deals with measuring mental traits, capacities and processes. There is a plethora of tools in use and there are strict guidelines that inform the use of these tools and

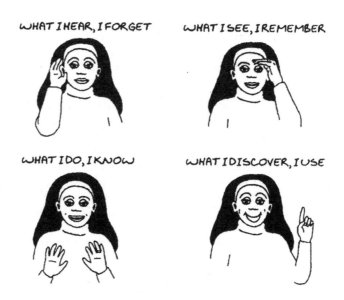

Figure 21.2 Adult learning
Source: Rowe et al. (1997: 10)
© Copyright Liverpool John Moores University/Premier Health NHS Trust

which practitioners administering them must adhere to in order to preserve confidentiality and maintain the integrity and quality of the experience. Psychometric tools are all different, but fall mostly into two categories of either measuring traits (illustrating how much of something you have, often against a range or scale of 'normative values') or measuring preference.

The Myers Briggs Type Indicator is one of the most commonly applied, respected and valuable tools which is used specifically to develop personal and interpersonal awareness. The tool is employed worldwide and culturally sensitive versions are available. The tool identifies personality type and was developed by a mother and daughter team who based it on the work of Carl Jung, a Swiss psychologist (Myers 2000). The tool focuses on preference across eight dimensions:

1 *Where you prefer to get your energy from. Extraverts* have a preference for drawing energy from the world around them through people and doing. *Introverts* are energised from their internal world through reflection, time alone and thinking.
2 *What type of information you pay attention to and how you like to take it in.* People with a preference for *sensing* prefer specific facts and like to focus on what is actually happening. Those with a preference for *intuition* are interested in connections, the big picture and the art of the possible.
3 *How you make decisions. Thinking* is about taking decisions in a logical, objective way, removed from the situation. *Feeling* is concerned with making decisions in a value–driven way that seeks to understand and empathise from the perspective of a situation.
4 *How you prefer to live your life. Judging* is a preference for living in a structured, organised, planned way. *Perceiving* is a preference for living in a more flexible way that keeps options open until the last minute. (Adapted from Cameron and Green 2004: 44.)

The tool is not about strengths, knowledge, skills or abilities and as such there are no right or wrong preferences. Using the tool should give individuals an insight and understanding into their own preferences and the behaviour of others. Each preference is valid, but it is the understanding and valuing of difference that is crucial for effective relationships.

Another tool to consider is Fundamental Interpersonal Relations Orientation-Behaviour (Firo B). This measures how you usually behave towards other people and how you expect them to behave towards you in return (Waterman and Rogers 2000). The tool helps heighten awareness in order to further understand what we want, what we need and importantly how we communicate this (or perhaps not).

Emotional intelligence

Perhaps the whole self-awareness arena is best characterised by the work on emotional intelligence by Daniel Goleman (1998a), who explored the ability to understand and manage how you impact upon others emotionally. Goleman's work looked at 181 different management competence models that originated from 121 organisations across the world. The research illustrated that 67% of the abilities perceived as essential management competence were emotional competencies (Cameron and Green 2004). Goleman's (1998b) research challenged traditional thinking and views about effective leadership by arguing that although technical skills and intelligence are important, they are not wholly sufficient to develop truly effective leaders, who are characterised by a high level of emotional intelligence, including self-awareness, self-regulation, motivation, empathy and social skill.

Self-management

The previous section focused on the importance of self-awareness for effective leadership, but awareness is not enough, as the work of Goleman (1998a) highlights. You need to be able to commit to develop and learn to manage yourself if you are to be truly effective. For example, if you know you react badly to undue pressure caused by tight deadlines, then plan to manage not just the deadline (Goleman 1998a) but yourself, your attitude and behaviour. If you get anxious about certain issues, then understand what makes you anxious and commit to try and reduce your anxiety, because anxiety is destructive and saps energy and confidence. If you get nervous about presenting, then undertake to develop your presentation skills, which will not just be about the content of the session but about how to develop your image and stance to improve both confidence and performance.

Developing confidence and reducing anxiety are key skills for effective management of self. The confidence to say no is crucial, as is the confidence to be clear about your limitations. Having the confidence and knowledge as to when to ask for help is a hallmark of self-awareness (Goleman 1998b), and not the sign of weakness that some people still persist in believing. Not everyone can be good at everything and the key to managing self is an understanding of your strengths and weaknesses and taking the time to plan and consider what you need to do in given situations.

Time management

Managing time effectively is perhaps one of the biggest challenges for health service managers and an area that many people struggle with. It is important to remember that you can do almost anything, but there will never be enough time to do everything. The real skill is knowing how to use time optimally. It is an important career and life skill and an essential attribute of really successful people.

'The bad thing is that time flies – the good thing is you are the pilot' (Michael Altshuler 2005). This comment illustrates that time, as in most areas of life, is an area over which you can take control if you have the commitment and the will. It is important to recognise the impact and cost of poor time management upon managers, their teams and organisations. But the answer is not to work ever-increasing hours, for there are clear associations between a long hours culture and lower productivity, poor performance, health problems and low motivation (Kodz et al. 2003). Different countries adopt different cultural approaches to working hours, with a long hours culture being more common in the UK than in many other European Union countries, but quite similar to working patterns in the USA, Australia and Japan (Kodz et al. 2003).

Covey (1999) identifies that there have been different approaches or 'waves' over the years in respect of time management, these having built upon previous approaches and become increasingly sophisticated and different in their focus. These waves have developed from systems that identified demands upon time to a recognition that people need to manage themselves and not time. The time management matrix (Figure 21.3) is a useful tool for considering how time is spent and encourages individuals to think about what is important as opposed to urgent or perceived to be urgent. We all have some crisis moments (Quadrant I), but really effective people try to minimise time spent in dealing with the issues raised by Quadrants III and IV and focus more on Quadrant II,

	URGENT	NOT URGENT
I m p o r t a n t	**I** **ACTIVITIES** Crises Pressing problems Deadline driven projects	**II** **ACTIVITIES** Prevention Developing production capability Relationship building Recognising new opportunities Planning, recreation
N o t i m p o r t a n t	**III** **ACTIVITIES** Interruptions, some calls Some mail, some reports, Some meetings Proximate, pressing matters Popular activities	**IV** **ACTIVITIES** Trivia, busy work Some mail Some phone calls Time wasters Pleasant activities

Figure 21.3   The time management matrix
Source: adapted from Covey (1999: 151)

which in turn becomes a way of reducing elements associated with Quadrant I as attention has been paid to issues that are important (Covey 1999: 151).

The word 'urgent' will have different meanings to people dependent upon their on background and profession. This is worth understanding as a healthcare manager for it can be a cause of real discontent in the clinician–manager relationship. The word is often misused and perhaps demands over-response because of a lack of understanding of what urgent really means in given situations. Thus it can be a real barrier to managing time effectively. However, the healthcare workforce is not just charged with being reactive – increasingly the whole workforce is being encouraged to be ever more creative and innovative in the approaches it adopts to service delivery. Claxton (2001) cautions that a climate where decisions are often made as fast as possible will mitigate against quality of thinking which is sometimes compromised by decisions being made under pressure. In an increasingly pressurised environment, understanding real priorities is fundamental to being effective. In reality, however, many things get in the way of good intentions and individuals are easily distracted, preferring to focus on familiar tasks. It is important to reflect upon what happens when we are deemed to be working really effectively, perhaps before going on holiday, and deciphering what happens in that situation. We are not always aware of how we really spend our time and the reality is often very different to perception. It is worth investing in taking the time to develop a time log, to demonstrate the reality of our use of time (See Self-test Exercise 2.).

Another important aspect of time management is to consider the boundaries of roles and responsibilities. It is pertinent at this point to refer to earlier chapters in this book which affirm that leadership and management styles are changing worldwide. Leading with and through others is the current zeitgeist and it is worth considering what this really means for leaders. In many situations, this will mean not doing, and instead letting go and delegating – a considerable change in role and practice to which many people find it difficult to adjust. Often this adjustment is not made and leaders and mangers end up carrying out roles and tasks that others really should be doing, which compounds the demands on their time. Effective leadership is often about negotiation and self-management is essential if you are to be confident about your own role and abilities and thus able to work successfully with others.

Working successfully with others

Really effective managers are able to work at all levels of organisations and be comfortable when working across boundaries – the key is connecting with people. Healthcare is no longer delivered in isolation from other organisations, agencies and services. There is a new and very real interdependence and networks are a way of establishing and developing connections that will enhance service development and delivery (the issue of working in partnership with other agencies is explored in more depth in Chapter 17). Building and reviewing networks is essential to understanding links and connections, although networking has become a bit of a 'buzz word' and is in danger of losing its credibility without consideration being given to what it means.

Networking

Colleen Wedderburn Tate (1999: 80) argues: 'leaders understand the power of networks, and use them appropriately. Networking is a key element in the process of continuous learning. They understand the value of knowing who is doing what, where, when, and with what result.' Goodwin (2005) argues that the real key to effective networking is the development of interpersonal relationships which need time and energy to develop. Therefore to be an effective leader it is worth taking time to consider your present networks and consider whether you need to further enhance them. A useful exercise can be the development of a network map, whereby you identify and write down your networks and connections and review them regularly to see how they are changing and growing. (See Self-test Exercise 3.)

Communication

When discussing networks, Goodwin (2005) identifies the importance of interpersonal skills, with communication being perhaps the most essential of those skills. There are many influences upon communication, including: socialisation associated with families, organisations and their systems; culture and individual teams; personal preferences; gender; power. Effective managers need to be able to communicate with a diverse range of people within and across organisations, people who will all see the world differently and who will perhaps associate different language and meaning with issues, thus creating immense potential for misinterpretation. It is pertinent to recognise that the worldwide growth in international recruitment is compounding this issue, making it even more essential that individuals consider the messages they are sending and how they are sending them.

Communication is at the heart of many of the issues that have risen to prominence in relation to poor practice in health and social care, which have often had terrible consequences for patients: 'I cannot account for the way other people interpreted what I said. It was not the way I would have liked it to have been interpreted' (Laming 2003: 9). This is a quote from an inquiry following the death of a child, but illustrates perfectly the issues associated with sending and receiving messages. It is perhaps worth remembering that when communicating the verbal word accounts for

7% of the message, whilst 38% of the message is in the way that it is said and non-verbal (body language) communication accounts for 55% of the message (Mehrabian 1972).

In England, the third most common cause of NHS patient complaints is about both written and oral communication, with attitudes of staff being the second highest cause of complaint (Health and Social Care Information Centre 2005). Arguably, these two issues are different sides of the same coin in that they are about the way messages are delivered and received. Technology is playing an increasing role in communication with, for example, the growth of emails and text messaging, but there is perhaps an over-reliance on these systems of communication. Effective managers really do need to take the time to reflect upon communication styles, systems and processes, and to consider how they can be improved. Individuals will always differ in their preferences for communication styles and systems, and this in turn will influence responses. Recognising and tuning in to individual preferences is a key element of personal effectiveness and considered a vital political skill.

Political skill

Mintzberg (1979) was one of the first people to use the phrase 'political skill' and many people believe that organisations can be viewed as political arenas (Perrewé and Nelson 2004). It therefore follows that leaders need the skills to operate effectively in those political arenas. Perrewé and Nelson (2004) argue that in political environments the reality of competing interest groups and scarce resources demands that individuals develop their influencing skills and tactics in order to succeed and thrive. These authors assert (p. 239) that political skill 'is characterised by social perceptiveness and the ability to adjust one's behaviour to different and changing situational needs to influence others'. Key to influencing others is an understanding of your own style and how it impacts upon those you are working with and a useful self-assessment tool can be found in the leadership toolkit developed by Hardacre (2003). Fundamental to developing influencing skills is a careful reflection upon your own actions, a subject upon which the next section of this chapter will focus.

Reflective practitioner

Whilst there are many uncertainties in healthcare today, what is certain is that the pace of change is and will remain unrelenting. It takes considerable time and investment to develop academic courses and competency frameworks and therefore traditional methods of learning and acquiring knowledge are not able to keep up with the pace of change. We need to value and embed other ways of learning, especially as there may not be answers to given situations and problems. Reflective practice is key to this.

Historically, reflective practice has not been valued in the same way as traditional training methods. Schon (1987) argues that technical and academic training is too limiting for professionals, who in reality face complex problems and dilemmas in their everyday lives. Redmond (2004) agrees and posits that a focus on academic rigour and role-related competencies has meant that, although learners are technically and theoretically skilled, they do not always have the skills critically to review and reflect upon their own practice, which often demands a change in perspective and thinking. Johns (2004: 3) clarifies that what is needed is not an 'either/or' situation, but a need to integrate the more traditional ways of learning with reflective practice, resulting in holistic practice that:

- focuses on the whole experience and then seeks to understand its significance within the whole
- is grounded in the meaning the individual practitioner gives to the particular experience and seeks to facilitate such understanding
- acknowledges that the practitioner is ultimately self-determining and responsible for his or her own destiny and seeks to facilitate such growth.

Redmond (2004) argues that the work of Argyris and Schön (1974) identifies that the concept of reflective practice has encouraged professionals to adopt a 'less expert stance' with clients. This concept is surely transferable to healthcare managers for whom patients' and service users' views are fundamental to healthcare in the twenty-first century.

Action learning

One way of practising a reflective approach to one's management activity is through the discipline of action learning. Increasingly, action learning is being used by organisations and individuals across the world to facilitate the resolution of complex problems and to support the development of teams, individuals and organisations (Waddill and Marquardt 2003). Action learning was developed by Revans in the middle of the twentieth century and many different approaches now exist. Core to all action learning approaches, however, is the importance of people taking time to work and reflect upon problems in small groups of supportive but challenging colleagues and to learn whilst doing so (Waddill and Marquardt 2003). For Revans, learning required action, and this action had to be informed by reflection. Thus he developed the learning equation $L = P + Q$ in which L is Learning, P is Programmed Knowledge and Q is Questioning to facilitate insight. (Revans 1998: 4). Weinstein concurs: 'One of the beliefs of action learning is that we learn best when we are committed to undertaking some action; another is that without action, there is no real evidence of learning. Thus the emphasis in action learning is as much on actions, as on gaining learning' (1998: 159). It is the taking action that distinguishes this approach from other learning approaches. Additional core elements of action learning are:

- the small group or set of people who work together – ideally six to eight
- the task, problem or project that each of the members brings to the set to work upon
- the processes the team adopts to work together – for example, each person has air time to present their issue and to be open to questioning and feedback
- a facilitator/advisor who helps the set to work together (adapted from Weinstein 1999; Waddill and Marquardt 2003).

Action learning is about groups of people working together in a reciprocal way, a feature that differs from another reflective approach – coaching – which is about one-to-one relationships.

Coaching

There is increasing and international interest in coaching and the profession of coaching is gaining ever greater legitimacy as evidence grows that investment in coaching can make a difference to the individual and to the organisation through improved performance (Latham et al. 2005). The origins of coaching can be found in different aspects of psychology (Wright 2005). It is not a form of therapy, although at times the boundaries between therapy and coaching can appear blurred. Coaches work with individuals to help them to grow, develop, see the world differently and realise more than they believed to be the limits of their potential (Goldsmith et al. 2000). The relationship between a coach and the person being coached is one of reciprocity and demands commitment from both partners. Goldsmith et al. (2000) argue that coaching is the leadership approach of the twenty-first century as today's leaders need to learn how to work with and through people in order to succeed.

The differences between coaching and mentoring are arguable and the focus of much debate in the literature (see D'Abate et al. 2003). A mentor is often perceived as an expert who can guide, signpost alternatives, advise and perhaps teach. A coach fundamentally differs in that he or she does not give answers, is interested in what the individual thinks and why, and often disappoints by not taking responsibility for providing answers and solutions (Goldsmith et al. 2000). A coach's prime motivation is to work with individuals on negotiated areas that the individual will take forward. To do this, coaches need to be able to question, give and receive feedback, motivate, empathise, listen, tolerate silence and structure conversations through informed dialogue (Lyons 2000).

Whichever developmental system individuals choose to or are able to access to support them in their management roles, it is essential that they recognise the importance of taking control over their own development and learning. Personal development plans are key to this, whereby individuals identify their learning needs and the associated skills and knowledge to gain both confidence and competence to support their ever-changing roles. It is a hallmark of an effective, reflective, practitioner to have a tangible and realistic personal development plan.

Conclusion

Traditional training and teaching methods will not give managers everything they need to function as optimally as possible in complex and changing healthcare environments. Training courses will help with the acquisition of skills, knowledge and competence, but leaders and managers really need to develop self-awareness and confidence, and to be able to value learning from a range of experiences. Understanding self, learning to develop and accept skills and perhaps unlearn others is essential if you are to develop as an effective healthcare leader and manager, and the responsibility for making this happen lies with each individual.

Personal effectiveness demands personal investment and perhaps a change of mindset. You need to commit to developing yourself and be kind to yourself in order to develop. This means recognising that you and your development needs are important and that time taken for such activities is a legitimate use of time even in very pressurised environments. If you can distance yourself from day-to-day pressures and take time to learn and to think, then evidence suggests that your performance will be enhanced (West 2000). If you value personal development and model it, then others are more likely to feel comfortable and empowered to follow you, and hence an even greater organisational change may take place.

Summary box

- Learning more about yourself and associated attitudes and behaviours is key to understanding yourself, and thus undertaking changes to act and behave differently.
- Learning about self is not always comfortable, but it is valuable learning nevertheless.
- Being clear about your strengths and limitations and learning to say no are crucial management skills.
- Taking control of learning by having clear personal development plans is vital to a process of ongoing development.
- Acting as a role model will enhance best practice in others and facilitate greater organisational performance.
- Using the support of others is crucial, for it is not a sign of weakness to ask for help – the best leaders always do!
- Valuing and respecting experience and intuition is vital to effective heathcare management.

Self-test exercises

1 *Learning experience.* Take time to think about your most *memorable* learning experience. Reflect upon and try and identify what made it such a memorable powerful experience for you and consider:

   • What did you enjoy or dislike about the experience and why?
   • Who else was involved and what role did they play?
   • How has it influenced how you react or respond in certain situations?

2 *Time management exercise.* We all think we know how we spend our time at work, but the rhetoric and reality are often different. Undertake to keep a diary/log at work for at least a whole day. Record all activities, interruptions, meetings, calls and planned work, and then find time to truly reflect upon what you have written and consider changes that you need to make.

3 *Networks exercise.* Building and reviewing networks and connections is essential to developing effectively as a leader. This exercise is about identifying your networks and connections and reviewing them regularly to see how they are changing and growing. Draw three circles and write in the three circles the people and organisations that make up your network:

   • *Inner circle*: people you see or have contact with daily
   • *Middle circle*: people you see or have contact with weekly
   • *Outer circle*: people you see or have contact with one–three monthly.

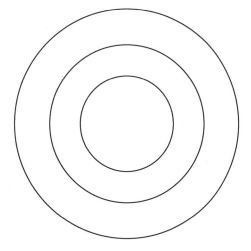

Source: Wedderburn Tate (1999: 84). Copyright: Elsevier Ltd (1999).

When completing the circles think about:

- personal
- professional
- organisational
- strategic
- international.

References and further reading

Altshuler, M. (2005) *www.time-management-guide.com* (accessed 16 December 2005).

Argyris, C. and Schön, D. (1974) *Theory in Practice: Increasing Professional Effectiveness*. San Francisco: Jossey-Bass.

Bolles, R. (2004) *What Color is Your Parachute? A Practical Manual for Job-Hunters and Career Changers*. Berkeley: Ten Speed Press.

Buzan, T. (2003) *Use Your head*. London: BBC Books.

Cameron, E. and Green, M. (2004) *Making Sense of Change Management*. London: Kogan Page.

Carvel, J. (2005) NHS Criticised for not heeding complaints. *The Guardian*, 31 October: 5.

Chapman, A. (2005) *www.businessballs.com* (accessed 16 December 2005).

Claxton, G. (2001) The innovative mind: Becoming smarter by thinking less. In J. Henry *Creative Management*, 2nd edn. London: Sage.

Covey, S. (1999) *The 7 Habits of Highly Effective People*. London: Simon and Schuster.

Covey, S. (2005) *The 7 Habits of Highly Effective People Personal Workbook*. London: Simon and Schuster.

D'Abate, C., Eddy, E. and Tannenbaum, S. (2003) What's in a name? A literature-based approach to understanding mentoring, coaching, and other constructs that describe developmental interactions. *Human Resource Development Review*, 2(4): 360–84.

Goldsmith, M., Lyons, L. and Freas, A. (eds) (2000) *Coaching for Leadership: How the World's Greatest Coaches Help Leaders Learn*. San Francisco: Jossey-Bass.

Goleman, D. (1998a) *Working with Emotional Intelligence*. London: Bloomsbury.

Goleman, D. (1998b) What makes a leader? *Harvard Business Review*, November–December: 94–9.

Goodwin, N. (2005) *Leadership in Healthcare: A European Perspective*. London: Routledge.

Grote, D. (1995) *Discipline Without Punishment*. New York: AMACOM.

Hardacre, J. (2003) *Leadership at Every Level – A Practical Guide for Managers and Clinicians*, 2nd edn. London: Emap Public Sector Management.

Health and Social Care Information Centre (2005) *Data on Written Complaints in the NHS 2004–2005*. London: Health and Social Care Information Centre.

Henry, J. (2001) *Creative Management*, 2nd edn. London: Sage.

Honey, P. and Mumford, A. (1992) *The Manual of Learning Styles*. Maidenhead: Peter Honey Publications.

Honey, P. and Mumford, A. (2000) *The Learning Styles Questionnaire – 80 item Version*. Maidenhead: Peter Honey Publications.

Iles, V. and Cranfield, S. (2004) *Developing Change Management Skills*. London: NHS Service Delivery and Organisation (SDO) R&D Programme.

Johns, C. (2004) *Becoming a Reflective Practitioner*, 2nd edn. Oxford: Blackwell.

Jones, R. (1992) Getting better: Education and the primary healthcare team. *British Medical Journal*, 305(6852): 506–8.

Kodz, J. et al. (2003) *Working Long Hours: A Review of the Evidence, Volume 1 – Main Report*. London: Department of Trade and Industry.

Kolb, D. (1984) *Experiential Learning*. New York: Prentice-Hall.

Laming, H. (2003) *The Victoria Climbié Inquiry*. Norwich: The Stationery Office.

Latham, G., Almost, J., Mann, S. and Moore, C. (2005) New developments in performance management. *Organizational Dynamics*, 34(1): 77–87.

Lyons, L. (2000) Coaching at the heart of strategy. In M. Goldsmith, L. Lyons and A. Freas (eds) *Coaching for Leadership: How the World's Greatest Coaches Help Leaders Learn*. San Francisco: Jossey-Bass.

Mehrabian, A. (1972) *Nonverbal Communication*. Chicago: Aldine-Atherton.

Mintzberg, H. (1979) *The Structure of Organizations: A Synthesis of the Research*. Englewood Cliffs, NJ: Prentice-Hall.

Modernisation Agency (2005) LQF 360 degree assessment tool. Available at *www.lqf360modern.nhs.uk* (accessed 16 December 2005).

Myers, I. (2000) *Introduction to Type*, 6th edn. Oxford: OPP.

Norman, R. (2001) *Reframing Business – When the Map Changes the Landscape*. Chichester: Wiley.

Pedlar, M. (1996) *Action Learning for Managers*. London: Lemos and Crane.

Perrewé, P. and Nelson, D. (2004) The facilitative role of political skill. *Organizational Dynamics*, 33(4): 366–78.

Perrewé, P., Zellars, K., Rossi, A., Ferris, G., Kacmar, C., Zinko, R., Liu, Y. and Hochwarter, W. (2005) Political skill: An antidote in the role overload-strain relationship. *Journal of Occupational Health Psychology*, 10(3): 239–50.

Redmond, B. (2004) *Reflection in Action: Developing Reflective Practice in Health and Social Workers*. Aldershot: Ashgate.

Revans, R. (1982) *The Origins and Growth of Action Learning*. Bromley: Chartwell-Bratt.

Revans, R. (1998) *ABC of Action Learning*, 3rd edn. London: Lemos and Crane.

Rogers, J. (2001) *Adults Learning*, 4th edn. Maidenhead: Open University Press.

Rogers, J. (2004) *Coaching Skills: A Handbook*. Maidenhead: Open University Press.

Rowe, A., Mitchinson, S., Morgan, M. and Carey, L. (1997) *Health Profiling – All You Need to Know*. Liverpool: John Moores University and Premier Health NHS Trust.

Schon, D. A. (1983) *The Reflective Practitioner*. New York: Basic Books.

Schon, D.A. (1987) *Educating the Reflective Practitioner: Towards a New Design for Teaching and Learning in the Professions*. San Francisco: Jossey-Bass.

Waddill, D. and Marquardt, M. (2003) Adult learning orientations and action learning. *Human Resource Development Review*, 2(4): 406–29.

Waterman, J. and Rogers, J. (2000) *Introduction to the Firo B*. Oxford: OPP.

Wedderburn Tate, C. (1999) *Leadership in Nursing*. London: Churchill Livingstone.

Weinstein, K. (1999) *Action Learning – A Practical Guide*. Aldershot: Gower.

West, M. (2000) Reflexivity, revolution and innovation in work teams. In M. Beyerlain, D. Johnson and S. Beyerlain (eds) *Product Development Teams*. Stamford, CT: JAI Press.

Wright, J. (2005) Workplace coaching: What is it all about? *Work*, 24: 325–8.

Websites and resources

Action Learning, Action Research and Process Management Association (ALARPM). A network of people who use action learning and action research and participatory process facilitation to generate collaborative learning: *www.alarpm.org.au*

Businessballs. Free website which has a wealth of material, tools and articles to support both personal and organisational development: *www.businessballs.co.uk*

Chartered Institute of Personnel and Development (CIPD). The UK's leading professional body for those involved in the management and development of people. Many selected resources, papers and tools are free: *www.cipd.co.uk*

Coaching network. Coaching and mentoring information. It is primarily aimed at coaches and people looking for coaches, but has a good resource centre which is freely available containing full text articles, case studies and up-to-date news: *www.coachingnetwork.org.uk*

EffectiveMeetings. Practical advice, support and resources for improving meetings, including presentation skills: *www.effectivemeetings.com*

Emotional Intelligence Consortium. Facilitates the advancement of research and practice relevant to emotional intelligence in organisations. The website contains full text articles, research papers, reports and guidelines: *www.eiconsortium.org*

International Coach Federation (ICF). Non-profit professional organisation that represents personal and business coaches: *www.coachfederation.org.uk*

Knowledge Exchange. Web-based community where health and social care managers connect to share information and exchange ideas: *www.theknowledgeexchange.co.uk*

Meeting Wizard. Wide range of ideas and techniques to enhance meetings: *www.meetingwizard.org*

Mind Tools. Contains a broad range of life, career training and management training skills, many freely available and supported by articles and exercises: *www.mindtools.com*

NHS Leadership Centre (NHSLC). This website contains the 360-degree assessment tool which has been designed to enable individuals to: manage the set-up and completion of 360-degree assessment entirely online: complete questionnaires as a participant in colleagues' 360-degree review: *www.lqf360.modern.nhs.uk*

NHS Networks. Aims to connect leaders in the NHS across geography, sectors, professions and government, to share new thinking and practice: *www.nhsnetworks.nhs.uk*

UK Positive Psychology Network. Promotes research, training, education and the dissemination and application of positive psychology and gives access to articles, questionnaires and personal development resources: *www.positivepsychology.org*

22 | Appreciating the challenge of change

Ann Shacklady-Smith

A hospital replaced a notice to outpatients that simply said: 'Wait here', with a notice that said: 'We promise to see you as soon as we can. Please take a seat here until a doctor is free.' The print bill might have risen fractionally, but patient morale soared. (Elliot 1999)

Introduction

This chapter is written for healthcare managers, who want to learn more about managing change in the workplace. Rather than a prescription or description of change, Collins (1998) encourages a 'thinking practitioner' approach to the subject. His advice is taken and the chapter is written with the aim of helping managers to find their own perspective and approach to the change process. The chapter aims to give managers an appreciation of the context driving change, change-theory frameworks and methods, models of change and managers' roles in change.

As the illusion that there can be a 'stable' environment fades and as organisations are embracing the challenge of thriving in a world of constant change, the impact on organisational change theory and practice has been profound (Watkins and Mohr 2001: xxxi). Charles Handy (1989) speaks of entering an age of 'unreason' where the future is there to be shaped by us and for us, where the only prediction that will hold true is that no predictions will hold true, 'Change is not what it used to be.' The time for new approaches to thinking about and approaching organisational change has clearly arrived.

In the following discussion the established typologies of 'planned' and 'emergent' change are explained and Ackerman's (1997) model is used to show the lack of a clear boundary between them. Transformational change is discussed in reference to the 'emerging paradigm' literature referring to the influence of new science (quantum physics, neurosciences, chaos and complexity theory) in shaping organisational change theory and methods and the challenge it poses to classical scientific versions of change (Watkins and Mohr 2001; Table 22.1).

Three change examples are discussed to illustrate the main themes of

Table 22.1 Current and emerging paradigms

Current scientific paradigm	Emerging paradigm
Newtonian mechanics; reductionist and dichotomous thinking	Quantum physics and new sciences: self-organising systems; chaos theory: complexity theory
We search for a model or method of objectively perceiving the world.	We accept the complexity and subjectivity of the world.
We engage in complex planning for a world we expect to be predictable.	Planning is understood to be a process of constant re-evaluation.
We understand language as the descriptor of reality: I'll believe it when I see it.	We understand language as the creator of reality: I'll see it when I believe it.
We see information as power.	We see information as a primal creative force.
We believe in reductionism, i.e. things can be best understood when they are broken into parts.	We seek to understand wholeness and the interconnectedness of all things.
We engage in dichotomous thinking.	We search for harmony and the common threads of our dialogue.
We believe that there is only one truth for which we must search.	We understand truth to be dependent on the context and the current reality.
We believe that influence occurs as a direct result of force exerted from one person to another, i.e. cause and effect.	We understand that influence occurs as a natural part of human interaction.
We live in a linear and hierarchical world.	We live in a circular world of relationships and cooperation.

Source: Watkins and Mohr (2001).

the chapter: the introduction of service-level financial management; enhancing the patient experience by reducing waiting time for medical appointments; generating 'an exceptional' twenty-first century global organisation. Reflective questions follow the case examples and a summary of the key points raised in the chapter is given at the end.

Context driving change

Much has been said in Chapter 1 of this book concerning the wide-ranging structural changes that are occurring throughout the health sector in many countries. These changes represent a shift in vision from one premised on provision of person-centred care to one located in improving the system and context of care (Peck: 2005).

Recognising that change is an ever-present and routine aspect of organisational life (Tichy 1983), there is little that is new about the fact of organisational change. What is new perhaps is the pace and complexity of change initiatives that are being introduced throughout the public sector, and the requirement for all affected by the change to have some part in its implementation.

Public sector transformation is also geared toward achieving broad socio-economic outcomes such as: reducing health inequalities; improving a sense of well-being; improving employment prospects; creating sustainable communities. This also presents some unique challenges to change agents, not least in finding multi-agency change solutions. Taking health as an example, there are many determinants involved in producing 'health and well-being' as Wanless's model attempts to show (see Figure 22.1). It follows therefore that the solutions do not reside within any single organisation. Change efforts will require the active collaboration of all agencies and organisations who have a role to play in influencing outcomes.

Transformational change involves altering the overall orientation of the organisation (Tichy 1983: 17). It is based on new paradigm thinking and the values that underpin it and represents the most important type of change facing the 'new public sector' (Lovell 1994: 4). The changes proposed are aimed at transforming the core aspects of an organisation's purpose, structures, image and work activity; or, as described (Beckhard and Pritchard 1992), as shifting the very 'essence' of the organisation, embracing its:

• purpose
• identity or image

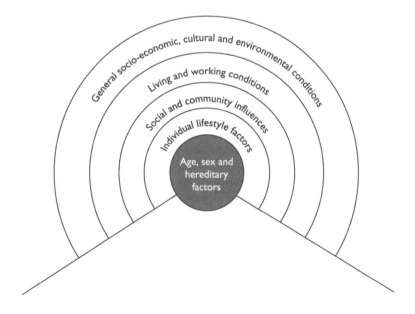

Figure 22.1   The determinants of health
Source: Adapted from Wanless (2004: 25)

- type of work
- roles, skills and employment paradigms
- relationship to stakeholders
- ways of working
- culture and values
- organisational processes.

The changes being managed within the health sector are extensive in their reach and impact. They involve a quantum shift in thinking as well as in practice and call for approaches to change management that are capable of handling the multiple dimensions of change involved.

Change theory

It is important to introduce some theoretical consideration of change, not least because implicit or explicit theories of change often lie behind the policies and strategies that managers are attempting to implement (Bolman and Deal 1991: 9). As they observed: 'Behind every effort to improve organizations lies a set of assumptions, or theories, about how organizations work and what might make them work better.' However, to point the reader to a body of literature on organisational change is not an easy task. The subject matter crosses many theoretical, philosophical and applied scholarly disciplines within the social and natural sciences (Burnes 1996).

Although it is outside the scope of this chapter to review the many theories and models of change available, the references that follow, whilst not exhaustive, will serve to guide the reader to further discussion. To gain a sense of the history relating to the various intellectual antecedents in the developing field of organisational change, see for instance: Pugh (1971); Silverman (1970) Pfeffer (1982); Tichy (1983); Reed (1992); Reed and Hughes (1992); Burnes (1996); Collins (1998) for analytical and critical accounts.

Readers are advised to be mindful also of the historical context in which particular theories were developed. The social, economic and political conditions involved in creating the markets in which organisations must operate are important factors in understanding the task of and literature concerning change management (Alvesson and Wilmott 1996). Change is a complex business and its study is best guided by seeking to understand the unfolding complexities involved and the research that sheds light on this (Collins 1998; Iles and Sutherland 2001). There is no one right theory or approach to change management, rather there are multiple perspectives and lenses through which to view organisations and from which to develop ideas, actions and technologies for approaching change (see, for instance, Pettigrew et al. (1992); Collins 1998; Iles and Sutherland (2001); Peck 2005.

Change management has been popularised somewhat in recent years by what are known as the 'how to' or 'guru' texts, which despite their appeal are not necessarily based on ideas that demonstrate a sound methodological or empirical base (Huczynski 1993). Whilst offering practical advice to managers who are attempting to introduce 'new visions, paradigms, and empowerment strategies', the anecdotal solutions offered are criticised by some for using 'the language of liberation and innovation, yet being more firmly wedded to refurbishing the status quo' (Alvesson and Wilmott 1996).

Collins (1998) similarly found amongst the 'practitioner genre' a tendency to offer a simplistic and prescriptive 'n-step' approach to change and an over-reliance on practical advice. Meanwhile Dawson (1994) identifies an over-emphasis of a planned model of change at the neglect of a 'processual approach'. According to Collins, authors neglect to relate their advice to the theory or research from which it is derived, and competing theories and explanations of change were not (if at all) fully evaluated or explored.

With this in mind, it is helpful to draw upon theoretical and diagnostic models (Iles and Sutherland 2001) which have been developed to reveal the motivational elements involved in formulating strategy, and in driving and managing change. For example, Porter's (1980) model of competitive analysis is used to help determine the forces that influence market position and strategy. Tichy (1983) makes the case for integrating technical, political, social and cultural dimensions of organisational reality when managing strategic change. Checkland and Scholes's (1999) soft systems methodology helps to identify the complex social processes involved in change.

Studies of change implementation (Pettigrew 1987; Buchanan and Boddy 1992; Pettigrew et al. 1992; Peppard and Preece 1995) have investigated the factors that contribute to providing 'receptive contexts for change'. Guidance on the crafting of strategy for change can be found in the analysis of ten approaches offered by Mintzberg et al. (1998). They provide a helpful critique of the different 'schools of thought' and the limitations and contributions that each intellectual tradition brings to a consideration of strategic change.

Typologies of change

Attempts to characterise the change process have tended to polarise change either as a mechanistic and planned event (Lewin 1958) or as an emergent process (Burnes 1996). Change is also commonly presented as a stable and linear process consisting of a one-off event or a series of single episodes, while emerging paradigms promise an approach that is grounded in the moment with stakeholders guiding its direction. A summary of each follows.

Planned change

Models of planned change rest on the assumption that change is a rational process. The presenting 'problem' can be observed or revealed through organisational data. Solutions arise from the diagnosis and change outcomes can be specified in advance. The language of change also tends towards a reification of the goals and objects of change, as something that lies outside the experience of people who make up the organisation.

Various models are proposed to characterise a planned change process. Many have drawn inspiration from Lewin's three-phase characterisation of planned change. This involves: *unfreezing* the organisation from a presumed steady and stable state, *moving* towards new goals and view of the future and *refreezing* or stabilising the norms, values, behaviours and culture representing a desired end state. Lewin also found in his fieldwork that strategies for reducing resistance, rather than exaggerating forces for change, were more effective for garnering support for change.

There are many criticisms of the planned approach, not least that it is assumed 'that we can differentiate between states of change and stability' (Tichy 1983: 17). The organisation is also assumed to represent a harmonious system made up of functional elements that cohere around common goals and shared interests (Alvesson and Willmott 1996). In practice, the tensions provoked by change inevitably impact on the experience of the women and men who are intended to embody them and becomes a significant part of what needs to be managed within change programmes.

Emergent change

It is widely accepted that change involves both 'planned for' and 'emergent from the situation' elements and that change outcomes cannot always be predetermined. Studies have shown that effective communication with and involvement of those most affected by change can help to reduce emotional tensions and fear of change, and prevent unnecessary conflict and resistance to change (Burnes 1996: 187–95).

Ackerman's three perspectives on change, although illustrating an essentially linear paradigm (Figure 22.2), does avoid the planned/emergent change duality that is evident in many typologies. Instead, our attention is drawn to the extent to which change outcomes can be known in advance of the change. This includes: developmental change, characterised by continuously improving on an existing situation; and transitional change where the organisation is transiting from a known old to known new state.

The third perspective offered by Ackerman (1997) refers to transformational change. In this case, the emergence of a new state is unknown until its shape emerges from the old. The change examples discussed later in the chapter also illustrate how different perspectives on change influence method choice and can limit the aims and outcomes of change.

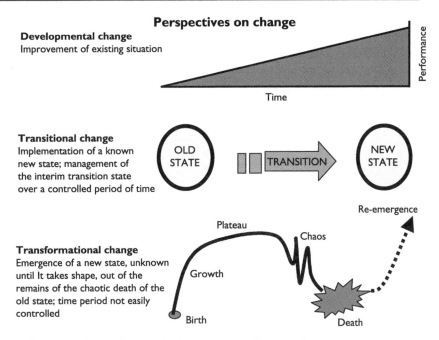

Figure 22.2   Ackerman's three perspectives on change
Source: Adapted from Ackerman (1997) in Iles and Sutherland (2001).

Emerging paradigms of change

Within the 'emerging paradigm' literature, a linear approach to change is abandoned in favour of a more relational interpretation. Emphasis is placed on the complex dynamics of the components of an interconnected social system and the chaotic nature of change (Bartram 2001; Wheatley 2001; Sweeney 2005) Knowledge about how and what to change is generated in the moment of change through social interaction with others. Organisations are therefore urged to become instruments for continuous learning. This involves embedding processes within the organisation for 'learning how to learn' (Argyris and Schon 1978, 1996) and for generating from the learning visions, mindsets and strategies for becoming the change they seek.

Models that attempt to show a generative and non-linear version of the change process tend to be cyclical in character and promote learning as the key to change. There are various influential contributions to this approach to change and notable amongst them are: the learning cycle (Kolb 1984); action research (ironically,[1] Lewin 1946); action learning (Revans 1980); appreciative inquiry (Cooperrider and Srivastva 1987); and the learning organisation (Pedler et al. 1989; Senge 1990; Argyris and Schon 1978, 1996). Fundamentally, all share a view that learning and change are inextricably interconnected.

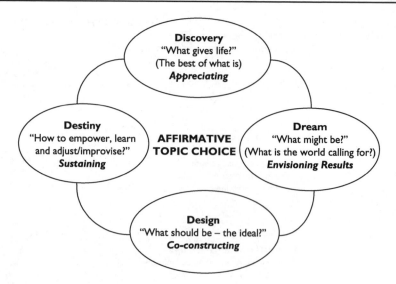

Figure 22.3   Appreciative inquiry 4-D cycle
Source: Cooperrider et al. (2000: 7).

The appreciative inquiry cycle (Figure 22.3) is one example of the models cited here which relies on generative learning. It is also used later in the case examples to illustrate emerging paradigm approach to transformational change. In the change cycle illustrated in Figure 22.3, change is generated by the social actors involved in the change process rather than being something that emerges from the planned and unintended consequences of change.

Choosing change methods

Change methods are derived from particular theories or assumptions about human or organisational behaviour. They are chosen with particular aims of change in mind, and their use in the change effort is designed to remedy diagnosed problems and produce specific outcomes. The challenge for change managers lies in revealing the different assumptions being made about the 'nature of the problem' as well as in providing a basis for assessing the efficacy of the proposed remedy.

There are several major schools of thought within social sciences[2] that have evolved, each with its own ideas. For example, Bolman and Deal (1991) suggest four influential frames of reference. Rational systems theorists will emphasise organisational goals, roles and technology and ways to align structure and process. Human relations theorists will stress the functional interdependence between people and organisations and look to match people's skills, values and aspirations with organisational roles and relationships. Political theorists see power, conflict and the equitable distribution of resources as the central issues, which are resolved through the use or manipulation of influence, power, conflict and bargaining. Symbolic theorists, on the other hand, emphasise meaning and rely on images, drama and storytelling as means for understanding the organisation. The same organisational situation can therefore be viewed in at least four different ways, depending upon how it is framed (Bolman and Deal 1991: 9).

An alternative approach proposed by Allen (2002) is to accept that people in organisations understand and navigate change in different ways. Thus there are multiple change journeys at work. People, she argues, can go on different journeys, yet arrive at the same destination. What is important is 'leveraging the reciprocal influence of individual and organisational transformation to achieve common goals' (p. 9). By this she means to focus on helping 'clients' to find their own unique solutions for integrating and synchronising the diverse initiatives occurring.

A vital part of the change management task involves selecting the methods whose focus matches the purpose and aims of the proposed change. Utilising Kaplan's (1964) quote 'I have found that if you give a little boy a hammer, he will find that everything needs pounding', Tichy (1983: 294–295) cautions managers to avoid faddism in choosing change technologies and what he calls the 'panacea hammers'. Change methods, Tichy advises, should be chosen on the basis of a robust diagnosis, a strategic change plan and an understanding of the variety, scope and contribution of potential methods available.

Speaking of change in relation to management development, Molander and Winterton (1994) propose that method selection should be based on whether change is pitched at individuals, groups or the organisation. How change is implemented, using either a prescriptive or consultative style, can also impact on outcomes. Behavioural change, for example, is perceived as the most common aspect of change management and is usually tackled through individualised training. To target change remedies at behaviour and neglect other influencing variables such as the impact of the environment, culture and work teams is, however, likely to provide only a partial change solution.

Design led by experts can also be problematic, particularly where the involvement of those subject to the change has been minimal. Appraisal, job rotation and mentoring require the active participation of learners and are paramount to their successful implementation: 'the obvious option is to involve them in the design of the development experience' (Molander and Winterton 1994: 89).

It is estimated that two out of three change programmes only partially realise their specified aims and potential (Kotter, 1994: Higgs and Dulewicz 2000; Higgs and Rowland 2001). Some of the reasons cited for this include:

• choosing the wrong approach
• generating little buy-in or commitment
• a lack of resources to implement change

- ignoring the politics and emotions associated with change
- the tendency to focus on a limited number of dimensions of change
- overlooking the strategic aspects of change
- viewing change as a one-time event that starts and stops.

Manager as change agent

That the manager's role in leading change is crucial seems widely accepted among scholars and practitioners in the field (Higgs 2002). Managers are also likely to find themselves occupying any one of several roles as *change strategists* concerned with end results; as *change implementers* concerned with the means of change and overcoming resistance; and as *change recipients* making the means fit the end while developing personal benefits (Kanter et al. 1992).

Adapting to new organic structures and ways of working also requires managers to incorporate values-based strategies and to develop more 'soft skills' in people management. They may need to take on a more facilitative role to empower workers and emphasise a solutions rather than problems focus in managing change. Consistent with emerging paradigm thinking, managers also need to develop a more inclusive approach to interpreting 'reality' and to embrace the realities of others (Pascale 1990: 32).

Leaving aside the debate as to whether the task of change management demands leaders not managers, Higgs attempts to identify a model of leadership that is relevant to the context and complexity of change facing organisations in the early twenty-first century.

Summarising a review of the leadership literature and borrowing from Goffee and Jones (2000), he concludes that leading change is about '*being yourself with skill*'. Comparing models of leadership (Alimo Metcalfe 1995; Bass 1985; Bennis 1989; Goffee and Jones 2000; Higgs and Dulewicz 2000; Kotter 1994; Kouzes and Posner 1988) he sees common agreement on the need for managers to be authentic and to demonstrate emotional intelligence in their approach to change. Whilst the models differ in emphasis, there are some common themes:

1 Reach a shared understanding with stakeholders about source, content and direction of change.
2 Engage stakeholders throughout in devising and implementing the change strategy.
3 Respect diversity of contribution and approach in handling and managing change.
4 Build trusting relationships.
5 Seek to learn continuously from the change and share new learning.
6 Own the change process and see that all goes well.

Case studies in change management

What can be said with some certainty about change management is that there is no 'one best approach' or one single change method that will be capable of tackling the range of problems and situations that arise. Rather, as Iles and Sutherland conclude: 'Managers in the NHS need to be adept at diagnosing organisational situations and skilled at choosing those tools that are best suited to the particular circumstances that confront them' (2001: 19). Here we use three change examples to explore the issues of theory, method and outcomes (Boxes 22.1, 22.2, 22.3).

The second change example (Box 22.2) is funded as a common problem in the health sector (Maher and Penny 2005) and contains

---

Box 22.1   Change example: Devolving financial management decision to service areas

Context driving change: Overspending and lack of accountability at service level.
Change example: Devolving financial management decision to service areas.
Change assumption: Skills gap issue, managers needed training in the new financial information management system (FIMS) through which they could monitor and manage their devolved budgets.
Predicted outcomes: More responsible financial accounting, budget control at source of spends/overspends kept within limits and savings accruing.
Change theory: There is no explicit theory of change operating. This is common in training solutions to change problems. The training solution may rest on one or more cognitive, experiential or adult learning theories that are designed into a learning event to equip learners with new knowledge and skills and lead to behaviour change (see for instance Galbraith 1991 for a summary of adult learning theory). Clearly, as the case shows, transferring learning to behavioural outcomes is a voluntary exercise.
Method: Training for all managers in the use of the new FIMS.
Analysis: The planned-for outcomes of the training did not produce the changes expected. Managers attended training but continued to refer decisions upwards and held off using the system on the grounds that the information contained within it did not match service reality. It emerged that managers collectively were anxious about managing overspends and the potential unpalatable tasks of cutting services and staffing, for which they were unprepared.

The focus of the change programme shifted from providing technical training to uncovering the emotions and blocks that prevented proper budgetary control. A new strategy emerged which involved managers in service planning and budget profiling which were based on customer, stakeholder surveys and employee consultation. Managers became accountable and responsible for the costing and delivery of user-led services they had consulted on and planned and budgeted for. The revised change strategy emerged from the expressed needs, values and emotions of those subject to the change and who helped shape the new approach.

Box 22.2   Change example: Reducing patient waiting times

Context driving change: Government-led improvement agenda.
Change example: Reducing patient waiting times.
Change assumptions: Change is driven by and grounded in data in and about the system not unfounded ideas or visions.
Predicted outcomes: Data provide basis for realistic measures of process improvement. People engaged in the process implicitly derive empowerment and control from their work since it is they who are involved in and assume responsibility for their contribution to continuous improvement.
Change theory: Derived from the application of principles of statistical variance originating from Shewart (1931) and Juran (1964) and incorporated in Deming's (1981) system of profound knowledge of management. Deming's approach to quality improvement draws on a theoretical mix that incorporates a systems view of organisation, knowledge about variation and theory of knowledge and psychology.

Deming's continuous cycle for process improvement involves four steps: a *plan* to improve, *do* what is planned, *study* the results and *act* on what has been learned. The degree to which the founding principles advocated by Deming are designed into some CI processes will impact on outcomes.
Method: Continuous improvement (CI) process mapping.
Staff are trained in CI philosophy – 'plan, do, study, act' – and process mapping. Customer surveys and interviews are also used to generate qualitative data.
Analysis: In this case a process mapping approach was used to scope out the 'patient journey' involved in making an appointment with a specialist consultant. The opening quotation to this chapter captures the essence of the patient-led focus that emerged. Other outcomes were: waiting times cut, a better appreciation of clinical and non-clinical roles and steps involved in the process; time savings; more efficient and patient-friendly processes introduced.[3]

---

aspects of both planned for and emergent change. It corresponds to Ackerman's developmental model in Figure 22.2.

The discussion of the appreciative inquiry example that follows in Figure 22.3 is grounded in the values of emerging paradigm thinking which encourages managers and change agents responsible for implementing change to 'shift their perspective' rather than their tools of practice (Watkins and Mohr 2001). As shown, the methodologies involved could equally be used within planned or emergent change scenarios. What is vital is the focus on the appreciative stance, the constructionist theory and the democratising values that are designed into their use. The example shown in Box 22.3 is based on the well-documented case study of Avon Mexico (Schiller, in Watkins and Mohr 2001: 123–6).

Methods that emanate from emerging paradigm thinking are beginning to be used effectively across all business, government and public sectors, for generating whole system change (see Elliott 1999; Cooper-

Box 22.3

Context: Corporate drive for gender equity in global company.

Change example: Valuing gender diversity.

Change assumptions: That organisations move in the direction of the questions that are asked. The more positive the question asked, the more sustainable the change (Cooperrider et al. 2000).

Predicted outcomes: The outcomes will be generated through the process of inquiry. Stakeholders must trust the process to produce positive outcomes of change (Elliott 1999).

Change theory: Social constructionist theory of change (Berger and Luckman 1977; Cooperrider and Srivastva 1999; Gergen 1992, 1999) provides the foundation to AI. Central to AI is the idea that we 'see what we believe', that reality is created through the language we use and there are multiple realities. The act of asking questions of an organisation or group influences the group in some way. Change begins at the moment the question is posed. Organisations are holistic 'social systems' that evolve towards the most positive images they hold of themselves.

   Change occurs less through the 'official voice' of meetings, committees and exhortations than through inner dialogues that are carried through stories and narratives which people tell themselves and each other (Bushe 2000). Organisational stakeholders are encouraged to pay attention to the 'best there is or can be' in the organisation rather than to problems, which involves a fundamental shift in thinking as well as in associated behaviours.

Method: Appreciative inquiry. Change is generated through an appreciative inquiry research process, which follows a cycle of activities and processes and the creation of new positive images through dialogue. This involves discovering 'the best of what is', dreaming what might be, designing, planning for and co-constructing the ideal future and destiny: empowering, learning, adjusting and improving, and sustaining the new futures. There are several illustrations of this fundamental process in Watkins and Mohr 2001.

Analysis: Workshops were held to introduce the AI theory and protocols to a 'pioneer' group made up of employees and stakeholders who were to conduct the AI interviews. They aimed to identify compelling stories about what gave vitality to the ways women and men worked together within the organisation.

   These inspirational stories revealed best practices and formed the basis for developing a future vision of the company. Reports were drafted, a stakeholder futures conference (summit) was held, consensus was built to capture the best stories, which were grounded in what was currently happening, and to clarify images of the organisation at its best.

   The new vision was activated via co-gender work committees through whom the new culture and values were expressed in employment policies and practices with the intention of creating an 'exceptional twenty-first century organisation'. As important was maintaining the spirit of inquiry, the positivity and solution focused orientation that characterised the approach (Schiller in Watkins and Mohr 2001).

> The appreciative inquiry intervention was credited with helping a successful company become even more successful. Profits were increased and the company won a Catalyst Award for its policies and practices that benefit women in the corporation. The first woman officer made it to the executive committee within six months of the project. The spirit of appreciative inquiry continued to be sustained four years after the inquiry and is part of the alignment with the mission, goals and values of the company (Schiller).

rider et al. 2000; Watkins and Mohr 2001 for examples of appreciative inquiry, and variants of it).

Conclusion

As we see from the examples above, change in the real world does not always correspond to a linear model of change, stable in character, with a beginning, middle and an end. More often what starts off as a seemingly one-off episode or event can become something more complex and transformational. Drawing together the key themes of the chapter, it is evident that the manager's role in change will depend upon the way the change is framed, the scope of change involved and the philosophical orientation that is 'designed into' the change process.

Summary box

- Much of the change agenda faced by a modernising health sector is intentionally transformational. Its reach extends beyond the boundaries of any single organisation and requires change methods and approaches that are up to the scale of this task.
- Intentional transformational change is usually premised on some view, theory or vision about why the change is necessary, which may be externally or internally driven.
- The purpose of much of the transformational change agenda is to produce socio-economic outcomes as well as specific organisational improvements and changes. Collaboration with all stakeholders is vital.
- Transformational change involves making paradigm shifts that involve values and the thinking which underpins them. Change models that emphasise learning are central to this approach.
- There is no single method capable of achieving multilevel, multistakeholder, multidimensional change. A multimethod approach is advised. Aligning method to change theory and paradigm is vital.
- Emerging paradigms based on complexity theory and systems thinking more adequately reflect the level and complexity of contemporary organisational change than do established planned and emergent approaches.
- Although there are plenty of resources on change management, approaches that emphasise analysis rather than prescription offer more credible accounts of change.
- We are all potential change agents.

Self-test exercises

1 Recall a change programme that you have been involved with, and tackle the following questions about what happened, how it worked, and what you learned from it:

- What were the memorable moments? And why?
- What best aspects of the change would you want to see more of?
- Who was involved and how can the 'best of' be extended?

2 How would you assess your current role and contribution to the change agenda in your organisation? What models of change are used and how is change managed? What opportunities are there to help stretch mindsets and achieve change? What can you do to achieve the best that can be?

Notes

1 Although often cited as primary advocate of the planned change method, it should be acknowledged also that Lewin's pioneering work in using action research to help tackle social and organisational problems means his influential legacy can be seen in all three of the paradigms discussed here. See Burnes (1996) for a fuller discussion on this point.
2 Other critiques which show the relationship between ideas about how change occurs and the technology to use to effect change can be found in the typology offered in Tichy (1983: 302–3) and the discussions throughout Pfeffer (1982) and Burrell and Morgan (1980).
3 See case studies by Iles and Sutherland (2001) and Elliott (1999), each citing outcomes similar to those mentioned in this chapter.

References and further reading

Ackerman, L, (1997) Development, transition or transformation: The question of change in organizations. In D. Van Eynde, J. Hoy and D. Van Eynde (eds) *Organisation Development Classics*. San Francisco: Jossey-Bass.

Alimo-Metcalfe, B. (1995) An investigation of female and male constructs of leadership. *Women in Management Review*.

Allen, R.C. (2002) *Guiding Change Journeys. A Synergistic Approach to Organization Transformation*. San Francisco: Jossey-Bass.

Alvesson, M. and Willmott, H. (1996) *Making Sense of Management: A Critical Introduction*. London: Sage.

Ansoff, H.I. (1965) *Corporate Strategy: An Analytic Approach to Business Policy for Growth and Expansion*. New York: McGraw-Hill.

Argyris, C. and Schon D (1978) *Organisational Learning: A Theory of Action Perspective*. Reading, MA: Addison-Wesley.

Argyris, C. and Schon D. (1996) *Organisational Learning II: A Theory Method and Practice*, Reading, Mass: Addison-Wesley

Auster, E.R., Wylie, K.K. and Valente, M. (2005) *Building Capabilities in your Organization*, Basingstoke: Palgrave Macmillan.

Bartram, A. (2001) *Navigating Complexity. The Essential Guide to Complexity Theory in Business Management.* London: The Industrial Society.

Bass, M.B. (1985) *Leadership and Performance beyond Expectations.* New York: Free Press.

Beckhard, R. and Pritchard, W. (1992) *Changing The Essence. The Art of Creating and Leading Fundamental Change in Organizations.* San Francisco: Jossey-Bass.

Bennis, W. (1989) *On Becoming a Leader.* London: Hutchinson.

Berger, P.L. and Luckman, T. (1977), *The Social Construction of Reality. A Treatise in the Sociology of Knowledge*, Harmondsworth: Penguin

Bolman, L.G. and Deal, T. E. (1991) *Reframing Organizations, Artistry, Choice, and Leadership.* San Francisco: Jossey-Bass

Buchanan, D.A. and Boddy, D (1992) *The Expertise of the Change Agent.* Harlow: Prentice Hall.

Burnes, B. (1996) *Managing Change. A Strategic Approach to Organisational Dynamics*, 2nd edn. London: Pitman.

Burrell, G. and Morgan, G. (1980) *Sociological Paradigms and Organisational Analysis: Elements of the Sociology of Corporate Life.* London: Heinemann

Bushe, G.R. (2000) Five theories of change embedded in appreciative inquiry. In D.L. Cooperrider, P.F. Sorensen, D. Whiteney and T. Yaeger (eds) *Appreciative Inquiry. Rethinking Human Organization Toward A Positive Theory of Change.* Champaign, IL: Stipes.

Checkland, P. (1981) *Systems Thinking, Systems Practice.* New York: Wiley.

Checkland, P. and Scholes, (1999) *Soft Systems Methodology in Action.* Chichester: Wiley.

Collins, D. (1998) *Organizational Change Sociological Perspectives.* London: Routledge.

Cooperrider, C. and Srivastva, S. (1987) Appreciative inquiry in organizaional life. *Research in Organizational Change and Development*, 1: 129–69.

Cooperrider, D.L. and Srivastva, S. (1999) *Appreciative Management and Leadership. The Power of Positive Thought and Action in Organizations.* Euclid, OH: Williams Custom publishing.

Cooperrider, D.L., Sorensen, P.F., Whitney, D. and Yaeger, T. (eds) (2000) *Appreciative Inquiry. Rethinking Human Organization Toward A Positive Theory of Change.* Champaign, IL: Stipes.

Dawson, P. (1994) *Organizational Change: A Processual Approach.* London: Paul Chapman.

Deming, W. (1981) *Out of the Crisis.* Cambridge, MA: Massachusetts Institute of Technology.

Dulewicz, V. and Higgs, J.J. (2000) Emotional intelligence: A review and evaluation study. *Journal of Managerial Psychology*, 15(4): 341–68.

Elliott, C. (1999) *Locating the Energy for Change: An Introduction to Appreciative Inquiry.* Winnipeg: International Institute for Sustainable Development.

Fineman, D. (2000) *Emotion in Organisation.* London: Sage.

Galbraith, M.W. (1991) *Facilitating Adult Learning, A Transactional Process.* Malabar, FL: Krieger.

Gergen, K.J. (1992) Organization theory in the postmodern era. In M. Reed and M. Hughes (eds) *Rethinking Organization. New Directions in Organization Theory and Analysis.* London: Sage.

Gergen, K.J. (1999) *An Invitation to Social Construction*. London: Sage.

Goffee, R. and Jones, G. (2000) Why should anyone be led by you? *Harvard Business Review*, September–October: 63–70.

Goleman, D. (1996), *Emotional Intelligence*. London: Bloomsbury.

Handy, C. (1989) *The Age of Unreason*. London: Arrow.

Harwood, A. (2005), Reaching the parts: The use of narrative and storytelling in organizational development. In E. Peck *Organisational Development in Healthcare: Approaches, innovations, achievements*. Oxford: Radcliffe.

Higgs, M. J. (2002) *Leadership – The Long Line: A View on How We Can Make Sense of Leadership in the 21st Century*. Henley: Henley Management College.

Higgs, M.J. and Dulewicz, S.V. (2000) Emotional intelligence, leadership and culture. Paper presented at Emotional Inteligence Conference, London.

Higgs, M.J. and Rowland, D. (2001) Building change leadership capacity: The quest for change competence. *Journal of Change Management*, 1(2): 116–31.

Huczynski, A. A. (1993), *Management Gurus: What Makes Them and How to Become One*. London: Routledge.

Iles, V. and Sutherland, K. (2001) *Managing Change in the NHS*. London: NCCSDO.

Juran, J. (1964) *Managerial Breakthrough*, New York: McGraw-Hill.

Kanter, R.M., Stein, B. and Jick, T. (1992) *The Challenge of Organisational Change*. London: Free Press.

Kaplan, A. (1964) *The Conduct of Inquiry*. San Francisco: Chandler.

Kolb, D. A. (1984) *Experiential Learning: Experience as the Source of Learning and Development*. New York: Prentice-Hall.

Kotter, J. (1994) Leading change: Why transformation efforts fail. *Harvard Business Review*, May–June: 11–16.

Kouzes, J. and Posner, B. (1988) *Encouraging the Heart*. San Francisco: Jossey-Bass.

Lewin, K. (1946) Action research and minority problems. *Journal of Social Issues*, 2: 34–46.

Lewin, K. (1958) Group decisions and social change. In G.E., Swanson T.M. Newcomb and E.L. Hartley (eds) *Readings in Social Psychology*. New York: Holt, Rhinehart and Winston.

Lovell, R. (1994) *Managing Change in the New Public Sector*. Harlow: Longman Civil Services College.

Maher, L. and Penny J. (2005) Service improvement. In E. Peck *Organisational Development in Healthcare: Approaches, Innovations, Achievements*. Oxford: Radcliffe.

Mintzberg, H., Lampel, J. and Anisbrand, B. (1998) *Strategy Safari*. San Francisco: Jossey-Bass.

Molander, C.F. (1986) *Management Development. Key Concepts for Managers and Trainers*. Bromley: Chartwell-Bratt.

Molander, C.F. and Winterton, J. (1994) *Managing Human Resources*. London: Routledge.

Oliver, C. (2005) Critical appreciative inquiry as intervention in organizational discourse. In E. Peck *Organisational Development in Healthcare: Approaches, Innovations, Achievements*. Oxford: Radcliffe.

Pascale, R. (1990) *Managing on the Edge*. Harmondsworth: Penguin.

Peck, E. (2005) *Organisational Development in Healthcare: Approaches, Innovations, Achievements*. Oxford: Radcliffe.

Pedler, J., Boydell, M. and Burgoyne, J. (1989) Towards the learning company. *Management Education and Development*, 20(1):

Pfeffer, J. (1982) *Organizations and Organization Theory*. London: Pitman.

Peppard, J. and Preece, I. (1995) The content, context and process of business process re-engineering. In G. Burke and J. Peppard (eds) *Examining Business Process Re-engineering*. London: Kogan Page.

Pettigrew, A. (1987) *The Management of Strategic Change*. Oxford: Blackwell.

Pettigrew, A., Ferlie, E. and McKee, L. (1992) *Shaping Strategic Change*. London: Sage.

Porter, M (1980) *Competitive Strategy: Techniques for Analyzing Industries and Competitors*. London: Macmillan.

Pugh, D. S. (ed.) (1971) *Organization Theory*. Harmondsworth: Penguin.

Reed, M.I. (1989) *The Sociology of Management*. Hemel Hempstead: Simon and Schuster.

Reed, M. I. (1992) *The Sociology of Organizations Themes, Perspectives and Prospects*. Hemel Hempstead: Simon and Schuster.

Reed, M.I. and Hughes, M. (eds) (1992) *Rethinking Organization. New Directions in Organization Theory and Analysis*. London: Sage.

Revans, R.W. (1980) *Action Learning: New Techniques for Management*. London: Blond and Briggs.

Salovey, P. and Mayer, J.D. (1990) Emotional intellivence. *Imagination, Cognition and Personality*, 9: 185–211.

Schein, E.H. (1969) *Process Consultation: Its Role in Organization Development*. Reading, MA: Addison-Wesley.

Schein, E.H. (1987) Initiating and managing change. In E. H. Schein *Process Consultation. Vol II: Lessons for Managers and Consultants*. Reading, MA: Addison-Wesley.

Senge, P, (1990) *The Fifth Discipline*. London: Doubleday.

Shewart W. (1931) *Economic Control of Quality of Manufactured Product*. Princeton, NJ: Van Nostrand Reinhold.

Silverman, D. (1970) *The Theory of Organisations*. London: Heinemann.

Sweeney, K. (2005) Emergence, complexity and organizational development. In E. Peck *Organisational Development in Healthcare: Approaches, Innovations, Achievements*. Oxford: Radcliffe.

Tichy, N.M. (1983) *Managing Strategic Change. Technical, Political and Cultural Dynamics*. New York: Wiley.

Wanless, D. (2004) *Securing Good Health for the Whole Population. Final Report*. London: HM Treasury.

Watkins, J.M. and Mohr, B.J. (2001) *Appreciative Inquiry. Change at the Speed of Imagination*. San Francisco: Jossey-Bass/Pfeiffer.

Wheatley, M. (2001) *Leadership and the New Science*. San Francisco: Berrett-Koehler.

Websites and resources

Appreciative Inquiry Commons. Devoted to sharing academic resources and practice tools. Includes case studies (see practice and management section): *http://appreciativeinquiry.cwru.edu/*

AI practitioner: *http://aradford@appreciativeinquiry.uk*

www.PositiveEmotions.org

23

Managing resources

Anne Tofts

There are three types of organisation: those who make things happen; those who watch things happen; those who wonder what happened. (Anonymous)

Introduction

The process of planning is essential in all health and care organisations and departments and is as relevant to health and care professionals as to managers. In health systems the world over there is a need to become cost conscious to ensure that increasing health needs and expectations can be met within the limitation of available resources. Resources are becoming scarce (e.g. funding and skilled people) or expensive (e.g. buildings and equipment), whilst an increasing and ageing population is creating greater healthcare need. As expectations within affluent populations also increase there will be a greater need to make choices about the use of funding and between different healthcare treatments. Governments are continuously making choices on public expenditure, for example, between health and education. There may also come a time in affluent societies when individual citizens will need to make personal choices on how they spend disposable income; for instance, choosing between buying a new car or a joint replacement for a member of the family.

Two critical skills that health managers must develop are business planning and budget management. Service priorities must be set to ensure the effective and efficient allocation of resources to meet the most important health needs of populations. A business planning approach builds on the identification of service needs and objectives, planning how best to allocate available resources to achieve those objectives. Health managers can work within agreed business plans if they are able to understand, monitor and manage costs using a budget as a framework for so doing.

This topic is also essential reading for health clinicians and professionals who play a role in managing a service or team. Anybody who has a responsibility for resources including people, equipment and buildings as well as money, should work in partnership with managers and accountants to contribute to the planning and shaping of the resources required for the future delivery of healthcare services.

As with all professions, resource and business planning has built its own terminology and language. This gives a false impression that it is an 'exclusive club' which is attempting to restrict entry. If health systems are to innovate and improve as resources become ever scarce and demands throughout the world ever greater, then all clinical leaders and managers have a responsibility to learn the language of business planning to be able to become active members of 'the club'.

Business planning is the process by which service heads and unit managers plan how best to use available resources to meet the strategic plan. The two main categories of resources that the business plan will address in a health context are people and finance. In turn the business plan should be used to inform the appraisal process – agreeing and reviewing individual objectives. This chapter explores concepts of business planning, financial planning, cost management and preparation of business cases. A list of further reading is also provided as an opportunity to understand issues of resource management in more depth beyond what is possible within this chapter.

Business planning and performance management processes

'Business planning' is a term not often used in healthcare settings. However, a business plan is as relevant in all parts of a health service as it is in the world of business. It is a tool that helps health professionals and managers to plan and communicate future intentions and developments. It is sometimes perceived as not fitting with public sector values and ethos, and instead managers talk about service or development plans. In effect, these are all part of the business planning process. A business plan can be defined as follows:

> A list of actions so ordered as to attain, over a particular time period, certain desired objectives derived from a careful analysis of internal and external factors likely to affect the organisation, which will move the organisation from where it is now to where it wants to be.
> (Puffit 1993: 9)

The attributes of a good plan should be:

- to set out the objectives of the department or unit in relation to the overall organisational goals
- to provide a structured analysis of the current strengths, weaknesses, opportunities and threats in relation to its goals
- to develop a detailed action plan to build on the strengths, address the weaknesses, optimise the opportunities and respond to the threats to achieve the objectives
- to include a budget for the level of financial resource needed to achieve the objectives
- to include a workforce development plan to enable the staff to achieve the objectives.

Where many organisations fail is in the integration of all business or service plans developed by constituent departments or service areas into a single organisation–wide planning framework: a framework that has a cohesive set of broader strategic objectives owned not only by all health professionals and managers within that organisation but also by partner agencies and stakeholders such as patient groups, commissioners and local government.

Business planning framework

The following simple but effective framework for a business plan is often used by health professionals and managers with their teams and stakeholders as a means of fully engaging them from the start. Weak business planning processes can result in faulty assumptions and costly errors in the development of new services and approaches to healthcare (Figure 23.1).

Stakeholder involvement

Every service or department involves a group of individual clinicians and managers contributing to its running and success. Each will have a specific view of the direction that the service or department should be moving in and the best way of doing it. The process of producing a business plan enables everybody to contribute their experience and ideas, providing a common agreement on where the service is going and how to get there. An effective and inclusive business planning process can therefore prove to be a very effective tool for team building, providing a common view of the future and commitment to achieving it. It goes without saying that it is important for all health organisations to engage their stakeholders in the process of service and business planning, stakeholders being those people likely to have an interest in, be affected by, or be able to influence the outcome of the proposed service improvement or business development.

Professionals and managers should be planning a service that meets the needs of their patients, service users and carers. The commissioners or purchasers of the service will also have expectations and views, as will the organisation's own board or senior management team. These are all stakeholders. No single department or service within a health organisation can work in isolation. There is always some level of interdependence. For instance, clinical services rely on non-clinical departments to be able to function effectively. All departments rely on the personnel or human resources department to recruit and retain their staff. Wards are dependent on an efficient service from the hospital porters, patient information and records departments. The list is endless, but the principle is the same – to be effective planning must involve and be owned by all stakeholders who have expectations of that service and will either performance manage it or be in a position to express views on its effectiveness. Planning

---

Where we have been and where we are now

A full analysis of the current services, organisation and its
environment identifying:

- Service and patient needs
- Strengths and weaknesses of the organisation, current service and
  resources
- Opportunities for and threats to the service
- Drivers and barriers to change

Where we want to be

Determining the future direction and goals with key stakeholders
including patients and staff, and identifying:

- Tangible and specific service objectives
- Financial targets
- The workforce and ways of working that will be needed to
  deliver the service objectives
- Infrastructure needed, e.g. information and communication
  systems, buildings and equipment

How we are going to get there

A detailed resource and action plan to achieve the vision and goals
including a gap analysis (what is needed to move from the current
position to the desired future position):

- Service improvements or redesign
- Changes in ways of working and practice
- Staff education and training
- Patient education
- Change management plan
- Equipment requirements
- Building requirements
- Systems changes
- Financial planning

**How will we know how we are doing and when we have got
there?**

Regular monitoring of progress against agreed timescales and
milestones

Ongoing review and refinement of the plan to reflect progress and
changing circumstances

Figure 23.1   Framework for business planning

within one department or service must involve and be owned by the departments that it serves, or upon which it is reliant.

Public sector scorecard

One useful framework to coordinate the expectations and views of a wide range of stakeholders within the business planning process is Moullin's (2002) public sector scorecard approach (Figure 23.2).

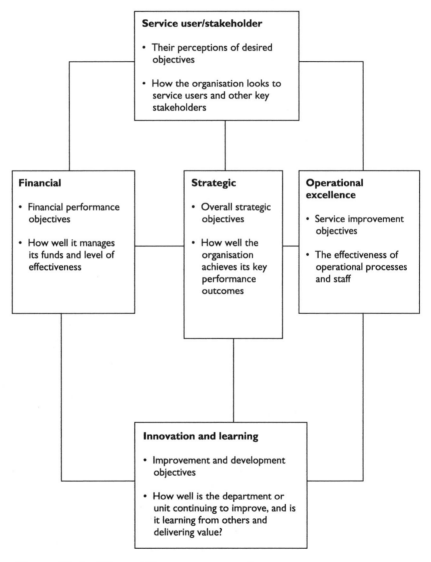

Figure 23.2 The public sector scorecard
Source: Adapted from Moullin 2002

Moullin has developed the ideas of Kaplan and Norton's (1992) balanced scorecard to make it more relevant to the public sector and use of this framework explicitly recognises the increasing importance of the interests of a key stakeholder group: service users and carers. The use of the scorecard can similarly assist managers to work together with professionals to develop multiple objectives that reflect internal organisational and external stakeholder expectations, balancing the need for both quality and financial performance. The scorecard is often used both in the context of performance development and performance measurement. For performance development it provides a framework for a focused review of how well the organisation or department is doing, along with an organisational development plan needed to achieve the agreed objectives. The framework likewise enables tangible objectives to be set and measured in the context of performance management.

If the interests of service users and patients are not met then it is unlikely that the organisation will be able to meet the needs of other stakeholders. In health systems that are adopting an internal market approach that encourages competition and contestability between service providers such as England and the US, it is increasingly important for business planning processes to recognise the relationship between different stakeholder perceptions and the need to meet them all. For instance, a hospital in England that fails to satisfy patients' expectations of the quality of service is unlikely to meet its financial targets as patients choose an alternative service provider. In an urban area with a high density of hospitals and over-supply of beds this could have a significant impact as hospitals find activity levels decreasing.

The public sector scorecard is a useful framework to help teams to analyse how well they are doing against a range of expectations and objectives. It can also be used to shape discussion with stakeholders in determining future objectives. The scorecard approach can likewise be used to determine the purpose of the organisation or department. How closely the service or business purpose is defined will determine how effective the business planning process is and there can be advantage in leaving the purpose very open or flexible, although it is then difficult to plan effectively.

Use of the balanced scorecard enables the organisation to develop and communicate a clear purpose and establish objectives that are aligned with its need to respond to the health needs and expectations of the local population, to meet clinical and service quality standards and to work within financial constraints.

Tangible and achievable objectives

The stated objectives should be SMART – Specific, Measurable, Achievable (i.e. challenging but not unobtainable), Realistic (explicit about constraints) and Time-related (identifying target dates and milestones along the way). An example of an objective that is not SMART would be 'to improve access to services for older people'. If this objective applied to the building of a new unit for older people then it could be restated in SMART objective terms as 'to open a new elderly care unit with 100 daily places in the XX city by 1 January 2008 within a budget of YY'.

A long-term business plan should include both long-term and shorter term SMART objectives. The short-term objectives or milestones should take the service or department in the direction needed to achieve the long-term objective. Regular monitoring and review against short-term objectives allow the manager to review progress towards the long-term objective, adjusting plans accordingly. Short-term objectives should be achievable within the given resources, thus providing staff with a sense of achievement motivating them to continue to strive to achieve the long-term goal.

Analysis of the current service and its environment

Having defined the purpose and long-term goal, the manager should undertake an analysis of the internal and external issues that will impact on the organisation's or department's ability to achieve its objectives. A common and simple model to aid this analysis is SWOT (Strengths, Weaknesses, Opportunities, Threats). What can seem at first glance to be a simple, straightforward analysis can be used as an inclusive process involving staff and other key stakeholders. Some people may perceive strengths as weaknesses, and opportunities as threats, and vice versa and hence the dialogue that the manager engages in will help staff and stakeholders to share their hopes and concerns. A common understanding of objectives and the current situation can also be built through such a dialogue. During the SWOT analysis, all resources should be analysed: staff; financial; equipment; facilities; estates; transport; systems, etc. The SWOT analysis is undertaken in relation to its purpose and objectives and a resource is only a strength if it is 'fit for purpose' to achieve the stated objectives, taking advantage of opportunities and overcoming threats. For example, a health unit that has stated its purpose as specialising in ortho-paedic care will perceive staff with appropriate clinical skills as a strength but staff highly skilled in diabetic care as a weakness. Many business plans include a SWOT analysis but few contain a detailed action plan that addresses this analysis. The action plan should demonstrate how the organisation or department plans to:

- build on its strengths
- overcome its weaknesses
- take advantage of opportunities
- minimise the risk from threats.

The process of scanning the external environment can be further strengthened using the PEST environmental analysis tool (sometimes known as STEP). PEST stands for: Political; Economic; Sociological; Technological.

- *Political*: e.g. national and local government initiatives that may advance or hinder the service/organisational objectives; or patient lobby groups that may have an influence on service developments.
- *Economic*: e.g. budgetary or funding issues at national, local or organisational level that might impact positively or negatively.
- *Sociological*: e.g. demographic trends that may impact on service needs; the organisation's ability to attract the workforce needed to achieve its objectives; or local population growth trends.
- *Technological*: e.g. technological advances in clinical equipment that may assist in the organisation's ability to achieve its service objectives; or advances in information technology.

PEST can help the manager to assess external pressures and influences on their service area or department that may be perceived as opportunities or threats within the SWOT analysis. Short-term objectives can be agreed with staff and other stakeholders which they feel are achievable, address the issues raised within the SWOT analysis and take the organisation or department in the direction of travel required to achieve the long-term goal.

Resource planning

Most of us do not have the luxury of planning from scratch or from a 'clean sheet of paper'. We are normally working with an 'envelope' of resources that has been built up over a period of time. These resources may, for example, be existing buildings, equipment and people with specific sets of skills, knowledge and attitudes. Our ability to change these will be limited by the availability of money and time for investment. Possibly the most important factor to consider is the time period within which a service development must be achieved balanced against the complexity and scale of change required and the existing resource envelope. Can the development realistically be achieved whilst maintaining the existing service? Resource factors must be considered at all stages of the planning process if planning is to be an exercise based in reality and not just the production of a 'wish list' of what it would be nice to do given unlimited resources. It is easy to demotivate staff and service users by setting expectations during the planning process that cannot be met within available timescales or financial resources. An essential part of the planning process is to assess the ability:

- of current resources to be used in new and different ways to meet changing needs
- to increase the productivity of existing resources
- to acquire new resources.

It should always be remembered that within the resource package are included staff (clinical and non-clinical), equipment and buildings as well as money.

Budget and cost management

Budget setting process

A key element of any business planning process is to estimate the level of income and expenditure that will be needed to achieve the objectives and allocate this to specific activities. This is the process of budget setting. A budget is a financial plan that details:

1 *Income*: funding available for a service or department.
2 *Expenditure*: how it is planned to allocate funding.

The process of setting and monitoring budgets should be an important part of both the planning and performance management cycle. Involvement by managers and health professionals at an early stage encourages them to take ownership of a budget that reflects the real needs of their service area. The process of negotiating a budget at the beginning of the financial year is often rushed, resulting in cost–cutting decisions that do not reflect service priorities. Equally, a flawed budget setting and monitoring process at the beginning of the year can lead to unplanned service cuts towards the end of the financial year to quickly reduce expenditure to be able to 'balance the books'. In a well-planned process that fully involves health professionals at all stages, department and service heads would work together to identify areas where cost-effectiveness improvements can be made that will have least effect on the quality of services and patient care. Equally, more effective use will be made of surpluses identified late in the financial year.

Three main types of budget

There are three main techniques of budget setting used in health organisations:

- zero based budgeting
- incremental budgeting
- activity based budgeting.

The *zero based* approach to budgeting is most frequently associated with the business planning process. A zero based budget assumes that the budget is calculated from scratch for each activity needed to achieve the business plan objectives. It starts from zero and re-evaluates all resource assumptions to create a plan for the future.

The *incremental* approach is the most commonly used in many health organisations. It builds on the historical budget, the budget that was in place the previous year. This forms the base line for the following period, usually being uplifted by an agreed percentage for inflation and adjusted for other known factors such as planned savings or growth.

Activity based budgeting provides a detailed budget for each specific activity involved in delivering a service or within a department or organisation. It is only feasible where clear separation between activities can be identified. Activity based budgeting has been used in the National Health Service in the UK to develop 'standard' costs for each unit of activity, for example, consultant episodes or outpatient attendances.

Some of the advantages and disadvantages of each approach are summarised in Table 23.1

Capital and revenue

Financial expenditure is distinguished as capital or revenue and within the public sector each of these is normally funded from different sources. Capital expenditure relates to expenditure that has an ongoing value to the business such as fixed assets including land, buildings, furniture and equipment. To be categorised as capital, items usually have to have a life of more than a year and organisations will typically determine a minimum level of expenditure that is required per item for an asset to be determined as capital. Revenue is expenditure on items that continually recur, or the ongoing costs of running a service or department. Revenue will include employee costs, rent, rates, utilities, consumables and training.

Table 23.1   Advantages and disadvantages of approaches to budgeting

Budget approach	Advantages	Disadvantages
Zero based	• A realistic achievable budget is set • It is proactive and forward looking • Links to business plans • Transparency about the relationship between cost and activity	• Very time consuming to prepare • Requires clear objectives • Can be difficult to implement
Incremental	• A quick process to complete • Accurate if there is little change in activity • Simple to calculate • Builds from a known and proven base	• Use of historical information can lead to inaccuracies • Inefficiencies can be hidden • No relationship between funding, cost and actual activity
Activity based	• Links finance to specific activity • Allows a budget that can flex • Simple to adjust to reflect changing activity levels	• Income may not flex with the budget • Difficult to allocate resources shared by different activities • Changes to standard costs may not be recognised

Budget monitoring

Middle managers and health professionals are usually responsible for the monitoring and control of revenue budgets for their service area or department. Effective budget management is dependent on the effectiveness of the initial budget setting process and the service/department manager and senior health professional should have worked in collaboration with the management accountant at the beginning of the financial year to ensure that a realistic budget was set. To be realistic, a budget should reflect the resources and activity needed to meet the agreed business plan objectives. The manager's monitoring role is then to investigate budget variances during the year, identifying why the variance occurred and taking management action to bring the budget back in line. A budget variance is the difference between planned and actual expenditure. There can be many reasons for variance to occur; it is not always an indication of poor management performance. In time, unforeseen circumstances may mean that the budget no longer reflects reality and should be adjusted for new and changing circumstances – for example, changed levels of service activity, new price discounts negotiated with suppliers, and staff absence resulting in increased use of agency staff.

The designated budget holder should be given responsibility and accountability to be able to control spending in terms of the major expenditure items. They may also be given authority to vire between budgets. Virement is the process by which funds can be moved from one budget heading to another – for example, changes in service activity in a day centre for older people may mean that catering costs are going to be higher than planned, whilst the usage of transport was overestimated and will not cost as much as originally planned. A proportion of the funds allocated to transport can be moved or vired to the catering budget to meet the additional costs. Virement is a way of managing budgets more efficiently when changes in activity or circumstances result in overspends in some areas and underspends in others. In practice, it makes the budget setting and monitoring process more meaningful. When the budget is being renegotiated at the beginning of the following year any virement should be analysed and the proposed budget adjusted to better reflect planned activity and expected costs.

Elements of cost and cost behaviour

Within most organisations, budgets are split between cost centres – an area of activity, department or function might be designated as a cost centre.

Cost classification

Costs can be classified in a number of different ways. The most common used in health settings are:

- *Fixed costs*. These do not vary within a given period of time with the level of use or service activity. They would still have to be paid if a service or department was closed for a short period of time – examples include equipment hire costs and rent.
- *Variable costs*. These vary in direct relation to the level of use or service activity. They do not have to be paid if the level of activity stops – examples include the cost of food consumed by patients and drugs used.
- *Semi-Variable costs*. It is difficult to classify some costs as either fixed or variable – for example, the cost of staff wages on a ward. If the ward closed then it may be possible to move some staff to other wards, but some staff may still have to be paid over a period of time before they could be redeployed. These are classed as semi-variable costs.

Additionally costs can be categorised as direct or indirect: *Direct costs* are those directly related to the department or service, whilst *indirect costs or overheads* are incurred in running the organisation within which the service or department is located. Using a ward as an example, direct costs would include: ward staff costs; bed linen costs; catering costs for the ward's patients. Indirect costs would include: the costs of the hospital having a personnel and finance department to support the ward manager; the sterile supplies department that services the ward. Both direct and indirect costs can be fixed or variable.

The way that indirect costs are allocated to service areas and departments will vary within each organisation. It is important for the service manager to understand how these costs have been allocated as they can have a major impact on unit costs and affect the manager's ability to manage costs and budgets within their area of responsibility.

The concepts of *stepped costs* and *opportunity costs* are also important for a manager to understand. Stepped costs occur when an additional unit of service results in an additional fixed cost. An example of stepped cost would be within an occupational therapy unit where it has been decided that one therapist can safely work with ten patients. At present the unit is only servicing eight patients and there are two spare places – if these two places are filled then there is no increase in the fixed staff cost, although there may be increases in variable costs such as catering. However, if the unit is instead asked to take three additional patients to fill the vacancies then this would require the appointment of an additional member of staff as it would take the unit above the safe ratio of ten patients to one staff. There is a significant increase in the fixed cost; this would be classed as a stepped cost.

Resources are always limited. Therefore using resources in one way is always at the expense of another option. This is the concept of opportunity cost. If a manager has limited development money and has two or more development proposals to consider, then the opportunity cost of funding one proposal is that the resources cannot be used to develop the other proposals. In relation to their own service area or department it is important for all managers:

- to know and understand the indirect and fixed costs
- to control and manage the direct and variable costs.

Developing a business case

A business case is a management tool that supports planning and decision making. Its purpose is to demonstrate how a preferred course of action best meets service needs and provides key decision makers with sufficient information on costs, benefits and risks to be able to assess proposals for service or business developments. A well-prepared business case should provide decision makers with the evidence needed when making choices between different health treatments or approaches. One example drawn from the NHS prison health service is the 'tale of the toenails'. A prison health service was funding a qualified and highly skilled podiatrist to trim the toenails of prisoners on a regular basis as prisoners are not permitted access to scissors on security grounds. A health manager newly recruited to the prison thought that this was an expensive way of providing an essential service and undertook an option appraisal. The manager identified a number of alternative ways of providing this service including training other members of staff who are paid less, and allowing prisoners to use toenail clippers under close supervision of prison officers. Both of these alternative approaches used existing resources differently and the latter involved minimal expenditure on equipment. Each alternative released an expensive resource in the form of the qualified podiatrist for more appropriate work. This may seem to be a simple case study, but every health organisation will have similar examples which if reviewed using business case techniques will release resources which can be used more effectively without involving complex changes.

Framework for a business case

A business case should include:

1 *Scoping the need*:

- Identification of the service or development need and strategic context.
- Strategic assessment of the internal and external environment that impact on the proposed service development using appropriate tools such as SWOT and PEST.
- Implications for maintaining existing services.

- Anticipated outcomes and benefits of the proposed development.
- SMART objectives.

2 *Option appraisal.* This section of the business case identifies at least three different options to achieve the SMART objectives. The options usually include a status quo or 'do nothing' option as a benchmark. The following should be included for *each* option:

- analysis of costs and benefits:
  - — financial
  - — non-financial
- analysis of the feasibility of achieving the SMART objectives
- risk assessment of feasible options.

This section will end with the identification of a *preferred* option after assessing each against agreed criteria.

3 *Implementation plan for the preferred option.* This section provides a detailed analysis and implementation plan for the *preferred* option which includes the following:

- project implementation plan including key milestones and timelines
- benefits realisation plan
- funding strategy – with a detailed cost appraisal (including opportunity costs) and identification of sources of funding
- staff and equipment plan
- change management strategy
- risk management plan
- communication plan
- monitoring and evaluation plan.

The identification and assessment of a range of options should involve a wide range of stakeholders. An inclusive process provides an opportunity to be creative and innovative, to challenge the status quo and constraints, and to ensure that stakeholders understand and are committed to the process of change.

4 *Identification and realisation of benefits.* The definition of SMART objectives to meet the specific service need at the beginning of the process will ensure that options can be evaluated against explicit criteria that are agreed by all stakeholders. Objectives should focus on the desired outcome of the service development; the 'what', and not on the process of achieving that outcome; the 'how'. In the private sector the identification of return on investment (ROI) is a key part of the business case. This is translated in the public sector into identification of quantifiable benefits for the investment made. Benefits may include:

- clinical outcomes
- improvement to the patient experience
- improved quality of life for the patient
- increased capacity to meet demand

- improvements for the workforce
- economic benefits such as efficiency in service delivery, cost savings, increased productivity
- economic benefits gained by returning the patient to work early.

In 2005 the UK government established the Healthcare Industries Task Force. In Figure 23.3 Sir Chris O'Donnell, the Task Force Chairman, explains the role of the task force in seeking to quantify the benefits of using increasingly expensive medical equipment and procedures

A scoring system agreed with stakeholders should be used to ensure an objective evaluation of options and identification of the preferred option. Each option is assessed against each of the agreed benefit criteria. Benefit criteria that might be used to appraise options for introducing a new system of admitting patients for elective surgery might include:

- reduction of waiting times for admission
- improved waiting list management
- patient comfort and safety
- improved utilisation of theatre space
- improved productivity of theatre staff
- improved working environment.

A detailed implementation plan for the preferred option forms part of the business case. This includes a benefits realisation plan which expands on each of the anticipated benefits identified in the option appraisal:

- how will they be achieved
- who will be responsible for ensuring they are achieved
- timescales
- stakeholder involvement
- monitoring and review process.

We are trying to raise the profile of the benefits of innovative medical technology in the NHS, but it's a long, hard struggle because there are countervailing forces of cost pressures and healthcare funding challenges.

They are looking at purchase price only. They're not looking at the benefit side of the equation, the value to the patient of improvement in their quality of life and in fact the value to the system of doing things properly.
What we have got to demonstrate is that [our products] actually help society by having an economic benefit model as well as a clinical benefit model. We can speed up the operation to make our products easy, consistent and fast to implant. We have more than halved the time it takes to implant a knee.

That means you can put more patients through and the waiting list falls. There's less anaesthetic, fewer side effects and you save on bed days. (Sir Chris O'Donnell)

Figure 23.3   The purpose of the UK healthcare industries task force

Source: Extract from 'A healthcare chief shoots from the hip over patient choices' *Daily Telegraph*, 3 January 2006: B5

Risk assessment

An important part of the business case is the identification and assessment of risks associated with the implementation of the preferred option. Once again, it is useful to involve stakeholders in this process. Figure 23.4 provides a simple matrix that can be used. All potential risks, however small or unlikely, are listed and these are then plotted on the matrix according to the likelihood of their occurrence – from rare to certain, along with the impact they will have on the project, from minor to catastrophic.

A risk management strategy must be developed for all risks that fall into the shaded quadrant. A decision will need to be taken on how other risks are to be addressed. It may be decided to ignore those that fall into the 'rare to unlikely' and 'minor to moderate' quadrant. The cost of managing these less likely risks will need to be weighed up against the cost and likelihood of their occurrence.

Conclusion

This chapter has emphasised the need for all health and care managers and professionals to develop an understanding and competence in planning the effective use of the resources of their service. This involves interpretation and management of budgets, understanding the costs of the service and identifying those that can be managed in line with activity, implementing an inclusive and continual business planning process to align available resources with current priorities, and ensuring that investment in service improvement and growth is supported with a

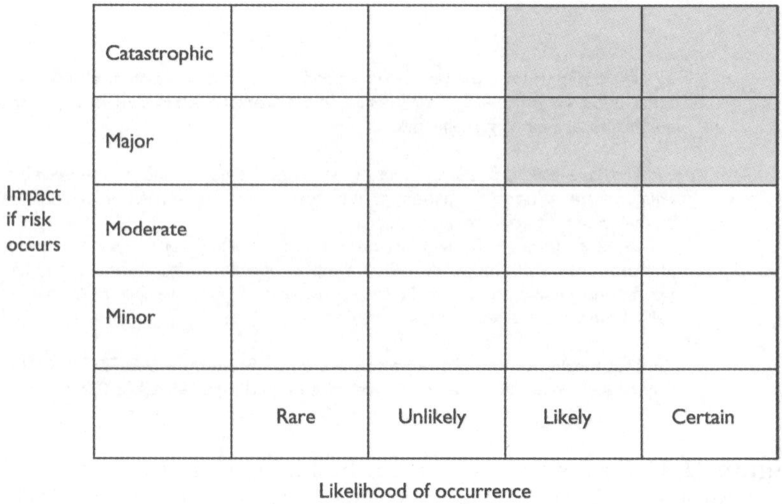

Impact if risk occurs		Rare	Unlikely	Likely	Certain
	Catastrophic				
	Major				
	Moderate				
	Minor				

Likelihood of occurrence

Figure 23.4   Risk assessment framework

robust business case. The key points raised in this chapter are shown in the Summary Box.

Summary box

- Involvement of all key stakeholders from the initial stages of business planning through to implementation will help to gain their commitment to the objectives and change needed to achieve them.
- Managers can and should monitor and control the direct and variable costs of their service area or department.
- Historical and incremental budget setting is unlikely to reflect the true costs of services that are changing.
- Whilst zero based budgeting is preferable to reflect the true activity of a service, it can be a time-consuming and therefore costly exercise.
- Time spent clarifying and quantifying anticipated benefits and objectives of proposed service improvements will help to manage expectations.
- It is important to undertake a full cost-benefit exercise for all proposed service improvements or changes to confirm that the anticipated benefits outweigh the costs.
- Planning within a framework of reality, i.e. working with the available resources or realistic expectations of increased resources, will mean that plans can be realised.
- Business planning is a continuous process in which objectives and plans must be constantly and regularly revisited to ensure they meet changing needs, opportunities and challenges.

Self-test exercises

1 Using the framework in Figure 23.1, reflect on a plan that you or a colleague have written recently for your department or service. Analyse your plan against each of the four stages. Do you think that you have included all aspects? How do you think your plan could be improved?

2 If you currently manage a budget, reflect on how that budget is set? Using the information in Table 23.1, analyse the advantages and disadvantages of the approach that is taken to set your budget currently. Do you think that it is the most effective approach? What recommendations would you make for setting the budget in the following year?

3 Using the concepts of cost and cost behaviour (pp. 411–13), analyse the costs of your service or department identifying those that you can control and those that are out of your control. Are you effectively managing the direct and variable costs within your control? Make recommendations to improve management of those costs.

4 Consider whether the objectives for your service or department are SMART. If they are not, rewrite them as SMART objectives.

5 Reflect on the process of business planning for your service or department. Are all key stakeholders involved in the process? What would you do differently next year to ensure their involvement in and ownership of the process?

References and further reading

Bailey, D. (2002) *The NHS Budget Holders Survival Guide.* London: Royal Society of Medicine Press.

Bean, J. and Hussey, L. (1997a) *Business Planning in the Public Sector.* London: HB Publications.

Bean, J. and Hussey, L. (1997b) *Finance for Non Financial Public Sector Managers.* London: HB Publications.

Brambleby, P. (1995) A survivor's guide to programme budgeting. *Health Policy,* 33(2): 127–45.

Calpin-Davies, P. (1998) A comprehensive business planning approach applied to healthcare. *Nursing Standard,* 12(46): 35–41.

Currie, G. (1999) The influence of middle managers in the business planning process: A case study in the UK NHS. *British Journal of Management,* 10(2): 141.

Dye, J. (2002) Business planning: A template for success. *Clinical Leadership and Management Review,* 16(1): 39–43.

Eagar, K., Grant, P. and Lin, V. (2002) *Health Planning: Australian Perspectives.* London: Allen and Unwin.

Finkler, S. (2005) Cost containment. In A. Kovner and J. Knickman (eds) *Health Care Delivery in the United States,* 8th edn. New York: Springer.

Finkler, S. A. and Kovner, C. T. (2000). *Financial Management for Nurse Managers and Executives,* 2nd edn. Philadelphia: W B Saunders.

Finkler, S. and Ward, D. (1999) *Cost Accounting for Health Care Organisations: Concepts and Applications,* 2nd edn. New York: Aspen.

Harrison, J., Thompson, D., Flanagan, H. and Tonks, P. (1994) Beyond the business plan. *Journal of Health, Organisation and Management,* 8(1): 38–45

Jacobs, K. (1998) Costing healthcare: A study of the introduction of cost and budget reports into a GP association. *Management Accounting Research,* 8(3).

Kaplan, R. and Norton, D. (1992) The balanced scorecard: Measures that drive performance. *Harvard Business Review on Measuring Corporate Performance,* 70(1): 71–9.

Mitton, C. and Donaldson, C. (2004) Health care priority setting: Principles, practice and challenges. *Cost Effectiveness and Resource Allocation,* 2(3).

Moullin, M. (2002) *Delivering Excellence in Health and Social Care: Quality Excellence and Performance Measurement.* Maidenhead: Open University Press.

O'Donnell, C. (2006) A healthcare chief shoots from the hip over patient choices. *Daily Telegraph,* 3 January: B5.

Piggot, C.S. (1996) *Business Planning for NHS Management.* London: Kogan Page.

Puffit, R. (1993) *Business Planning and Marketing: A Guide for the Local Government Cost Centre Manager.* London: Longman.

Ratcliffe, J., Donaldson, C. and Macphee, S. (1996) Programme budgeting and marginal analysis: A case study of maternity services. *Journal of Public Health Medicine,* 18(2): 175–82.

Thompson, D. (1996) Business planning in Hong Kong hospitals: The emergence of a seamless health care management process. *Health Services Management Research*, 9(3): 192–207.

Twaddle, S. and Walker, A. (1995) Programme budgeting and marginal analysis – application within programmes to assist purchasing in Greater Glasgow Health Board. *Health Policy*, 33(2): 91–105.

Worthern, J.C. (1992) Business planning: Who, what, when, where, why and how. *Top Health Care Finance*, 18(3): 1–8.

Websites and resources

Business case template: *www.phac-aspc.gc.ca/pau-uap/fitness/work/case_template_e.html*
www.hfma.org
www.pocketbook.co.uk
www.resource-allocation.com
www.solutionmatrix.com

24

Managing people: the dynamics of teamwork

Helen Parker

Introduction

The workforce or 'people factor' is recognised as an important organisational asset in contributing to performance at an individual, team or organisational level (Senior 1997; Handy 1999). The role of the individual managing and developing this asset is distinct from the human resource (HR) function of organisations, described by Farnham and Horton (1996) as the 'professionalization of people management'. Whilst the HR department provides specialist advice and support to managers in ensuring good employment practice, workforce development and personnel support, the direct management responsibility of teams and individuals is a much closer relationship between the team and the manager and, unlike the HR function, the overall performance of a team is a management responsibility.

The role requires an equal mix of management and leadership skills that on a day-to-day basis are inextricably linked, but in certain situations will require an increased emphasis of one or the other. Working with teams and becoming an effective people manager also requires the individual manager to have an awareness of their own personal effectiveness and leadership style and these concepts are explored in earlier chapters.

Healthcare systems undergoing major reform of structures, systems and workforce, as in the English NHS (DH 2000), require line managers to have the theoretical understanding and practical skills to lead and manage teams to work effectively and efficiently. This is on account of the devolution of corporate objectives to teams of staff across a wider organisation or service. Barber and Strack (2005) sum this up well by stating that 'human resource management is no longer a support function but a core process for line managers' and yet investment in training for these skills is often lacking (Corby 1996; Martinez and Martineau 1998).

Healthcare systems are also complex environments and this is reflected in their diverse structures, cultures and services. Managing this complexity through the development of teamwork is considered an effective and efficient model (Ingram and Desombre 1999; West and Markievicz

2004). Managers at all levels will find themselves working in and with teams that include members from different professional, organisational and cultural backgrounds and successfully managing these potential tensions can be challenging. In addition, most healthcare professionals also belong to more than one team and can face the pressures of competing agendas and demands on their time and therefore the management of the individual requires sensitivity and understanding.

An online search or visit to most academic libraries will reveal the vast amount of literature now available relating to the theory and practice of managing or leading teams. Within this literature are interesting management debates relating to the difference between leadership and management (Kotter 1990) and between groups and teams (Belbin 2000; Clegg et al. 2005) and further reading on these issues is recommended. This chapter examines the broad theoretical concepts of team working and the role of the manager in supporting team development, performance and delivery of agreed objectives.

What is a team?

A simple definition of teams comes from the work of Mohrman et al. (1995) who assert that a team is a 'group of individuals who work together to produce products or deliver services for which they are mutually accountable'. Higgs (1999) in a literature review of definitions of teamworking suggests there is a consensus of opinion that teams have seven common elements and these are outlined in Box 24.1. The element of interdependence of team members in achieving team objectives is an important distinction between a team and a group. A group, as defined by Clegg et al. (2005), can involve two or more people with common goals, but they have no shared responsibility and achieving the goals is less dependent on the members working together. Allen and Hecht (2004) suggest a group of individuals working together under the title of a team do not necessarily achieve more than could be achieved by a group of competent individuals working alone and that empirical evidence shows

---

Box 24.1   Common elements of team definitions

- Common purpose.
- Interdependence.
- Clarity of roles and contribution.
- Satisfaction from mutual working.
- Mutual and individual accountability.
- Realisation of synergies.
- Empowerment.

Source: Higgs (1999).

it is the psychological benefits or the 'romance of teams' that lead people to assume their team is high performing. Belbin (2000) puts forward the view that size is the key differentiator between a team and a group and that when a team reaches a size of more than six to eight then the spread of individual contributions becomes uneven and other factors play a part in the team dynamics such as seniority and professional status. Of course, an appropriately sized team for the task does not automatically create an effective team. This depends on the quality of the development and review process explored below.

There is evidence, however, that teams who do work together effectively produce better outcomes for patients, staff and the organisation (Senior 1997; Borill et al. 2001; Mickan 2005). Examples of this are health maintenance organisations in America that have moved to a team-based model of working and developed strategies for empowering their providers, resulting in significant improvements in the quality and outcomes of their service both for customers and staff (Wade and Kleiner 1998). These teams can be seen to display all the elements described in Box 24.1, but in particular the mutual accountability for performance and patient satisfaction which provides the motivation of members to maximise their individual contribution.

As with many other service industries, healthcare professionals have increasingly needed to work together because of skill specialisation and complex agendas. Team-based working has implications for those with a traditional management background where direct one-to-one management of all individuals within a management portfolio is the norm. Those who take the nature of team-based working seriously understand the concept of teams looking after the individuals within the team, and the organisations being responsible for enabling the teams. In this way, direct responsibility for the day-to-day management of individuals is devolved to a team level enabling them to have greater responsibility for the way in which they work and utilise resources (see West and Markiewicz 2004 for further reading on team-based working).

Characteristics of an effective team

So what is it that sets apart an effective team from other teams and what factors contribute to success or failure? Much has been written on this subject and warrants more detailed study than can be provided here (Hackman 1990; West 2003; Belbin 2004; West and Markiewicz 2004) but is summed up by Parker and Williams (2001: 23) as a team that 'promotes organisational benefits as well as individual mental health and job satisfaction'. This recognises that an effective team is not one that just delivers the organisational objectives but sees team goals and development as equal priorities. Research has also demonstrated that effective teams use healthcare services more efficiently due to effective communication, processes and use of team and organisational resources (Mickan 2005). This reflects the consensus within the literature of the key

---

Box 24.2   Key characteristics of effective teams

• Support from the organisation for team-based working.
• A shared sense of purpose and common goals.
• A shared ownership and accountability for achieving goals.
• A clear and accepted shared leadership model.
• Consensus in decision-making processes.
• A team composition with appropriate skills, resources and experience.
• Mature conflict resolution strategies.
• Clearly defined team roles.
• Clear process for performance management and review.
• A climate of trust, learning and mutual support.

---

characteristics displayed by effective teams summarised in Box 24.2. A significant role for managers is to create an environment where these characteristics can develop and flourish in order to ensure effective team working is achievable and sustainable. This is discussed further below.

The team as an organisational asset

Teams have an important role and function within the organisation as a system. Modernist organisation theory includes a conceptual model of an open system that transforms organisational 'inputs' into 'outputs' (Hatch 1997). Teams can be described as the 'transformers'. Figure 24.1

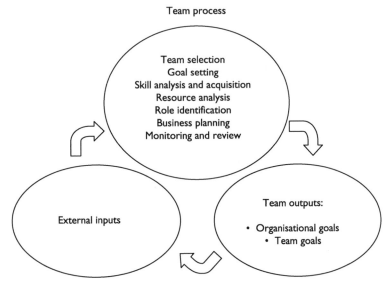

Figure 24.1   The team as transformers

illustrates how teams translate external inputs into agreed objectives and implementation strategies to successfully deliver organisational outputs. To do this, each team needs to be equipped with the skills and expertise to:

- understand the bigger picture of the organisation's vision, values, principles and objectives
- understand other external inputs influencing their environment in which they operate, including national and local political and economic contexts, available resources and different professional and organisational cultures
- translate the external inputs into a team strategy with agreed goals using tools such as business planning, skills and resource analysis and identified team roles
- action a team implementation plan that makes best use of their internal and external resources, recognising individual skills and competencies
- deliver, monitor and review the team outputs within a performance management framework.

The team development process

The theory and concepts of team development are well served in the literature (Adair 1986; Sheard and Kakabadse 2002; West and Markiewicz 2004; Wheelan 2005) with a general consensus that excellent leadership and management skills are required for teams to become highly effective and perform well. The team development process takes teams through various stages that lead to greater autonomy and accountability and the speed with which teams can move through the various stages depends on the individuals involved, the team model (see below) and the nature of management support available. Given the common elements defining teams, it would be unrealistic to expect a group of people immediately and confidently to display these elements without some form of managed development process having occurred. The 'hands-on' role of the manager will be determined largely by how far the team has advanced through the development process, and the extent to which management responsibilities have been devolved to the team. A skill for managers is not only to resist the temptation to 'over-manage' individuals within the team but also to ensure that those with delegated team leadership or management responsibilities have the necessary resources and skills to undertake this role in an effective manner.

The predictable five stages of team development most commonly described in the literature were developed by Tuckman (West and Markiewicz 2004; see Figure 24.2). Tuckman describes the transition through each stage as a continuum but there is some argument which suggests that the process is not necessarily sequential and that a team can move back and forth between the different stages as it responds to

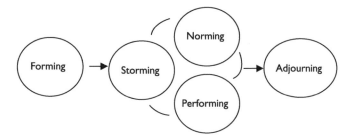

Figure 24.2   Tuckman's stages of team development
Source: Adapted from West and Markiewicz (2004).

external and internal influences (Shaw and Barrett-Power 1998; Sheard and Kakabadse 2002). These stages acknowledge that, like individuals, teams need to mature and develop their collective and emotional competency before they can perform effectively. The behaviour displayed by teams during each phase will provide some insight into the appropriate management support that should be made available to enable teams to move towards performing well and this is described below.

Forming

This stage is characterised by team anxiety, with individual members making initial judgements of each other based on background, skills and personal qualities. They may be reluctant to give much away about themselves but spend time eliciting information about other team members at both personal and professional levels. This is the time when the team collects information on the external inputs available to them and in particular the initial leadership role and management responsibilities expected of them. It could be described as the 'honeymoon period' and individuals are careful not to create conflict or challenge the status quo.

Specific management role

During this stage, the manager should create opportunities for team-building activities that allow the team to get to know and understand one another. There should be a clear management brief that clarifies the team purpose and corporate objectives to be delivered. In supporting the development of a business plan, the manager should indicate the resources available and support the allocation of team roles and responsibilities.

Storming

The honeymoon is over and the team begin to seek clarification of roles and objectives. Conflict can arise as hidden tensions emerge and team members begin to feel comfortable enough to challenge individual behaviours. The team may question some of the initial assumptions made in the forming stage, particularly in relation to allocated roles and the team purpose. Some 'cliques' may develop as team members seek out those with similar views. This is not an unhealthy stage of development and can help the team to build an environment of trust that allows honest exchange but needs to be managed in a timely and sensitive manner in order for the team to move onto the next stage.

Specific management role

This is a stage when a manager may need to employ specific conflict resolution strategies (see Fritchie and Leary 1998). Support will be required in gaining consensus about team direction, roles and ground rules. The manager can facilitate meetings that allow honest discussions and encourage equal participation of all members.

Norming

Having weathered the storm, the team behaviour displays an acceptance of individual roles and responsibilities and cooperation with each other. The levels of trust and commitment to the team increase and communication between members becomes more open. The team settles into an accepted working pattern, positively contributing to a consensus on team strategies and goals. Some conflict may still occur but the team manage it more effectively with clarity in the decision-making process.

Specific management role

The manager needs to ensure that the team behaviour is congruent with organisational objectives as it is possible for teams to establish a working pattern that begins to neglect the corporate objectives. At this stage the manager can agree and facilitate further devolution of management responsibilities, facilitating the ability for the team to be self-managing. The manager can also support and encourage innovation by allowing managed risks to be taken within the team to support learning and professional development.

Performing

The team demonstrates a strong cohesion and team identity. All roles are being performed effectively to achieve organisational and team goals. The team displays the characteristics of an effective team with team members developing roles flexibly to support innovation and are comfortable with self-management. It values the contribution and interdependence of each member and spends time planning and reviewing team outcomes. The team will have also developed effective networks and working relationships with other teams.

Specific management role

At this stage the manager should have very little active management input, moving from a supervising to coaching role. The manager should also be expecting regular feedback of performance and encouraging the team to influence organisational strategies and policies.

Adjourning

This stage applies to teams whose purpose is time-limited such as project teams and can be a result of the task being completed or having been curtailed. Team members may feel a sense of loss or even 'mourn' the ending of the team and can sometimes display behaviour typical of the storming stage, particularly if the ending is not the result of a successful conclusion.

Specific management role

The manager facilitates a formal closure allowing team members to celebrate success or manage feelings of disappointment or failure. The manager should also support individuals in moving on if there is no further role for them within the organisation.

Team models

Within an organisation, or across a healthcare economy, different team models can be observed and should be designed with the team purpose in mind. The basic and most common models in healthcare can be classified into three types: project teams, cross-functional teams and work teams. However, the development and use of information technology within healthcare is now seeing an increase in the number of virtual teams, in both clinical and management settings, in a drive to reduce unnecessary costs associated with face-to-face meetings.

Project teams

Project teams are established with the remit of working on one particular problem or topic and as such they tend to be non-repetitive in nature and focused. These teams generally include members from different organisational functions that take time away from their 'day job' to bring their specific area of expertise to the team collective. As health systems develop to include more partner organisations the membership of these teams can represent a variety of professional and organisational cultures that requires sensitive and capable management to reduce the potential for conflict, demotivation and inability to achieve the agreed objectives. A differentiating factor between these and other teams is that they are time-limited and therefore there is a management responsibility to ensure that the team follows a clear brief and has a system of review in place that clearly identifies when the job is done. If not, there is a danger that the team drifts on without any formal closure. Typically, these teams move through the development process more quickly than other teams in order to achieve the team objective within a given timescale.

Work teams

These are perhaps the team model most people think about when referring to team working. They are typically comprised of individuals with a strong team identity as they work together in that team for most of their working time and do not have an identified end point. Good examples of these in healthcare are clinical teams such as community nursing, therapy or ward teams. These teams can have a varying degree of self-direction and autonomy of decision making. If supported in their development, they can collectively take on the management responsibilities of a traditional line manager in determining allocation of roles and resources, undertaking responsibility for team selection, individual appraisal and regular monitoring and review of team performance.

Cross-functional teams

Cross-functional teams, as the name suggests, brings individuals together from the various functions within an organisation to share ideas, information and expertise. Typically, these teams are involved in strategic planning or overseeing organisational processes and can often represent one or more organisations. This, as Robbins (1984) observes, can mean the team takes longer to move through the forming and storming phase as team members take time to feel comfortable with the different professional and cultural backgrounds. However, this diversity can often mean these teams are highly influential in determining the corporate vision and objectives. A challenge in the management of these teams is agreeing the levels of authority that each team member has in contributing to team decisions on behalf of their organisation or functional department. Also, the success of the team can depend on the extent to which the individual functional departments legitimise the work of the team and are willing to share information and resources to help it achieve its objectives.

Virtual teams

The development of virtual teams in healthcare is on the increase and poses a unique set of challenges for the manager. These teams are described as 'geographically dispersed' but use information technology to achieve a common purpose through interdependent tasks (Lipnack and Stamps 1997). Commonly, they appear in health systems when members from different organisations working at the clinical interface using telemedicine or working on a project or task together find the model of communicating and sharing ideas electronically more efficient in time and other resources. A specific example is strategic planning across a health and social care economy where regular face-to-face contact is less crucial to team success than the sharing of expertise and knowledge. However, it has been identified that these teams still require a certain element of trust to perform effectively and therefore some face-to-face contact is required to achieve this (Panteli and Duncan 2004). It can be argued that because virtual teams are different in various ways, the traditional management theories do not easily transfer and managers need to find new methodologies for providing leadership and support (DeRosa et al. 2004).

These last three teams that are sometimes well established and long term in nature can often move back and forth between the stages of team development due to team and organisational changes. They may need external support to ensure that the development process does not become stifled, paralysing the team in a particular stage. This is particularly evident for a team stuck in the storming phase. Unable to manage conflict effectively, team members change frequently due to high levels of demotivation and job dissatisfaction and lead the team back to the forming/storming phase in a repetitive cycle. It is at this point that the team will need external management support to address the areas of conflict and move on to norm and perform successfully. A more positive characteristic of these teams is the opportunity they have over a longer period of time to develop individual professional roles in a way that leads to innovation and a high level of team competency.

Team roles

A managerial challenge when developing and recruiting teams is to ensure that they have the necessary collective skills and competencies to deliver not only the organisation's business objectives but also to establish effective teamwork. This is achieved by understanding and developing the roles acted out within teams. One of the leading researchers and writers on team roles is Belbin who suggests that each team member fulfils four different roles:

1 *Team role*: the tendency to behave, contribute and interrelate with other team members in a particular way.

2 *Functional role*: the expected duties and role of a team member according to their professional title, e.g. nurse, accountant, surgeon
3 *Professional role*: the professional qualifications and formal training that members bring to the team
4 *Work role*: the tasks and responsibilities, typically management based, that individuals or the team undertake.

Senior (1997) suggests that people's functional roles, whilst necessary for their expertise and knowledge, do not necessarily contribute to the way in which the team operates, makes decisions and implements them. This is related to their team role and the way in which they approach a problem or task. Belbin's research developed the theory that there are a limited number of ways in which individuals can contribute to team working in this way and produced a framework of nine different team roles (see Table 24.1). Belbin states that 'a well-balanced team will encompass all the team roles required for an effective performance' and that where team roles are absent the team will have a lower success rate (Belbin 2000: 114). This has an implication for the recruitment to teams and may not form part of a traditional recruitment process.

A management role in enabling individual participation in the team is ensuring that each member is clear about their role and the associated responsibilities. A lack of clarity about all the four roles each team member undertakes can lead to confusion, mistrust and conflict and potentially impact on corporate and clinical governance.

Belbin's research also identified that the positive characteristics for each team role had an opposite 'weakness', but that this was no more than 'the obverse side of the strength' (Belbin 2003: 49). This is an important observation for managers and other team members as what could be perceived as being a negative or obstructive attitude may indeed be a corresponding weakness that should be seen as a 'trade-off' for the strength. However, Belbin also suggests that some associated weaknesses can undermine the strength and contribute negatively to the effectiveness of the team and need to be managed appropriately (see Table 24.1). The management role is creating an opportunity for individuals to assess their strengths and weaknesses in this context and discover how to play to their strengths and develop strategies to manage their weaknesses.

Sustaining effective teams

No manager can make a team perform well but they can create a supportive environment and ensure the right conditions are in place to encourage the development of the characteristics of effective team working outlined above. Alongside support in progressing through the team development process, the manager can facilitate the team to reflect continually on their role as transformers – how well they are determining

Table 24.1 Belbin team roles

Team role	Weaknesses	
	Allowable	Not allowable
Plant Creative, imaginative, unorthodox. Solves difficult problems	Ignores details. Too preoccupied to communicate effectively	Strong 'ownership' of idea when co-operation with others would yield better results
Resource investigator Extrovert, enthusiastic, communicative. Explores opportunities. Develops contacts	Over-optimistic. Loses interest once initial enthusiasm has passed	Letting people down by not following up arrangements
Coordinator Mature, confident, a good chairperson. Clarifies goals, promotes decision making, delegates well	Can be seen as manipulative. Delegates personal work	Taking credit for the effort of the team
Shaper Challenging, dynamic, thrives on pressure. Has the drive and courage to overcome obstacles	Can provoke others. Hurts people's feelings	Inability to recover situation with good humour or apology
Monitor evaluator Sober, strategic and discerning. Sees all options. Judges accurately	Lacks drive and ability to inspire others. Overly critical	Cynicism without logic
Teamworker Co-operative, mild, perceptive and diplomatic. Listens, builds, averts friction, calms the waters	Indecisive in crunch situations. can be easily influenced	Avoiding situations that may entail pressure
Implementer Disciplined, reliable, conservative and efficient. Turns ideas into practical actions	Somewhat inflexible. Slow to respond to new possibilities	Obstructing change
Completer Painstaking, conscientious, anxious. Searches out errors and omissions. Delivers on time	Inclined to worry unduly. Reluctant to delegate. Can be a nitpicker	Obsessional behaviour
Specialist Single minded, self-starting, dedicated. Provides knowledge and skills in rare supply	Contributes on only a narrow front. Dwells on technicalities. Overlooks the 'big picture'	Ignoring factors outside own area of competence

Source: Belbin (2003).

their objectives, developing appropriate strategies and processes and reviewing their outputs. West and Markiewicz (2004) suggest that promoting a continual cycle of reflection, planning and action will stimulate innovation and improve the performance of the team more effectively than one-off team building events. However, for clinical and management teams with heavy workloads, creating the time and motivation for reflection can be the biggest challenge. It seems obvious to suggest that a team cannot develop the characteristics of effective teamworking without regularly setting time aside as a whole team, and yet this is often a neglected aspect of effective teamwork. Therefore, one of the conditions to be cultivated is that of 'organisational permission' – the explicit development of a culture where time out for team reflection, business planning and appraisal is valued as much as clinical practice and management tasks.

Focusing on the real issues

It is tempting for teams to spend time and effort focusing on those areas that are comfortable, avoid conflict and are working well, as opposed to the aspects of team performance that are the causes of ineffectiveness. Lencioni (2005) suggests that for teams to be sustainable and perform well on an ongoing basis, five common dysfunctions need to be overcome:

- absence of trust
- fear of conflict
- lack of commitment
- avoidance of accountability
- inattention to results.

In order for a team to understand which issues are relevant to them and causing dysfunction as an effective team, they need to have some method for analysing critically the way they function and behave. Team performance reviews enable teams to have constructive feedback and a recognised tool for assessing team performance is an audit questionnaire that can be repeated at regular intervals as a benchmark for improvement. A number of examples are available for use (see Kinlaw 1991; Wheelan 2005; West and Markiewicz 2004) and follow a similar format of Likert scales to assess individual member's agreement or disagreement with statements that reflect optimum team and organisation practices. The outcome of these questionnaires can then be used as a basis for a team action plan and can sometimes highlight tensions in the team that have not surfaced as illustrated in the case study (Box 24.3).

The outcome of the performance review can then inform a team development plan that is agreed by all team members and ensures the team are expending their effort and energies in the areas that will bring about most change and improve performance. The important role for the manager is to ensure that the team has the necessary resources to implement the plan and provide the leadership and support to prevent it becoming a one-off event that is never repeated.

> **Box 24.3   Implementing audit questionnaires: case study**
>
> The author worked with an established team of podiatrists to facilitate effective teamworking. The audit questionnaire (Team Climate Inventory, West and Markiewicz 2004) revealed a marked difference of opinion in how effectively different aspects of team working were performed. In particular, this related to: contribution to decision making; support for new ideas; and transfer of information. Initial thoughts were that this was a difference between grades within the team with senior members not communicating effectively with more junior members, but analysis demonstrated a difference in feelings between full-time and part-time staff. When this issue was worked through as part of a team development plan it transpired that most of the team meetings were held at times when part-time staff were unavailable and no one in the team had addressed this. More significantly, resentment in the part-time staff, previously unexpressed, was able to be managed constructively and a repeat exercise six months later identified a consensus of high performance.

Conclusion

The Summary Box draws together the key themes from this chapter. What cannot be overemphasised, however, is the significant role a manager plays in the development of competent individuals and teams. The 'human factor' within management is critical to success and yet too often the appropriate training and development for managers to equip them with the necessary skills to manage people effectively is neglected in favour of 'harder' management skills. Each manager should critically assess their own knowledge, skills and ability to facilitate effective teamwork and address any gaps through a personal development plan. Equally important is for a manager to recognise the importance of investing time in a team, to actively encourage teams to take time away from the workplace in order to reflect and grow. Valuing this component of teamwork contributes perhaps more than anything else to positive transformation within complex organisations.

> **Summary box**
>
> - The workforce is a significant organisational asset that needs to managed effectively if the organisation is to be successful.
> - Team-based working in organisations is considered an effective and efficient model for managing the complexity of healthcare services.
> - Teams are distinct from groups by their shared accountability for team performance and the interdependence of each member in achieving objectives.
> - Each team member has four distinct roles that form their individual contribution to the team.
> - The team development process and the associated management role are key factors in developing effective teams.
> - Sustaining effective teams is dependent on the organisation investing in time out for the team to regularly reflect on performance and review their business plans and team working processes.

Self-test exercises

1 Does your organisation support team working? Are the right conditions in place to ensure those teams are effective?
2 To which teams do you belong or have responsibility as a line manager? Are the roles and responsibilities within these teams clearly defined?
3 Within the teams can you observe the roles described by Belbin? Are the strengths or weaknesses predominant? What impact does this have on team performance?
4 Do you feel you have the necessary skills and knowledge to support team-based working? In what ways can you develop these skills?

References and further reading

Adair, J. (1986) *Effective Teambuilding*. Aldershot: Gower.

Allen, N. and Hecht, T. (2004) The 'romance' of teams: Toward an understanding of its psychological underpinnings and implications. *Journal of Occupational and Organizational Psychology*, 77: 439–61.

Barber, F. and Strack, R. (2005) The surprising economics of a 'people business'. *Harvard Business Review*, 83(6): 80–90.

Belbin, M. (2000) *Beyond the Team*. Oxford: Butterworth-Heinemann.

Belbin, M. (2003) *Team Roles at Work*. Oxford: Butterworth-Heinemann.

Belbin, R. (2004) *Management Teams: Why They Succeed or Fail*, 2nd edn. London: Elsevier.

Borill, C., West, M., Rees, A., Dawson, J., Shapiro, D., Richards, A., Carletta, J. and Garrard, S. (2001) *The Effectiveness of Health Care Teams in the National Health Service: Final Report for the Department of Health*. London: Department of Health.

Clegg, S., Kornberger, M. and Pitsis, T. (2005) *Managing and Organisations. An Introduction to Theory and Practice*. London: Sage.

Corby, S. (1996) The National Health Service. In D. Farnham and S. Horton *Managing People in the Public Services*. London: Macmillan.

Department of Health (DH, 2000) *The NHS Plan – A Modern and Dependable NHS*. London: Department of Health.

DeRosa, D., Hantula, D., Kock, N. and D'Arcy, J. (2004) Trust and leadership in virtual teamwork: A media naturalness perspective. *Human Resource Management*, 43: 219–32.

Farnham, D. and Horton, S. (1996) *Managing People in the Public Services*. London: Macmillan.

Fritchie, R. and Leary, M. (1998) *Resolving Conflicts in Organisations*. London: Lemos and Crane.

Hackman, J.R. (ed.) (1990) *Groups that Work (and those that don't): Creating Conditions for Effective Teamwork*. San Francisco: Jossey-Bass.

Handy, C. (1999) *Understanding Organisations*, 4th edn. Harmondsworth: Penguin.

Hatch, M. (1997) *Organization Theory: Modern Symbolic and Postmodern Perspectives*. Oxford: Oxford University Press.

Higgs, M. (1999) *Teams and Team Working: What Do We Know?* Henley Management College Report HWP 9911. Henley: Henley Management College.

Ingram, H. and Desombre, T. (1999) Teamwork in healthcare: Lessons from the literature and good practice around the world. *Journal of Management in Medicine*, 13: 15.

Kinlaw, D. (1991) *Developing Superior Work Teams: Building Quality and the Competitive Edge*. Lexington, MA: Lexington Books.

Kotter, J. (1990) *A Force for Change: How Leadership Differs From Management*. London: Free Press.

Lencioni, P. (2005) *Overcoming the Five Dysfunctions of a Team*. San Francisco: Jossey-Bass.

Lipnack, J. and Stamps, J. (1997) *Virtual Teams: Reaching Across Space, Time and Organisations with Technology*. New York. Wiley.

Martinez, J. and Martineau, T. (1998) Rethinking human resources: An agenda for the millennium. *Health Policy and Planning*, 13: 345–58.

Mickan, S. (2005) Evaluating the effectiveness of health care teams. *Australian Health Review*, 29(2): 211–18.

Mohrman, S.A., Cohen, S.G. and Mohrman, A.M. (1995) *Designing Team-Based Organisations*. San Francisco: Jossey-Bass.

Panteli, N. and Duncan, E. (2004) Trust and temporary virtual teams: Alternative explanations and dramaturgical relationships. *Information Technology and People*, 17(4): 423–40.

Parker, S. and Williams, H. (2001) *Effective Teamworking: Reducing the Psychosocial Risks*. Norwich: The Stationery Office.

Robbins, P.R (1984) *Essentials of Organisational Behaviour*. Harlow: Prentice Hall.

Senior, B. (1997) Team roles and team performance: Is there 'really' a link? *Journal of Occupational and Organizational Psychology*, 70(3): 241.

Sheard, A.G. and Kakabadse, A.P. (2002) From loose groups to effective teams: The nine key factors of the team landscape. *Journal of Management Development*, 21(2): 133–51.

Shaw, K. and Barratt-Power, E. (1998) The effects of diversity on small groups and performance. *Human Relations*, 51(10): 1307–25.

Wade, J. and Kleiner, B.H. (1998) Practices of excellent companies in the managed health care industry. *International Journal of Health Care Quality Assurance*, 11(1): 31–5.

West, M. (2003) *Effective Teamwork: Practical Lessons from Organisational Research.* Oxford: Blackwell.

West, M. and Markievicz, L. (2004) *Building Team-based Working – A Practical Guide to Organizational Transformation.* Oxford: Blackwell.

Wheelan, S.A. (2005) *Creating Effective Teams: A Guide for Members and Leaders,* 2nd edn. London: Sage.

Websites and resources

Belbin. Home to the team building work of Meredith Belbin and includes resources and access to online team role inventories: *www.belbin.com*

Businessballs. Free management and training templates, resources and tools: *www.businessballs.com*

EffectiveMeetings. An online resource centre with tools and techniques for effective meetings and also team development resources: *www.effectivemeetings.com*

Leadership through effective HR management. Good people management in healthcare is everybody's business – chief executives, board members and non-executives, HR professionals and staff, general managers, doctors, nurses, allied health professionals, line managers and frontline staff: *www.hrmdev.com*

Management Standards Centre. British government recognised standard-setting body for the management and leadership areas that has online resources outlining a range of management and leadership functions: *www.management-standards.org.uk*

25

User perspectives and user involvement

Shirley McIver

Introduction

The relationship between those who provide health services and the people who use them is a changing one. Most writers link this to other economic and social changes, such as a rise in consumerism associated with the growth of market-based societies which produces rising expectations in the context of scarce resources (Abercrombie 1994; Mechanic 1998; Mays 2000). Falling levels of public trust due to increased media coverage of healthcare scandals, such as the lack of appropriate screening of blood products in France in the 1980s or the Bristol cardiac surgeons in the UK, and greater explicitness about the way care is resourced or rationed have also been cited (Davies 1999). Within this context, many governments have introduced health policy that increases the importance of user perspectives and involving users in decisions. The form this health policy takes varies between countries but there are some common elements. For example, many European countries have developed policies for protecting patients' rights (e.g. Finland) although in some countries these rights are not enforced by legislation (e.g. the UK Patient's Charter). Other countries have carried out national consultation about health priorities (e.g. New Zealand, UK) or have citizen involvement on local health organisations (e.g. Israel, New Zealand, UK) and in most countries there have been surveys to find out users' views (Calnan 1995, 1998). Few countries make involvement in health decision making a legal requirement apart from the UK (Health and Social Care Act 2001).

The issue of user involvement is complex but in this chapter it will be broken down into four main areas. The first section examines evidence about whether user perspectives are different from those of the health professionals and managers and what is known about influences on these perspectives. It also considers the different aims and objectives of user involvement and the advantages in taking a strategic overview to ensure that involvement is integrated into the organisation. The second section looks at the involvement of users in choices about treatment and care, identifying the reasons why this is considered important and ways of helping users to make these decisions such as better information, decision aids and education programmes. The third section examines the involvement of users in service improvement, looking specifically at the involvement of users in clinical research, service planning and evaluation. The importance of the wider context of quality management is emphasised to overcome a common tendency to collect users' views without working out the implications for practice so that changes to services can be produced as a result. The fourth section concentrates on the involvement of the public or local communities and identifies a number of different approaches whilst arguing for the value of community involvement because it has a clearer conceptual foundation than other approaches and is supported by the World Health Organisation.

Identifying users and objectives

The first question important to address is 'why involve users?' This question can be answered in a number of ways. One argument is that health professionals and service users have different interests. Rudolf Klein, for example, argues that where there are scarce resources then different groups will come into conflict about how the resources should be shared out. Some healthcare systems institutionalise the power of the professional expert and so this voice is dominant and other voices become repressed, which results in the interests of users being overlooked (Klein 1984).

There is evidence that health professionals and service users have different views on what are the most important indicators of good quality care. For example, research by Wensing and colleagues (1996) with chronically ill patients and general practitioners, utilising panels, focus group discussions and a written consensus procedure, showed such differences. These included the finding that general practitioners stressed the importance of answering patients' needs, whereas patients wanted to be listened to and taken seriously. Patients valued involvement in decisions, whereas general practitioners thought that patients' capacities should not be overestimated. The findings led the researchers to comment about indicators that are relevant for patients but not for general practitioners:

> To use such indicators as part of quality improvement initiatives might therefore cause resistance among general practitioners and reduce the likelihood of achieving improvement. On the other hand, as many indicators as possible that patients consider relevant should be included to get a full picture of patients' views. Clearly a balance has to be found. (Wensing et al. 1996: 80)

Another argument is that healthcare decisions cannot be based on technical information alone but will also include values and beliefs. This means that those involved will weigh options differently. This can result in two doctors disagreeing about which treatment is best for a patient.

Rakow (2001) found that doctors treating children with congenital heart disease varied in their preferred management for the same patient, leading the researcher to comment: 'Ultimately, it is the outcome and time preferences of patients (or arguably, of parents when they act as proxy decision makers) that should determine choice' (p. 149).

A third argument is that patient involvement in decisions about treatment and care produces better health outcomes. Studies have shown that patients who are informed are more likely to comply with treatment and to have improved outcomes (Kaplan et al. 1989), although, as Angela Coulter (1997) noted, much of this evidence comes from North America and may not apply to publicly funded healthcare systems.

These arguments have a number of consequences. The first is that different interests and values can be found amongst different types of users, as well as between users and health professionals (and also amongst different types of health professionals). This suggests that there is value in distinguishing between regular and occasional users, current and potential users, user advocates and representatives, and carers. It also raises the importance of differential access to 'voice'. Disempowered and vulnerable people are less likely to be able to get their views across.

Another consequence is consideration of the degree of influence that users should have over decisions. This raises questions about the mechanisms and methods for listening to users and involving them in decisions. Clearly the implications will be different if the decision takes places at the micro level of an individual, the meso level of a health organisation, or the macro level of a health system. This presents a complicated set of issues to consider and so it is useful to summarise them into a framework. Various analytical frameworks are available (e.g. Charles and DeMaio 1993; Saltman 1994) but most make distinctions between the individual patient, service users in general and the local community, and between the different types or focus of involvement. There may also be a connection between the focus and the method. Table 25.1 provides a summary showing the connections between these different elements.

It is important that managers involved in health and social care organisations are clear about the three different strands of patient, user and community involvement, understand the arguments for and against involvement and are aware of some of the difficulties that can occur and how they might be overcome. These issues will be covered in more depth in the following three sections. It is also important that a manager new to the area of user involvement knows where to start. If an organisation does not have a user involvement strategy, it can be useful to develop one. (The self-test exercise on pp. 451–2 present some key stages to work through.)

Involving users in choices about treatment and care

There are two main arguments for the importance of involving users in treatment choices. The first relates to the ethical principle of autonomy

Table 25.1   Framework for examining public and patient involvement

Level	Focus	Methods
Micro	Patient information	Different media, link workers
	Patient education	Patient self-management programmes, self help groups
	Patient choice of provider	League tables and performance data, Facilitators
	Patient involvement in treatment and care decisions	Patient consultation aids Decision aids
	Voice (complaints) and redress	Complaints system Patient's advocates Patient's rights
Meso	Evaluation of local services	Patient surveys and other methods Inspection and scrutiny of services
	Planning changes to local services	Membership of decision making groups and organisations
	Allocating resources locally	
	Local accountability	Role of voluntary and community sector organisations Press
Macro	Influencing national health policy and government agenda	National voluntary sector organisations and patient committees and groups
	Input into clinical research agenda	Members of Parliament Lobbying, protest and direct action

which states that individuals have a right to exercise control over decisions which affect their lives. In many countries this had led to legislation to support the clinical duty to obtain informed consent for treatment and participation in research. This means that if users believe that health professionals have abused their right to make informed choices about their care they can seek redress in court. However, legal standards and procedures differ between countries. In the UK users can pursue a case for battery if they feel they have been touched without consent, or for negligence if they consider that they have received insufficient information. The standards are changing in the UK but they are relatively weak compared to some other countries and the professional view of what counts as reasonable information usually has precedence (Doyal 2001).

The second argument is that better information and greater involvement in decisions produces improved health outcomes. Most of the evidence for this has come from the USA and there have not been a large number of studies. The most well known research is that carried out by Kaplan and colleagues who ran a series of studies in which patients with chronic conditions were either given education about treatment options and helped to ask questions in the consultation, or were given only basic information. The patients who had received coaching and support were more involved in the consultation and had significantly better health outcomes using measures such as blood sugar or blood pressure levels, activities of daily living or subjective perceptions (Kaplan et al. 1989).

There is strong evidence that users value information. Lack of information and poor communication are a frequent source of patient dissatisfaction (McIver 1993). This means that the argument for improving information for patients is more straightforward than the argument for greater participation in treatment decisions. A number of authors have pointed out that the extent to which users desire involvement will vary depending on factors such as whether or not it is an emergency situation, or whether they have a chronic condition and have built up knowledge about it. Research has also shown that younger and more highly educated people express a greater desire to be involved in treatment decisions than older people (Coulter 1997; Charles et al. 1997).

The main arguments against providing patients with better information and giving them more opportunity to get involved in treatment and care decisions are the difficulties and the resource implications. As Angela Coulter points out:

> It is certainly asking a great deal of doctors to expect them to provide full information about the risks and benefits of all treatment options, given the short consultation times experienced in most busy general practice and outpatient clinics and the fact that they may not have all the facts at their fingertips anyway. (Coulter 1997: 116)

Difficulties lie not just in conveying complex information about the risks and benefits of one course of action over another, but also in establishing what is actually happening in a consultation and then changing patterns of established behaviour. For example, research carried out by Fiona Stevenson and colleagues (2000) showed that although the majority of patients in the study believed that talking to their doctors about the medicines they were taking was useful and that they were encouraged to do so, observations of the consultations showed that in reality this did not happen. Even when information was shared, patients' beliefs were not generally taken seriously. Solutions to these problems lie in creating standard treatment information packages that can be adapted for individual use, usually know as 'decision aids' and providing alternative methods of informing, educating and supporting users.

There has been an increase in the number of decision aids being constructed and tested. A systematic review identified 17 that had been subject to randomised controlled trials to assess the impact on health outcomes (O'Connor et al. 1999). A decision aid has the following features that distinguish it from more general patient information:

- information tailored to patients' health status
- values classification
- examples of other patients
- guidance or coaching in shared decision making

- different modes of delivery
- not educational materials that inform about health issues in general way
- not passive informed consent materials
- not designed to promote compliance with recommended option.

Although decision aids may not be useful in all situations, they are valuable when the options have major differences in outcomes or complications, decisions require trade-offs between short-term and long-term outcomes, one choice can result in a small chance of a grave outcome or there are marginal differences in outcomes between options. The systematic review found that trials were consistent in showing that decision aids do a better job than usual care in improving patients' knowledge about options, reducing their decision conflict, and stimulating patients to take a more active role in decision making without increasing their anxiety. The researchers concluded that 'the largest and most consistent benefit of decision aids over usual care is better knowledge of options and outcomes. . . . Decision aids increased active participation in decision making' (O'Connor et al. 1999: 733).

There have also been developments in providing alternative ways of educating and supporting patients. One of these is the chronic disease self-management programme developed by Professor Kate Lorig and colleagues at the University of Stanford in the USA. This is a community-based patient self-management education course that uses trained people who have a chronic condition to deliver the programme. It covers topics such as exercise and nutrition, use of cognitive symptom management techniques, fatigue and sleep management, dealing with emotions of anger, fear and depression, communication and problem solving and decision making. A randomised controlled trial showed that treatment subjects, when compared with controls, demonstrated improvements at six months in weekly minutes of exercise, frequency of cognitive symptom management, communications with physicians, self-reported health, health distress, fatigue, disability and social/role activities limitations. Also they had fewer hospitalisations and days in hospital, but no differences were found in physical/pain discomfort or psychological well-being (Lorig et al. 1999). One of the main ways in which managers can help in the development of greater user involvement in treatment and care decisions is to make sure that the organisation is helping clinicians to provide good quality information (see self-test exercises p. 451).

The linked task of making sure informed consent procedures are clear and monitoring the implementation of these procedures is also vital. Other important steps are providing advocates and interpreters to help vulnerable people and those who have difficulty communicating, facilitating access to self-help and support groups and providing resources to enable local access to chronic disease self-management programmes.

Involving users in service improvement

The literature on quality management emphasises the importance of focusing on the customer to achieve services that meet their needs. The health sector has adopted many of the approaches used in manufacturing and other sectors to manage and improve service quality, including carrying out market research to find out users' views. The most important point to be made about involving users in quality improvement initiatives such as service planning and evaluation is that this involvement must not be carried out as a separate activity. The quality management context, including the systems for assuring and accounting for quality in an organisation should be linked together. This principle has been promoted in many countries (for example, the system of clinical governance in the UK) and internationally by the World Health Organisation (WHO).

An example of this is the International Alliance for Patient Safety which has been established by the WHO. There is also evidence that the importance of the user's perspective on what comprises good quality care has gained widespread acceptance. A seminar entitled 'Through the Patient's Eyes', which was attended by 64 individuals from 29 countries in Salzburg in 1998, adopted the guiding principle of 'nothing about me without me' and created the country of PeoplePower. This set out a vision for the future that included the principles of production, governance and accountability created by patients and health professionals working closely together (Delbanco et al. 2001).

There are a number of stages in health and social care service development when users can be involved, but three are particularly important and have received most attention:

1 During research to find out which treatments and services are most effective.
2 During the planning, development and redesign of services.
3 During the evaluation of services.

This section will briefly examine each of these areas in turn before considering some of the particular difficulties encountered in this sector.

The value of consumer involvement in health research is a relatively recent activity but one that has been acknowledged internationally through organisations such as the Cochrane Collaboration, the Consumers Health Forum of Australia and the UK Health Technology Assessment Programme (Telford et al. 2004). This stretches beyond issues around the involvement of users as research subjects into their involvement at all stages in the design, conduct and dissemination of clinical and health services research.

As Charlotte Williamson has pointed out, consumer groups have for some time lobbied governments and professional bodies over their concerns about the lack of investigation of certain topics, of poorly designed and unsafe research and a disregard of research evidence from other countries, and this had some impact. Members of consumer groups have pressed research organisations to include consumers on their research committees, or they have initiated research themselves and invited clinicians and researchers to join them (Williamson 2001). Most countries have identified a need for the training of users if they are to be able to take part in research a meaningful way. A US course called LEAD (Leadership, Education and Advocacy Development) is now seen as a prerequisite for women participating in breast cancer research activities funded by the US Department of Defense and the National Cancer Institute, and this is being attended by consumers from other countries such as Australia (Goodare and Lockwood 1999). In the UK, the Department of Health has set up an organisation called Involve to support and promote public and user involvement in health and social care research and this funds research and produces a newsletter. In 2004 a project to assess training provision and participants' experiences was carried out and this confirmed the value of training, leading the researchers to comment: 'We recommend that training should be an integral, vital part of any research activity if service user involvement is to be effective and meaningful' (Lockey et al. 2004).

User involvement in the planning and development of health services is also a relatively recent activity. A systematic review of the literature on this subject identified reports going back to the 1980s (Crawford et al. 2002). Very few of these assessed the subsequent impact on quality of care although the researchers were careful to point out that the absence of evidence should not be mistaken for the absence of effect and they were able to identify a number of improvements to services that resulted from user involvement (see Box 25.1).

Users can be involved either indirectly or directly in planning and development. They can be involved indirectly by providing their views through a market research technique such as focus group discussions, interviews or a questionnaire survey, which are then taken into consideration along with other information by health professionals making the planning decisions. Alternatively they can be directly involved on committees or in workshops where decisions are made. Little research has been carried out on which methods are the most effectives for involving users. One useful piece of research was carried out in the UK by the North of England evidence-based guideline development programme (van Wersch and Eccles 2001). Four different approaches were tried out:

- including individual patients in guideline development groups
- a 'one-off' meeting with patients
- a series of workshops with patients
- including a patient advocate in guideline development groups.

The researchers found that when individual patients were included in guideline development groups they contributed infrequently and had problems with the use of technical language. In the 'one-off' meeting the users again had problems with the medical terminology but the group were interested in the sections on patient education and self-management. The workshops enabled the patients to have explanations

Box 25.1   Summary of findings of systematic review on user involvement in planning and development of health services

- There was evidence of an impact upon the patients involved. Several papers commented that patients who participated in initiatives welcomed the opportunity to be involved and that their self-esteem improved as a result of their contributions, although there were also studies in which patients described dissatisfaction with the process.
- Among the most frequently reported effects of involving patients was the production of new or improved sources of information for patients.
- Other changes included making services more accessible, such as extending opening times, improving transport to treatment units, and improving access for people with disabilities.
- Several reports described new services being commissioned as a result of the requests of patients, including advocacy, initiatives aimed at improving opportunities for employment, complementary medicine, crisis services, and fertility treatments. Two reports describe how involving patients led to proposals to close hospitals being modified or abandoned.
- Eight reports stated that initiatives had a more general effect on organisational attitudes to involving patients, including comments that staff attitudes to involving patients became more favourable and that the culture of organisations changed in a way that made them more open to involving patients.
- Some projects resulted in further initiatives aimed at strengthening the involvement of patients.
- Concerns were also expressed by researchers who found evidence that involving patients was used to legitimise decisions that would have been made whether or not patients supported them.
- Attempts to gauge the overall impact of involving patients had been made by conducting surveys of participants and retrospectively examining records of meetings. A survey of the leaders of public involvement initiatives of Health Systems Agencies in the United States in 1980 asked respondents to judge the effects of involving patients and 75% of those who replied said that involving patients had improved the quality of health services and 46% (71) that it had led to improvements in people's health.
- Facilitated meetings between workers in primary care and patients with diabetes in 17 primary care centres in Stockholm in the mid–1980s generated 196 plans for improving patient care. Eighteen months later the extent to which plans had been implemented was evaluated and 70% (137) of plans had been implemented.

Source: Crawford et al (2002)

about the technical elements of the guideline development so patients could then make relevant suggestions but this was relatively resource intensive. The patient advocate within the guideline development group was familiar with the terminology, had the confidence to speak and was able to contribute.

The findings suggest that when users are involved directly on working groups or committees this should be someone who has either been trained to speak on behalf of patients or is experienced in doing so. It also reinforces the message delivered earlier about the importance of investing in training for users involved in health service activities. The findings about the effectiveness of patient advocates and representatives is interesting because there is a view amongst health professionals that such people lose their amateur status and so become unrepresentative of the majority of users. However, this is only a problem if the role of the user on the committee or group is unclear. Is the person speaking on behalf of a particular group of users (for example, they may have been elected by a voluntary sector organisation to represent the interests of that group), or are they bringing information summarised from research into users' views, or are they speaking from their own experience of using services?

There is evidence that patients like patient advocates to speak on their behalf. A questionnaire survey of patients carried out in Scotland by Entwistle and colleagues (2003) asked which of three methods – patient's representatives, telephone comments line or a feedback website – they preferred. Although many indicated they would be reluctant to approach their healthcare providers about perceived shortfalls in care because they lacked confidence that they would get any response, more supported the patient representative method than the other methods.

Of the three main stages of health and social care service development, the one with the longest history is that of user evaluation of services. Patient and user 'satisfaction' surveys have been carried out in many countries since the 1970s. Despite this, 'satisfaction' is a complex and little understood concept in the health sector. As Williams (1994) writes: 'We do not currently know how patients evaluate and, because of this, inferences made from many satisfaction surveys may not accurately embody the true beliefs of service users.'

Some of this complexity is due to the different types of information that can be collected from users. Wensing and Elwyn (2002) summarise this along two dimensions: whether users are evaluating their own health outcome or whether they are evaluating the service provided, and whether they are reporting their experiences or rating them in some way. There has been progress in recent years, however. A systematic review of the literature on the measurement of satisfaction with healthcare and the implications for practice was carried out by Crow et al. (2002) This provides a good summary of the key issues and makes a number of methodological recommendations. There is also a survey advice centre for the UK NHS patient survey programme run by Picker Institute Europe, an organisation that produces a newsletter dedicated to sharing good practice on improving the patient's experience.

One of the most important difficulties experienced in the health and social care sector is that of involving groups of people who are vulnerable or who have communication problems, such as those with learning disabilities, autism or dementia, but examples can be found:

- Researchers at the Norah Fry Research Centre at the University of Bristol, UK involved service users with learning difficulties in a project on gender issues in service provision that used a questionnaire survey approach (Towsley 2000).
- The Alzheimer's Society won an award in 2001 for its involvement of users in all aspects of its research programme using a Consumer Network approach.
- Potter and Whittaker (2001) explored the way in which children with a diagnosis of autism communicated and how the environment could enable them.

Tailoring approaches to capture the views of these groups of people is still a methodologically underdeveloped area but the research so far suggests that indirect approaches to questions using stimuli such as singing, pictures, reminiscence and questions during everyday activities work best, although advocates, interpreters and people with special skills may be needed (McIver 2005). A key task for managers lies in making sure that patient surveys and similar activities designed to get users' views about services are linked to other mechanisms to assure and improve the quality of services. A common failing of patient surveys has been an inability to use the findings to improve services (see self-test exercises p. 452).

Involving potential users and communities

This final section examines the involvement of 'the public' or local communities in health and social care decisions. This can encompass a range of different activities at both the national and local level such as: lay representation on professional bodies or national inspectorates; national consultation exercises; lay representation on the governing boards of local organisations; and consultation with local communities. Three main types of approaches can be identified: public representation on committees and governing boards; market research and opinion polls; and community involvement. These approaches have different aims and serve different purposes although there is a general lack of clarity around the role and function of involving the public in these different ways. The most developed approach is that of community involvement and several arguments can be put forward for why it is important.

First, it can be seen as a basic right for citizens. Many countries have signed up to the World Health Organisation Alma-Ata Declaration 1978 that stated: 'the people have the right and duty to participate individually and collectively in the planning and implementation of their health care'.

A second reason linked to this is that it gives people an enhanced sense of self-esteem and capacity to control their own lives and reaffirms the role of people in managing their own health (Annett and Nickson 1991). More typically, health services providers have seen community consultation as a way of finding out local needs and priorities for resource allocation. Associated with this is the fact that involvement can enhance accountability to local communities through more open decision making and participative democracy. Community involvement is a rather broad and general concept that can include a wide range of activities. A useful definition is provided by Zakus and Lysack (1998: 2):

> Community or public participation in health, sometimes called citizen or consumer involvement, may be defined as the process by which members of the community, either individually or collectively and with varying levels of commitment:
>
> (a) develop the capability to assume greater responsibility for assessing their health needs and problems
> (b) plan and then act to implement their solutions
> (c) create and maintain organisations in support of these efforts
> (d) evaluate the effects and bring about necessary adjustments in goals and programmes on an ongoing basis
>
> Community participation is therefore a strategy that provides people with the sense that they can solve their problems through careful reflection and collective action.

This is a helpful definition because it makes very clear the different stages involved. That is, it emphasises the fact that local communities are not necessarily aware of their own health needs and so health planners cannot expect to find out needs by just asking people. Public health doctors and others will have information that they can share with local communities to help inform their discussions. It also identifies the importance of establishing and resourcing community organisations that can support communities during the process of assessing, identifying and implementing solutions. Finally, it highlights the need for regular evaluation to assess the impact of activities and measure progress towards objectives.

One of the advantages of taking a community development approach is that it provides a framework that can encompass a range of methods for listening to the views of local people and can coordinate this information collection. A systematic literature review to establish evidence for what is successful in community involvement identified the following key elements (Home Office 2004):

1 Understand the geography and socio-demographic features of the local community, identify local circumstances that may present barriers (e.g. transport) and act to overcome these.
2 Engage the community in project management.
3 Develop targeted and universal strategies to reach all members of the local community.
4 Engage in training and capacity building.
5 Provide information and publicity.
6 Evaluate progress and identify barriers.
7 Work in partnership with local voluntary sector and other agencies.

The involvement of the public in priority setting and rationing in healthcare has become of particular interest in many countries in recent years.

A range of different methods has been used including surveys, meetings, focus groups and panels and rapid appraisal, as well as various techniques to elicit values or rank and rate different options (Mullen and Spurgeon 2000). A number of deliberative methods have also been piloted. The most well known is the citizens' jury or planning cell, an approach used in the USA, UK and Europe to involve citizens in planning decisions (Stewart et al. 1994). The key features of deliberative methods are: the provision of information to participants in a way that does not rely on a high literacy level (e.g. through presentations or role play); the opportunity for participants to ask questions to get the information they need; time for discussion and debate between participants to enable them to work through the implications of the information. The assumption is that this approach will enable participants to develop a more informed view and that this will be more stable than that produced in response to questions in a survey (Dolan et al. 1999). Box 25.2 summarises the findings of an evaluation of citizens' juries in the UK.

An important task for managers is to make sure that community involvement takes places within a framework that improves networking and coordination between different agencies in order to minimise the duplication of information collection and maximise the effective use of resources. A difficult but necessary aspect of this is to assess the impact

---

Box 25.2   Findings from an evaluation of citizens' juries in healthcare in the UK

The citizens' juries enabled local people to contribute to debates about funding priorities within service areas for five reasons:

1 *Clarity and focus:* The method requires a specific question. This ensures that there is a focus to the issue which enhances a person's ability to get to grips with it. Also jurors were given a definite task to perform so expectations were clear.
2 *Information provision:* Witness presentations enable jurors of all literacy levels to hear about the issues in an interesting and accessible way. Questioning of witnesses allows people to get information relevant to their needs.
3 *Discussion and deliberation:* Time allowed for discussion in small and large groups enabled people to exchange views, share ideas and work together as a team. This enhanced their understanding of issues, broadened their perspective and maintained their commitment to working hard on the task.
4 *Recommendations:* The process enabled local people to formulate a number of practical recommendations about what action the organisation should take to address the issue. This was useful for the organisation because the implications were clear and it facilitated project planning.
5 *Accountability:* The citizens' jury process made clear what was expected of the organisation. The recommendations went to a public board meeting and this made sure they got onto the organisation's agenda. Local publicity and observers ensured that the organisation had to respond.

Source: McIver (1998).

of community involvement activities to measure progress against goals and account for the use of resources (see self-test exercises p. 452 on measuring the impact of community involvement).

Conclusion

Managers can have an important role to play in facilitating the development of user involvement through making sure that a strategic approach is adopted that covers different aspects of involvement, including patient involvement in choice of treatment, user involvement in service improvement and community involvement in tackling local health problems. They can help to create an organisation that values the user's voice as an integral part of its activities and one which learns from its experiences and develops the skills of its staff by evaluating user involvement initiatives and mechanisms.

Self-test exercises

Stages in developing a user involvement strategy

1 Has there been any mapping of current user involvement activities? What kind of information is being produced for users? Is it co-ordinated? Is there user involvement in service improvement? Are there mechanisms to ensure users' views are heard at all levels in the organisation? How diverse is the range of views heard? Are some groups of users overlooked, such as the vulnerable, children or people with communication difficulties? What relationships exist with local communities? Are there networks linking different organisations representing users and community interests?
2 How would you analyse the internal environment? Who would you involve? What are the strengths and weaknesses of the current mechanisms to involve users?
3 How would you analyse the external environment? What are the pressures supporting user involvement or creating barriers to it?
4 What other information would be useful? Policy documents and/or evidence of what works? What are other similar organisations doing?
5 How would you identify priorities from the list of possible activities?
6 How would you develop a consensus amongst stakeholders on what are the priorities for action?
7 How would you identify the resources to address the priorities?
8 Who will lead on developing and overseeing the implementation of an action plan?

Summary box

- Different interests and values can be found amongst different types of users, as well as between users and health professionals so it is important to distinguish between groups of users to make sure that they are involved.
- Disempowered and vulnerable people are less likely to be able to get their views across.
- It is important that managers involved in health and social care organisations are clear about the three different strands of patient, user and community involvement, understand the arguments for and against involvement and are aware of some of the difficulties that can occur and how they might be overcome.
- There is strong evidence that users want better health information because lack of information and poor communication are a frequent source of patient dissatisfaction. This means that the argument for improving information for patients is clearer than the argument for greater participation in treatment decisions and is a good place to begin to develop patient choice.
- Decision aids and self-management programmes are ways of helping users to become more informed and better able to take part in decisions about choice of treatment.
- There are many examples of ways in which users have been involved in clinical research, service planning and evaluation, but it is important that this involvement is set within the wider context of quality management so that improvements in services can be produced as a result
- The public have been involved as members of committees and groups at both national and local level through market research techniques and opinion polls and through deliberative methods which are thought to facilitate the development of a more informed view.
- Many writers argue that a community involvement approach should be adopted because this is supported by the World Health Organisation and concentrates on the benefits brought by enabling people to solve their own problems through collective action.

---

9 Is there a way of reporting on the progress of the action plan to the governing board of the organisation?

10 When will progress against achievements be assessed?

Checklist for developing good quality information

1 Identify sources of up-to-date evidence that can be used in the information.

2 Find out from users what they want to know and when they need to know it.

3 Review what information is already available and look for sources that might be adapted or used.

4 Work with clinicians and users to develop draft information and test it

out on users, improving the clarity of the language and presentation as required.

5 Think about using a variety of different media to make it accessible to different types of users at different times.

6 Make sure that all professionals involved are referring to the same information and are consistent in what they say to users.

7 Consider whether the information could be taken further to educate patients to better manage their condition and if so look for or set up a self-management programme.

8 Consider whether users might benefit from information about sources of support.

9 Evaluate the effectiveness of the information in fulfilling the aims.

Using the findings of patient surveys to improve services

Your organisation wants to listen to the views of its service users in order to improve services and it recently carried out a self-completion questionnaire survey of patients about their satisfaction with services. Unfortunately the response rate was only 10% and the questionnaires have not been analysed as the project manager is on extended sick leave. You have been given the job of working out what to do next.

1 What might be reasons why the response rate was so low?
2 Would it be worth analysing the findings?
3 What could you do to increase the response rate in future surveys?
4 What other methods could you adopt to get users' views?
5 What other sources of information could you use together with the findings to help you identify areas that might be causing problems for users?
6 What would you do when you had identified a problem area? What method could you adopt to investigate the root cause of the problem?
7 How would you develop ideas for overcoming the problem? Who would you involve?
8 How would you report back to users about what had been the findings and impact of the survey?

Measuring the impact of community involvement activities

1 How would you measure the impact on services (e.g. changes in uptake, new services being offered, changes in location of services)?
2 How would you measure the impact on service users (e.g. greater or more appropriate use of services, more diverse range of users, greater willingness to get involved or provide their views)?
3 How would you measure the impact on staff (e.g. greater staff satisfaction, less sickness leave)?
4 How would you measure the effect on other agencies (e.g. better

networking, more appropriate referrals from and to other agencies, greater level of activities)?

5 How would you measure the impact on community health (e.g. greater uptake in screening programmes and other services; greater uptake of sport, leisure and recreation facilities; improvements to the local environment, decline in crime rates)?

References and further reading

Abercrombie, N. (1994) Authority and consumer society. In R. Keat, N. Whiteley and N. Abercrombie *The Authority of the Consumer*. London: Routledge.

Annett, H. and Nickson, P. (1991) Community involvement in health: Why is it necessary? *Tropical Doctor*, 21: 3–5.

Calnan, M. (1995) Citizens views on health care. *Journal of Management in Medicine*, 9(4): 17–23.

Calnan, M. (1998) The patient's perspective. *International Journal of Technology Assessment in Health Care*, 14(1): 24–34.

Charles, C. and DeMaio, S. (1993) Lay participation in health care decision making: A conceptual framework. *Journal of Health Politics, Policy and Law*, 18(4): 881–904.

Charles, C., Gafni, A. and Whelan, T. (1997) Shared decision-making in the medical encounter: What does it mean? (or it takes at least two to tango). *Social Science and Medicine*, 44: 681–92.

Coulter, A. (1997) Partnerships with patients: The pros and cons of shared clinical decision-making. *Journal of Health Services Research Policy*, 2(2): 112–21.

Crawford, M.J., Rutter, D., Manley, C., Weaver, T., Bhui, K., Fulop, N. and Tyrer, P. (2002) Systematic review of involving patients in the planning and development of healthcare. *British Medical Journal*, 325.

Crow, R., Gage, H., Hampson, S., Hart, J., Kimber, A., Storey, L. and Thomas, H. (2002) The measurement of satisfaction with healthcare: Implications for practice from a systematic review of the literature. *Health Technology Assessment*, 6(32).

Davies, H. (1999) Falling public trust in health services: Implications for accountability. *Journal of Health Services Research and Policy*, 4(4): 193–4.

Delbanco, T., Berwick, M. D., Boufford, J. I., Edgman-Levitan, S., Ollenschlager, G., Plamping, D. and Rockefeller, R. G. (2001) Healthcare in a land called PeoplePower: Nothing about me without me. *Health Expectations*, 4: 144–50.

Dolan, P., Cookson, R. and Ferguson, B. (1999) Effect of discussion and deliberation on the public's views of priority setting in health care: Focus group study. *British Medical Journal*, 318: 916–19.

Doyal, L. (2001) Informed consent: Moral necessity or illusion. *Quality in Health Care*, 10(suppl. I): I29–I33.

Entwistle, V., Andrew, J., Emslie, M., Walker, R., Dorrian, C., Angns, V. and Conniff, A. (2003) Patients' views on feedback to the NHS. *Quality and Safety in Healthcare*, 12: 435–42.

Goodare, H. and Lockwood, S. (1999) Involving patients in clinical research. *British Medical Journal*, 319: 724–5.

Home Office (2004) *Facilitating Community Involvement: Practical Guidance for*

Practitioners and Policy Makers. Home Office Development and Practice Report 27. London: Home Office (www.homeoffice.gov.uk).

Kaplan, S.H., Greenfield, S. and Ware, J.E. (1989) Assessing the effects of physician–patient interactions on the outcomes of chronic disease. *Medical Care*, 27(suppl): S110–S127.

Klein, R. (1984) The politics of participation. In R. Maxwell and N. Weaver (eds) *Public Participation in Health*. London: King Edward's Hospital Fund for London.

Lockey, R., Sitzia, J., Millyard, C. and colleagues (2004) *Report Summary. Training for Service User Involvement in Health and Social Care Research: A Study of Training Provision and Participants' Experiences*. Eastleigh: INVOLVE (www.invo.org.uk).

Lorig, K. R., Sobel, D. S., Stewart, A. L., Brown, B. W., Bandura, A. and Ritter, P. (1999) Evidence suggesting that a chronic disease self-management programme can improve health status while reducing hospitalization: A randomized trial. *Medical Care*, 37(1): 5–14.

McIver, S. (1993) *Obtaining the Views of Health Service Users about Quality of Information*. London: King's Fund.

McIver, S. (2005) Listening to 'quiet' voices. In J. Burr and P. Nicolson *Researching Health Care Consumers: Critical Approaches*. London: Palgrave Macmillan.

McIver, S. (1998) *Healthy Debate? An Independent Evaluation of Citizens' Juries in Health Settings*. London: King's Fund.

Mays, N. (2000) Legitimate decision making: The Achilles heel of solidaristic health care systems. *Journal of Health Services Research and Policy*, 5(2): 122–6.

Mechanic, D. (1998) Public trust and initiatives for new health care partnerships. *Milbank Quarterly*, 76(2): 281–302.

Mullen, P. and Spurgeon, P. (2000) *Priority Setting and the Public*. Oxford: Radcliffe.

O'Connor, A. (2001) Using patient decision aids to promote evidence-based decision making. *Evidence Based Medicine*, 6: 100–102.

O'Connor, A. Rastom, A. and Fiset, V. (1999) Decision aids for patients facing health treatment or screening decisions: A systematic review. *British Medical Journal*, 319: 731–4.

Potter, C. and Whittaker, C. (2001) *Enabling Communication in Children with Qutism*. London: Jessica Kingsley Publishers.

Rakow, T. (2001) Differences in belief about likely outcomes account for differences in doctors' treatment preferences: But what accounts for differences in belief? *Quality in Health Care*, 10(suppl.): 144–149.

Saltman, R.B. (1994) Patient choice and patient empowerment in Northern European Health Systems: A conceptual framework. *International Journal of Health Services*, 24(2): 201–29.

Stevenson, F.A., Barry, C.A., Britten, N., Barber, N. and Bradley, C.P. (2000) Doctor–patient communication about drugs: The evidence for shared decision making. *Social Science and Medicine*, 50: 829–40.

Stewart, J., Kendall, E. and Coote, A. (eds) (1994) *Citizens' Juries*. London: Institute for Public Policy Research.

Telford, R., Boote, J. D. and Cooper, C. L. (2004) What does it mean to involve consumers successfully in NHS research? A consensus study. *Health Expectations*, 7: 209–20.

Towsley, R. (2000) Archive – *Avon calling*. 5 June (communitycare.co.uk).

Van Wersch, A. and Eccles, M. (2001) Involvement of consumers in the development of evidence based clinical guidelines: practical experiences from the

North of England evidence based guideline development programme. *Quality in Health Care*, 10: 10–16.

Wensing, M., Grol, R., van Montfort, P. and Smits, A. (1996) Indicators of the quality of general practice care of patients with chronic illness: A step towards the real involvement of patients in the assessment of the quality of care. *Quality in Health Care*, 5: 73–80.

Wensing, M. and Elwyn, G. (2002) Research on patients' views in the evaluation and improvement of quality of care. *Quality and Safety in Health Care*, 11: 153–157.

Williams, B. (1994) Patient satisfaction: A valid concept? *Social Science and Medicine*, 38(4): 509–16.

Williamson, C. (2001) What does involving consumers in research mean? *Quarterly Journal of Medicine*, 94: 661–4.

Zakus, J. D. and Lysack, C. L. (1998) Revisiting community participation. *Health Policy and Planning*, 13(1): 1–12.

Websites and resources

INVOLVE. A national advisory group, funded by the Department of Health, which aims to promote and support active public involvement in NHS, public health and social care research: *www.invo.org.uk*

King's Fund. An independent charitable institution which researches and evaluates health and social care policy: *www.kingsfund.org.uk*

Public Involvement Programme. Consumers in NHS Research Support Unit: *www.pip.org.uk*

Standing Conference for Community Development. *www.com-dev.co.uk*

Strengthening Accountability. *www.nel-involve.org.uk*

26

Quality improvement in healthcare

Ruth Boaden

Introduction

'Quality' is a term widely used not only within healthcare but throughout society, with numerous references to the quality of care, commissioning, the use of the primary care 'Quality and Outcomes Framework', the regulation of quality of care and the impact of IT on quality and service user expectations of quality in this book alone. However, the study and development of quality is often hampered by lack of clarity of definition. Diverse meanings of the term make it both a 'seductive and slippery philosophy of management' (Wilkinson and Willmott 1995).

Within the healthcare field, the dominance of the medical profession with its own perspective on quality means that 'quality has become a battleground on which professions compete for ownership and definition of quality' (Øvretveit 1997). The medical profession has traditionally 'owned' quality and utilised its own professional approaches to assuring and regulating it. The rise of quality improvement as something that involves more than the clinical professions has therefore led to 'the quality movement being equated with a change in power or a bid for power by managers within European health care systems' (Øvretveit 1997).

One early pioneer of healthcare quality was Donabedian (1966) whose research and writings were important foundation for other developments, although some would argue that healthcare quality has been an issue since Florence Nightingale's time (Stiles and Mick 1994). Definitions of quality in healthcare abound (Reeves and Bednar 1994), and as the concept has been formalised within the healthcare field, a suite of healthcare-related definitions and 'dimensions of quality' have developed (see Table 26.1).

Quality can be viewed from various perspectives, and whilst patients may not feel qualified to judge the technical quality of healthcare 'they assess their healthcare by other dimensions which reflect what they personally value' (Kenagy et al. 1999). The concept of 'quality' outside healthcare was pioneered by Shewhart and his work on statistical process

Table 26.1   Definitions of healthcare quality

Donabedian (1987)	Maxwell (1984)	Langley et al. (1996)	Institute of Medicine and Committee on Quality Health Care in America (2001)
• Manner in which practitioner manages the personal interaction with the patient • Patient's own contribution to care • Amenities of the settings where care is provided • Facility in access to care • Social distribution of access • Social distribution of health improvements attributable to care	• Access to services • Relevance to need • Effectiveness • Equity • Social acceptability • Efficiency and economy.	• Performance • Features • Time • Reliability • Durability • Uniformity • Consistency • Serviceability; • Aesthetics • Personal interaction • Flexibility • Harmlessness • Perceived quality • Usability	• Safety • Effectiveness • Patient-centredness • Timeliness • Efficiency • Equity

control (SPC) in the 1930s (Shewhart 1931). However, many academic fields of study have contributed to the study of quality, including services marketing, organisation studies, human resource management and organisational behaviour. Recent developments into patient safety as one aspect of quality are also multidisciplinary in approach (Walshe and Boaden 2006).

There is no doubt that there is an increased focus on quality in all sectors, and particularly in healthcare. However, there is a wide variety of approaches that may be used to improve quality. While these may not be mutually exclusive, there is little guidance on which approaches may be appropriate in differing circumstances. It has been suggested that a number of approaches may be needed: 'give attention to many different factors and use multiple strategies' (Grol et al. 2004), and these are developed from very differing perspectives on organisational and individual behaviour (summarised by Grol et al. 2004). (See Table 26.2.)

The development of quality improvement

This section describes the development of the quality improvement 'movement' in general, with reference throughout to where the approaches have been applied to healthcare. These improvement approaches have been targeted at improving organisations and interactions within them.

Table 26.2   Approaches to quality improvement

Approaches to quality improvement may have a focus on changing:
- organisations
- professionals
- interactions between participants in the system

Quality may be controlled and improved by:
- self-regulation amongst professionals (see Chapter 19)
- external control, regulation and incentives (see Chapter 19)
- patient power, which may be exercised through market forces (see Chapter 25)
- reducing variation and waste in organisational processes

Quality may be improved from:
- the top down
- the bottom up
- the outside in (see Chapter 19)

The gurus

There are a number of key figures who contributed to the development of quality improvement in the west, often referred to as quality 'gurus' (Dale 2003).

- *W. E. Deming* was an American who first went to Japan in 1947 and developed a 14-point approach (Deming 1986) for his management philosophy for improving quality and changing organisational culture. He was also responsible for developing the concept of the Plan–Do–Check–Action (PDCA) cycle. It is argued that his ideas influenced the development of the field of strategic management both directly and indirectly (Vinzant and Vinzant 1999).
- *Joseph Juran* focused on the managerial aspects of implementing quality (Juran 1951). His approach can be summarised as: 'Quality, through a reduction in statistical variation, improves productivity and competitive position.' He promoted a trilogy of quality planning, quality control and quality improvement, and maintained that providing customer satisfaction must be the chief operating goal (Nielsen et al. 2004).
- *Philip Crosby* was a American management consultant whose philosophy is summarised as 'higher quality reduces costs and raises profit', and who defined quality as 'conformance to requirements'. He too had 14 steps to quality and his ideas were very appealing to both manufacturing and service organisations. He is best known for the concepts of 'do it right first time' and 'zero defects' and believed that management had to set the tone for quality within an organisation.
- *Armand Feigenbaum* defined quality as a way of managing (rather than a series of technical projects) and the responsibility of everyone. His major contribution was the categorisation of quality costs into three: appraisal, prevention and failure, and his insistence that management and leadership are essential for quality improvement. His work has been described as relevant to healthcare (Berwick 1989).

There are both similarities and differences between these approaches and there is no clear overarching philosophy of quality improvement, although the key points are as follows (Bendell et al. 1995):

1 Management commitment and employee awareness are essential (Deming).
2 Actions need to be planned and prioritised (Juran).
3 Teamwork plays a vital part (Ishikawa who pioneered the quality circle concept).
4 Tools and techniques are needed (e.g. seven quality control tools promoted by Ishikawa).
5 Management tools/approaches will also be needed (Feigenbaum).
6 Customer focus is needed (Deming).

Nielsen et al. (2004) asked the question 'Can the gurus' concepts cure healthcare?' Although their focus was on the overall philosophy rather than the use of individual tools, they concluded:

• Crosby would emphasise the role of leadership in pursuing zero defects.
• Deming would emphasise transformation (as he did in the fourteenth of his 14 points (1986) whilst being disappointed at the reactive behaviour of healthcare organisations and individuals with 'far too little pursuit of constant improvement' (Nielsen et al. 2004).
• Feigenbaum would focus on clearer identification of the customer and the application of evidence-based medicine.
• Juran's emphasis would be on building quality into processes from the start (what he termed 'quality planning').

Total quality management

The most popular term for an overall organisational approach to quality improvement is 'total quality management' (TQM), whose common themes may be summarised; (Berwick et al. 1992, Hackman and Wageman 1995) as follows:

• Organisational success depends on meeting customer needs, including internal customers.
• Quality is an effect caused by the processes within the organisation which are complex but understandable.
• Most human beings engaged in work are intrinsically motivated to try hard and do well.
• Simple statistical methods linked with careful data collection can yield powerful insights into the causes of problems within processes.

Just as the term 'quality' has a variety of meanings, there is a confusion of terminology in this area, with not only TQM used but also 'continuous quality improvement' (CQI; McLaughlin and Simpson 1999) and 'total quality improvement' (TQI; Iles and Sutherland 2001),

Table 26.3   Principles of quality management

1 Productive work is accomplished through processes.
2 Sound customer–supplier relationships are absolutely necessary for sound quality management.
3 The main source of quality defects is problems in the process.
4 Poor quality is costly.
5 Understanding the variability of processes is a key to improving quality.
6 Quality control should focus on the most vital processes.
7 The modern approach to quality is thoroughly grounded in scientific and statistical thinking.
8 Total employee involvement is crucial.
9 New organisational structures can help achieve quality improvement.
10 Quality management employs three basic, closely interrelated activities: quality planning, quality control and quality improvement.

although such terms appear to be interchangeable in practice. Another view with a specific healthcare focus is found in (Berwick et al. 1990/ 2002) who describe the principles of 'quality management' (see Table 26.3).

These principles of quality management have been applied in the US healthcare system (see Box 26.1 and Table 26.4).

Box 26.1   Influences on quality in healthcare: Institute for Health Improvement (IHI)

Established in 1991 as 'a not-for-profit organization driving the improvement of health by advancing the quality and value of health care . . . a reliable source of energy, knowledge, and support for a never-ending campaign to improve health care worldwide. The Institute helps accelerate change in health care by cultivating promising concepts for improving patient care and turning those ideas into action', IHI has had influence not only in the USA but also in the UK. Its work has developed since its establishment to educate, encourage healthcare staff to work together in collaboratives, to redesign processes and now to promote a quality improvement 'movement'. The president of IHI, Don Berwick, has authored a number of books and articles on quality improvement, including *Curing Health Care* (Berwick et al. 1990) which was reissued in 2002 with a Preface reflecting on 'ten things we know now that we wish we had known then'. These provide an interesting summary of the progress of thinking about quality improvement in healthcare over this period.

Widening the scope of quality improvement

Until the 1980s most of the emphasis on quality improvement was within manufacturing industry, but then the field of 'service quality' developed (Groonroos 1984; Berry et al. 1985), with the widespread use of the SERVQUAL questionnaire (Parasuraman et al. 1988), as well as

Table 26.4   If only we had known then what we know now

Ten key lessons for quality improvement (Berwick et al. 1990/2002)	*What we know now (Berwick et al. 1990/2002)*
Quality improvement tools can work in healthcare	• Spending too much time analysing processes can slow the pace of change. • Teams can enter the PDSA cycle in several places. • Tools are important in their place, but not a very good entry point for improvement: 'Teams can unconsciously use the tools as a way to delay or avoid the discomfort of taking action.'
Cross-functional teams are valuable in improving healthcare processes	• Getting action is more important than getting buy-in. • The process owner concept from industry is helpful here.
Improvement is a matter of changing the process, not blaming the people	• The shift of blame from individuals to processes is not 100%. • There are limits to a blame-free culture, but perhaps not to a process-minded culture.
Data useful for quality improvement abound in healthcare	• Measurement is very difficult for healthcare, and healthcare is far behind. • Balanced scorecards are helpful. • SPC has enormous potential with 'hundreds of as-yet-untapped applications'. • Medical records need modernising to enable better public health data. • IT is key.
Quality improvement methods are fun to use	• There need to be consequences for not being involved in improvement (not improving should not be an option).
Costs of poor quality are high and savings are within reach	• Waste is pervasive in healthcare; improvement is the best way to save money.
Involving doctors is difficult	• Balance is important. • Doctors are not well prepared to lead people. • Doctors can (and are) learning new skills to supplement their medical training, not to replace it.
Training needs arise early	• Healthcare lacks a training infrastructure. • The argument here refers to professional boundaries.
Non-clinical processes draw early attention	• Clinical outcomes are critical. • This is the 'core business' of healthcare and focus on them achieves buy-in from all health professionals.
Healthcare organisations may need a broader definition of quality	• Definitions of quality in healthcare must include the whole patient experience – not just clinical outcomes and costs. • The Institute of Medicine's six aims for improvement are cited here (2001).
In healthcare, as in industry, the fate of quality improvement is first of all in the hands of leaders	• The executive leader doesn't always have to be the driver of change. • This is especially true at the start of improvement, but achieving system-level improvement does require senior commitment.

promotion of the concept of the 'moment of truth' and an emphasis on service recovery. Many of these concepts are applicable to the provision of healthcare as a service, although they have not been extensively used.

However, a tension between 'hard' (systems) approaches and 'soft' (people/culture) issues (Wilkinson 1992) also developed at this time, partly in response to the apparent 'failure' of quality improvement (whichever term was used) to achieve sustained improvements in organisational performance. Criticism of the quality improvement literature came from those who described it as 'an evangelical line that excludes traditions and empirical data that fail to confirm its faith' (Kerfoot and Knights 1995); a view that could be justified because of much of the prescriptive research labelled as 'quality' (Wilkinson and Willmott 1995). However, this led to research from the 1990s that offers additional perspectives on quality (Hackman and Wageman 1995; Webb 1995) whose findings are perhaps more applicable to the complex world of healthcare and in particular focus on individuals, their motivation, behaviour and interaction and the way in which this affects quality.

Achievements in the area of quality improvement were increasingly the subject of national 'awards'. The Deming Application Prize (Japan) led to the development of the Malcolm Baldrige National Quality Award (USA) and the European Foundation for Quality Management (EFQM) Award/Excellence Model (Europe), with its associated national and sector-specific derivatives. Quality was increasingly assessed by organisations themselves (self-assessment) as a means of improvement, and these models attempted to integrate the 'hard' and 'soft' factors, with the term 'quality' being replaced by 'excellence'. There is specific guidance for US organisations in healthcare wishing to apply for the Baldrige Award (Baldrige National Quality Program 2005) and the European Excellence award has a 'public sector' category.

Quality improvement techniques

This section describes the most commonly used quality improvement techniques and their application in healthcare. Although there is considerable debate about whether techniques are any use on their own ('teaching tools very rarely results in a change to the system', Seddon 2005), the empirical evidence is that much quality improvement in healthcare has been carried out using these techniques.

Plan–Do–Study–Act model

The Plan–Do–Study–Act (PDSA) model was first formally proposed in healthcare by (Langley et al. 1996) as part of the 'Model for Improvement' (see Figure 26.1) to improve processes and therefore outcomes (Deming 1986). This links the PDSA cycle with three key questions and is often referred to as rapid-cycle improvement (Horton 2004), where a number of small PDSA cycles take place one after the other, similar to a learning approach (e.g. Kolb 1984; Schon 1988). The model for improvement can be regarded as a philosophy rather than an individual technique and one which can be used as an overarching framework within which other improvement techniques can be utilised. It is, however, a continuous (incremental) improvement approach, rather than a breakthrough (transformational) approach, and this may be in conflict with current management styles or past experience of improvement (Walley and Gowland 2004).

The PDSA cycle is a key part of the collaborative approach which was one of the first large-scale applications of PDSA in healthcare, initiated by IHI and then developed in the NHS. The approach involves a number of teams with a common interest (e.g. improving cancer services) working together in a structured way with a group of national experts for a period of around 12 to 18 months to plan, implement and monitor improvements in care. Use of the PDSA model with NHS collaboratives has been reported (Kerr et al. 2002) to facilitate the use of teamwork to make improvements, as well as provide a framework for the application of effective measurement and use of improvement tools. However, there is to date insufficient evidence to determine whether collaboratives are more or less cost effective in making and spreading improvements than other approaches (Øvretveit et al. 2002), or to assess spread and sustainability. The PDSA cycle is an adaptation of the Plan–Do–Check–Act (PDCA) cycle developed by Deming (Deming 1986) and termed by him the Shewhart cycle (Dale 2003).

Statistical process control

The roots of statistical process control (SPC) can be traced to work in the 1920s in Bell Laboratories (Shewhart 1931), where Shewhart sought to identify the difference between 'natural' variation in processes – termed 'common cause' – and that which could be controlled – 'special' or 'assignable' cause variation. Processes that exhibited only common cause variation were said to be in statistical control. One of the many significant features of this work, which is still used in basically the same form today, is that 'the management of quality acquired a scientific and statistical foundation' and in healthcare it is often regarded as a tool for measurement (Plsek 1999).

The statistical approach has been applied in a variety of healthcare areas (Benneyan et al. 2003), (Marshall et al. 2004a), although it is not promoted centrally within the NHS. The use of control charts (the way in which SPC data is displayed) is viewed as helping to decide how to improve – whether to search for special causes (if the process is out of control) or work on more fundamental process redesign (if the process is in control). Charts can also be used to monitor improvements over time (Benneyan et al. 2003). A study of the effect of presenting data as league tables or control charts for the purposes of decision making (Marshall et al. 2004b) concluded that fewer outliers for further investigation are identified when data is presented in control charts.

There is evidence that discussions about the applications of SPC in healthcare started in the early 1990s (Berwick 1991) and it is certain that there have been a number of applications in US healthcare for some while (Mohammed et al. 2001), as well as some debate (Benneyan and Kaminsky 1995). Mohammed (2004) reports the results of his search on Medline for 'statistical process control' to demonstrate the rapid growth in publications about SPC in healthcare. He was also involved in the widely publicised application of SPC to data about mortality in the light of the Shipman case (Mohammed et al. 2001, 2004), and this raised the profile of SPC amongst doctors. However, the fact that SPC was first used in manufacturing makes translation difficult: 'there is a reluctance, despite evidence to the contrary, to accept that an approach for improving the quality of "widgets" can be legitimately applied to healthcare' (Mohammed 2004).

Six sigma

Six sigma is an improvement approach which was initially established by Motorola in 1987. It represents the amount of variation in a process. The term 'six sigma' refers to a process that has at least six standard deviations (6σ) between the process mean and the nearest specification limit. Six sigma as an approach has a number of fundamental themes:

1 A genuine focus on the customer: six sigma measures start with customer satisfaction, and there is an emphasis on understanding customer expectations and requirements.
2 Data and fact-driven management: decisions based on fact, with the development of an understanding of internal processes.
3 Process focus, management and improvement: understanding the process is the key and controlling the inputs will improve the outputs.
4 Proactive management: developing an understanding of six sigma principles, defining the root causes of problems, challenging 'why' things are done this way.
5 'Boundaryless' collaboration: the approach is teamwork focused.
6 Drive for perfection, tolerance for failure: it is okay to fail during improvement, but the key is to understand why failure occurred and improve it next time.

There are a number of core six sigma methods/tools (many of which are also used in other improvement approaches), but the two key ones are generally agreed to be Define–Measure–Analyse–Improve–Control (DMAIC) and Define–Measure–Analyse–Design–Verify (DMADV; Brassard et al. 2002). DMAIC is the most commonly used methodology and claimed to be very robust and able to provide a framework and common language, enabling organisations and individuals to 'improve the way they improve' (Brassard et al. 2002).

The academic and theoretical underpinning of six sigma lags rather behind its practical application (Antony 2004). There is a 'paucity of studies that fundamentally critique the phenomena of six sigma in organisations from both people and process perspectives' (Erwin and Douglas 2000). An overview of healthcare applications can be found in Chassin (1998) and Sehwail and DeYong (2003), but it should be noted that 'six sigma has not been widely applied to patient care' (Revere et al. 2004).

Lean

The term 'lean' has been developed in the context of manufacturing from work carried out at Toyota, and like many other 'approaches' it consists of a number of tools, some of which are also used elsewhere: just-in-time (JIT), the kanban method of pull production and mistake proofing (Hines et al. 2004), with an overall focus on the elimination of waste. Over the early 1990s these principles were gradually extended so that system design was described as based on 'lean principles' (Womack and Jones 1996):

- identification of customer value
- management of the value stream
- developing the capability to flow production
- use of 'pull' mechanisms to support material flow
- pursuit of perfection through reducing all forms of waste in the system.

The lean approach is gradually being promoted both in the USA and UK with the implementation of the Toyota production system in a US health centre (Kaplan and Rona 2004) and lean in healthcare (Hill 2001; Bushell and Shelest 2002; Greenwood et al. 2002). There are no reports of outcomes apart from case studies and most of these are in conference papers rather than refereed journal articles.

Theory of constraints

The basic concepts of the theory of constraints (TOC) are:

- Every system has at least one constraint – anything that limits the system from achieving higher performance.
- The existence of constraints represents opportunities for improvement. Constraints are not viewed as negative, as traditional thinking might do, but as opportunities to improve.

It was developed by Elihu Goldratt who believed that theory of constraints (TOC) represented 'an overall theory for running an organisation' (Goldratt 1988). Although it had evolved from factory-floor concepts, it was applicable to the whole organisation; constraints might be managerial policy related rather than related to physical things. It claims to be designed for 'achieving breakthroughs in performance in large complex environments dominated by high uncertainty' (Goldratt Consulting Group 2005), which would seem to make it ideal for healthcare. One of its prerequisites is to establish the goal of the organisation, which is often contestable in the complex professionalised environment of healthcare. Its Five Focusing Steps describe how to reduce the impact of the constraint on the system.

A recent review of TOC across all sectors (Mabin and Balderstone 2003) states that over 400 articles and 45 books have been published on the subject since 1993, but without much systematic assessment of its impact. Where research results have been reported, the research is 'anecdotal and fragmented' (Lubitsh 2004) and mainly from the US. There is some work on the application of TOC in healthcare in the UK (Goldratt Consulting Group 2005), but the results are only reported by those who supported the work.

Other techniques

The term 'redesign' covers more than a single technique, although it can be described as 'thinking through from scratch the best process to achieve speedy and effective care from a patient perspective' (Locock 2003) – something which may involve many of the improvement techniques already described in this chapter. The basic principles of process redesign have been 'packaged' into an approach usually termed 'business process re-engineering', first coined by Hammer and Champy (1993), arguably as a response to the failure of the incremental improvement approach proposed by TQM. Its most publicised and studied application in healthcare was probably that at Leicester (McNulty and Ferlie 2002), although redesigning of healthcare at a whole system as well as at individual organisation level is an 'international preoccupation' (Locock 2003) and one which has led to increased discussion between IHI and the NHS (e.g. Locock 2003). Redesign was the driver for the initial establishment of a national body to promote quality improvement in England (see Box 26.2).

There are many other techniques claimed to be useful for quality improvement: a summary and basic description is shown in Table 26.5 (developed from Dale 2003).

Clinical approaches to improvement

There are some approaches to quality improvement which have been developed specifically within the clinical field. These include clinical governance, clinical guidelines and pathways and a number of approaches to reducing adverse events and focusing on patient safety, although these are not always exclusively clinical (Walshe and Boaden 2006).

Box 26.2   Promoting quality improvement in England: NHS Modernisation Agency (MA)

The NHS Modernisation Agency (MA) was established in 1991 'to support the NHS and its partner organisations in the task of modernising services and improving experiences and outcomes for patients' (2005) and has recently been superseded (in 2005) by the NHS Institute for Innovation and Improvement.

Many of the key staff in the NHS MA were drawn from the team involved with a large re-engineering project at a hospital in Leicester in the mid-1990s (Bowns and McNulty 1999) and were influenced by this experience. The original ambition of this project for rapid organisational transformation altered to one of continuous incremental change, resulting in a shift of timescales within which such change could be achieved from two years to five to ten years. This shift in philosophy was seen as accounting for the fact that the resulting changes in performance fell short of those aimed for, although they were generally sustainable. The learning from this project itself had influence:

- Some re-engineering techniques (particularly 'process thinking') were used successfully to improve patient care. This has been the basis of much of the subsequent work of the MA.
- External management consultants were shown to need a deep understanding of the NHS environment to support change effectively. Much process/quality improvement since this time within the NHS has been supported internally by trained staff, rather than by external organisations.
- Change was shown to be highly context specific and continuity of support by senior management 'necessary, though not sufficient' to re-engineer in an NHS setting; effective redesign needs sustained leadership and support of change by a critical mass of clinicians. The issue of clinical support for, and involvement in, improvement has not however always been at the forefront of improvement efforts (Degeling et al. 2003).

Clinical governance can be defined as the 'action, the system or the manner of governing clinical affairs' (Lugon and Secker-Walker 1999) and is a specified statutory duty of all NHS organisations. It was developed as an overall approach as part of policy on quality in the NHS (DH 1998) and it has led to the establishment of formal audit programmes, increased focus on clinical effectiveness and the formal management of risk, amongst other things. It can be viewed as an overall quality improvement process, but one which focuses specifically on clinical issues whilst still highlighting the importance of organisational culture, individual behaviour and interaction and may itself use a range of techniques for improvement.

Clinical guidelines/pathways are structured, multidisciplinary plans of care designed to support the implementation of clinical guidelines and protocols, providing guidance about each stage of the management of a patient with a particular condition, including details of both process and outcome. They aim to improve continuity and coordination of care and

Table 26.5 Quality improvement tools

Tool	Description	Source (where one identifiable)
Benchmarking	Learning from the experience of others by comparing products or processes – can be internal (within a company), competitive (with competitors), functional/generic (comparing processes with 'best in class')	Developed from the work at Rank Xerox in the 1980s, documented by (Camp 1989).
Brainstorming	Used with a variety of tools to generate ideas in groups.	Term now often replaced by 'thought showering' which is felt to be more politically correct, with some considering the original term to be offensive for those who have epilepsy.
Checklists	Lists of key features of a process, equipment, etc. to be checked.	Commonly used in a variety of situations.
Departmental purpose analysis	Tool used to facilitate internal customer relationships.	Originated at IBM in 1984.
Design of experiments (DOE)	A series of techniques which identify and control parameters which have a potential impact on performance, aiming to make the performance of the system immune to variation.	Dates back to agricultural research by Sir R. A. Fisher in the 1920s, later developed by Taguchi (1986) and adopted in both Japan and the west.
Failure mode and effects analysis (FMEA)	A planning tool used to 'build quality in' to a product or service, for either design or process. It looks at the ways in which the product or service might fail, and then modifies the design or process to avoid these or minimise them.	Developed in 1962 in the aerospace and defence industry as a means of reliability analysis, risk analysis and management. Termed 'Failure Mode Effect and Criticality Analysis' (FMECA) by Joint Commission on Accreditation of Healthcare Organisations (2005)
Flowcharts	A basis for the application of many other tools. A diagrammatic representation of the steps in a process, often using standard symbols. Many variations available.	Developed from industrial engineering methods but no one identifiable source. Widely used in systems analysis and business process re-engineering.
Housekeeping	Essentially about cleanliness, etc. in the production environment.	Based on what the Japanese refer to as the five 5s: • *seiri* – organisation • *seiton* – neatness • *seiso* – cleaning • *seiketsu* – standardisation • *shitsuke* – discipline
Mistake-proofing	Technique used to prevent errors turning into defects in the final product – based on the assumption that mistakes will occur, however 'careful' individuals are, unless preventative	Developed by Shingo (1986)

Table 26.5 continued

Tool	Description	Source (where one identifiable)
	measures are put in place. Statistical methods accept defects as inevitable, but the source of the mistake should be identified and prevented.	
Policy deployment	The western tradition of *hoshin kanri* – Japanese 'strategic planning and management process involving setting direction and deploying the means of achieving that direction' (Dale 2003). Used to communicate policy, goals and objectives through the hierarchy of the organisation, focusing on the key activities for success.	Developed in Japan in early 1960s, concept conceived by Bridgestone Tire Company, and adopted in the US from the early 1980s, with great popularity in large multinationals with Japanese subsidiaries.
Quality costing	Tools used to identify the costs of quality, often using the prevention–appraisal–failure (PAF) categorisation	PAF developed by Feigenbaum (1961). Cost of (non)conformance developed by Crosby (1979).
Quality function deployment	Tool to incorporate knowledge about needs of customers into all stages of design and manufacture/delivery process. Initially translates customer needs into design requirements, based on the concept of the voice of the customer. Closely related to FMEA and DOE.	Developed in Japan at Kobe shipyard.
Total productive maintenance	Can be considered as a method of management, combining principles of productive maintenance (PM) with TQM.	Developed by the Japanese from the planned approach to PM.
Seven quality control tools		
1 *Cause-and-effect diagram*	Diagram used to determine and break down the main causes of a given problem – sometimes called 'fishbone' diagrams. Used where there is one problem and the causes may be hierarchical in nature. Can be used by teams or individuals.	Ishikawa (1979).
2 *Checksheet*	Sheet or form used to collect data.	Can be similar to a checklist.
3 *Control chart*	The way in which SPC data is displayed, viewed as helping to decide how to improve – whether to search for special causes (if the process is out of control) or work on more fundamental process redesign (if the process is in control). Charts can also be use to monitor improvements over time (Benneyan et al. 2003a).	Control charts were used as the basis for SPC development but it is not clear exactly when they were first used.

Table 26.5   continued

Tool	Description	Source (where one identifiable)
4 *Graphs*	Any form of pictorial representation of data.	Basic mathematical technique.
5 *Histogram*	Developed from tally charts, basic statistical tool to describe the distribution of a series of data points.	Basic mathematical technique.
6 *Pareto diagram*	Technique for prioritising issues – a form of bar chart with a cumulative percentage curve overlaid on it. Sometimes referred to as the 80/20 rule.	Named after nineteenth-century Italian economist who observed that a large proportion of a country's wealth is held by a small proportion of the population.
7 *Scatter diagram*	Used to examine the possible relationship between two variables.	Basic mathematical technique.
Seven management tools (M7)	Generally used in design or sales/ marketing areas, where quantitative data is less easy to obtain.	Developed by the Japanese to collect and analyse qualitative and verbal data. Many have already been used in other TQM applications.
1 *Affinity diagrams*	Used to categorise verbal data/ language about previously unexplored vague issues.	
2 *Arrow diagrams*	Applies systematic thinking to the planning and execution of a set of complex tasks.	Used in project management as part of critical path analysis (CPA) and programme evaluation and review technique (PERT).
3 *Decision programme chart*	Used to select the best process to obtain the desired outcome by listing all possible events, contingencies and outcomes.	Similar to decision tree for unsafe acts culpability, based on decision trees presented in (Reason 1997).
4 *Matrix data analysis process*	Multivariate mathematical methods used to analyse the data from a matrix diagram.	
5 *Matrix diagrams*	Used to clarify the relationship between results and causes or objectives and methods, using codes to illustrate the direction and relative importance of the influence.	
6 *Relations diagrams*	Used to identify complex cause-and-effect relationships, where the causes are non-hierarchical and the 'effect' is complex.	
7 *Systematic diagrams*	Sometimes called a 'tree' diagram – used to examine the most effective means of planning to accomplish a task or solve a problem.	

enable more effective resource planning, as well as providing comparative data on many aspects of quality of care, and are increasingly being used in the UK as patient choice is introduced. They are claimed to reduce variation and improve outcomes (Middleton et al. 2001).

Patient safety is a vast area of study that has developed at least in part from quality improvement (Walshe and Boaden 2006) and cannot be covered in detail here.

Overview

Changing organisations and systems: the process view

Many of the quality improvement techniques described in this chapter are focused on organisational change and all are based on the process view of organisations (Slack et al. 2004). Process management is defined as entailing three practices: mapping processes, improving processes and adhering to systems of improved processes (Benner and Tushman 2003). It is argued that taking a process view is one of the key characteristics of organisations that are successful in improvement, along with adopting evidence-based practice, learning collaboratively and being ready and able to change (Plsek 1999).

The process view has also been the basis for the development of systems thinking, which developed into hard systems and soft systems (Checkland 1981), and has been more recently linked with organisational learning (Senge et al. 1994). It can be described as exploration of 'the properties which exist once the parts [of the system] have been combined into a whole' (Iles and Sutherland 2001) and is in some ways simply a combination of processes. Systems thinking has also been proposed as a means of understanding medical systems (Nolan 1998), based on the following principles:

- A system needs a purpose to aid people in managing inter-dependencies.
- The structure of a system significantly determines the performance of the system.
- Changes in the structure of a system have the potential for generating unintended consequences.
- The structure of a system dictates the benefits that accrue to various people working in the system.
- The size and scope of a system influence the potential for improvement.
- The need for cooperation is a logical extension of interdependencies within systems.
- Systems must be managed.
- Improvements in systems must be led.

This process view is therefore not only about changing organisations but also examining and improving the interaction between elements of the organisation, including the individuals who work within them. It can also be seen in the clinical emphasis on pathways and the use of clinical guidelines.

Taking a process view of organisations leads to consideration of other factors, which are reflected in varying degrees in the various quality improvement approaches available:

1 Variation within a process is inherent and it is argued that understanding and analysing the variation are keys to success in improvement (Snee 1990). This is especially true in healthcare (Haraden and Resar 2004) and is seen to be the result of clinical (patient) flow and professional variability (Institute for Healthcare Improvement 2003). Patient variability is 'random' and cannot be eliminated or reduced but must be managed, whereas non-random variability should be eliminated. It is argued (Institute for Healthcare Improvement 2003) that 'it is variation . . . that causes most of the flow problems in our hospital systems'.

2 Managing the flow of patients through a process is also important and can to some extent draw on approaches widely used in manufacturing (Brideau 2004). Understanding and evaluating flow requires more detailed understanding of demand and capacity than has often been the case in healthcare organisations (Horton 2004). Zimmerman (2004) proposes that studying and improving flow leads to a need to consider alignment within the whole healthcare system and within pre-hospital care of goals within the system, especially between healthcare organisations and clinicians. This will inevitably lead to whole systems approaches to improvement.

3 All approaches to quality improvement involved the identification of the customer, which may be internal or external to the organisation, and subsequently their needs. The purpose of the process has to be clear before improvement can take place. It is in this area that the issue of professionalism and the increasing role of the patient have an impact. Whilst much rhetoric about healthcare systems states that they are patient driven, this does not appear to be the case in practice. Whether the 'customer' can be defined as the patient is open to question but it is clear (Walley and Gowland 2004) that to date patient involvement in quality improvement has been limited, with lack of attention to the presence of the patient in processes (Shortell et al. 1995) and lack of consumer power also being cited as important (Zbabada et al. 1998). It is also argued that the market structure of healthcare in the UK does not enable 'consumers' to alter the behaviour of healthcare providers as there is no effective choice (Zbabada et al. 1998).

The application of many of these concepts is embodied in the ten 'high impact changes' (NHS Modernisation Agency 2005a) in the NHS (see Table 26.6), which now form a key part of the programme for public sector efficiency improvement (Gershon 2004).

Table 26.6 The ten high impact changes

Change No. 1	Treat day surgery as the norm for elective surgery.
Change No. 2	Improve access to key diagnostic tests.
Change No. 3	Manage variation in patient discharge.
Change No. 4	Manage variation in patient admission.
Change No. 5	Avoid unnecessary follow-ups.
Change No. 6	Increase the reliability of performing therapeutic interventions through a care bundle approach.
Change No. 7	Apply a systematic approach to care for people with long-term conditions.
Change No. 8	Improve patient access by reducing the number of queues.
Change No. 9	Optimise patient flow using process templates.
Change No. 10	Redesign and extend roles.

Source: NHS Modernisation Agency (2005)

The things that are different about healthcare

Much experience and evidence of organisational quality improvement has been in the private sector. Compared to the private sector, healthcare can be characterised (Pollitt 1993) by the following:

- the range and diversity of stakeholders
- its complex ownership and resourcing arrangements
- the professional autonomy of many of its staff.

Healthcare practitioners believe that healthcare systems are 'uniquely complex' (Benneyan and Kaminsky 1995), although many would argue that this should not mean that quality improvement approaches are not useful (Walley 2003). The extent to which knowledge, theories and models from the private sector can be transferred to healthcare/public sector organisations is described in the meta-analyses reported by Golembiewski et al. (1982) and Robertson and Seneviratne (1995) who show that public and private sector interventions had similar patterns of results.

Conclusions

Many believe that 'in matters of quality improvement, healthcare can indeed learn from industry – and perhaps, equally important, industry can also learn from healthcare. The fundamental principles of quality improvement apply to both' (Berwick et al. 1990/2002). However, given the variety of perspectives on quality improvement, especially those from an organisation/process perspective and those developed by professionals, there are challenges for all:

- Quality improvement needs to be demystified: 'much of it is common sense, accessible to all and not the preserve of a few. The tendency for each new quality improvement theory to generate its own jargon and esoteric knowledge must be resisted' (Locock 2003).

• Healthcare professionals need to recognise their role and responsibility to the wider system: 'the need to balance clinical autonomy with transparent accountability, to support the systematization of clinical work' (Degeling et al. 2003).

• Managers need to recognise the limits of their authority in improvement: 'there was no evidence that managers alone could produce . . . clinical buy-in' (Dopson and Fitzgerald 2005).

In the continually changing world of healthcare, quality is always going to be important and the differing perspectives and multidisciplinary approaches taken into account.

Summary box

• Quality is a widely used term with a variety of meanings attributed to it.
• Approaches to quality improvement may have a focus on changing organisations, professionals and interactions between participants in the system. Quality may be controlled and improvement by a variety of means, including reducing variation and waste in organisational processes.
• Quality improvement developed from the ideas of a series of gurus in manufacturing, with these concepts later translating to service organisations and to a more 'total' (i.e. organisationwide) approach to improvement.
• There is a wide variety of techniques and approaches available for quality improvement from other sectors, including the plan–do–study–act model, statistical process control, six sigma, lean, theory of constraints and process redesign.
• Clinically developed approaches to improvement include clinical governance, clinical pathways and some approaches to patient safety.
• Viewing organisations as processes is the basis of many improvement approaches and this links to wide whole system concepts.
• Improvement in processes can result from consideration of variation, flow and clarification of the goal of the system, taking into account what the customer(s) want.
• Healthcare is different from other sectors in terms of quality improvement primarily because of the professional autonomy of many of its staff, but improvement is a challenge for all parties who need to simplify concepts, recognise their responsibilities and the limits of their authority.

Self-test exercises

1 What were the influences on the development of the quality movement from its origins in both manufacturing and professional practice?
2 There are many quality improvement techniques available but which ones do you think would be most useful in improving quality:

- in a hospital emergency department?
- in a large organisation where multiple performance measures are used?
- in a pathology laboratory?
- in a primary care centre where there are often queues of patients waiting to see health professionals?

3 What are the challenges of getting clinicians to accept methods of improvement other than those developed as 'clinical governance'?
4 What needs to be in place if quality improvement in healthcare is to continue to develop?

References and further reading

Antony, J. (2004) Some pros and cons of six sigma: an academic perspective. *TQM Magazine,* 16(4): 303–6.

Baldrige National Quality Program (2005) Health care criteria for performance excellence. *http://www.quality.nist.gov/HealthCare_Criteria.htm* (accessed 12 December 2005).

Bendell, T., Penson, R. and Carr, S. (1995) The quality gurus–their approaches described and considered. *Managing Service Quality,* 5(6): 44–8.

Benner, M. J. and Tushman, M. L. (2003) Exploitation, Exploration and process management: The productivity dilemma revisited. *Academy of Management Review,* 26(2): 238–56.

Benneyan, J. C. and Kaminsky, F. C. (1995) Another view on how to measure health care quality. *Quality Progress,* 28(2): 120–25.

Benneyan, J. C., Lloyd, R. C. and Plsek, P. E. (2003) Statistical process control as a tool for research and healthcare improvement. *Quality Safety Health Care,* 12(6): 458–64.

Berry, L. L., Zeithaml, V. A. and Parasuraman, A. (1985) Quality counts in services too. *Business Horizons,* 28(3): 44–52.

Berwick, D. (1989) Continuous improvement as an ideal in healthcare. *New England Journal of Medicine,* 320: 53–6.

Berwick, D. (1991) Controlling variation in healthcare: A consultation from Walter Shewhart. *Medical Care,* 29: 1212–25.

Berwick, D., Endhoven, A. and Bunker, J. P. (1992) Quality management in the NHS: The doctor's role. *British Medical Journal,* 304: 235–9, 304–8.

Berwick, D., Godfrey, A. B. and Roessner, J. (1990/2002) *Curing Health Care.* San Francisco: Jossey-Bass.

Bowns, I. R. and McNulty, T. (1999) *Re-engineering Leicester Royal Infirmary: An Independent Evaluation of Implementation and Impact.* Sheffield: University of Sheffield

Brassard, M., Finn, L., Ginn, D. and Ritter, D. (2002) *The Six Sigma Memory Jogger.* Salem: GOAL/QPC.

Brideau, L. P. (2004) Flow: Why does it matter? *Frontiers of Health Services Management,* 20(4): 47–50.

Bushell, S. and Shelest, B. (2002) Discovering lean thinking at progressive healthcare, *Journal for Quality and Participation,* 25(2): 20.

Camp, R. C. (1989) *Benchmarking: The Search for Industry Best Practice that Leads to Superior Performance*. Milwaukee: ASQC Quality Press.

Chassin, M. (1998) Is health care ready for six sigma quality? *Milbank Quarterly*, 76(4): 565–91.

Checkland, P. (1981) *Systems Thinking, Systems Practice*. New York: Wiley.

Crosby, P. (1979) *Quality is Free*. New York: McGraw-Hill.

Dale, B. G. (ed.) (2003) *Managing Quality*. Oxford: Blackwell.

Degeling, P., Maxwell, S., Kennedy, J. and Coyle, B. (2003) Medicine, management, and modernisation: A 'danse macabre'? *British Medical Journal*, 326(7390): 649–52.

Deming, W. E. (1986) *Out of the Crisis*. Cambridge, MA: MIT, Centre of Advanced Engineering Study.

Department of Health (DH, 1998) *A First Class Service: Quality in the New NHS*. London: Department of Health.

Donabedian, A. (1966) Evaluating the quality of medical care. *Milbank Memorial Fund Quarterly*, 44(3): 166–206.

Donabedian, A. (1987) Commentary on some studies of the quality of care. *Health Care Financing Review*, annual supplement: 75–86.

Dopson, S. and Fitzgerald, L. (eds) (2005) *Knowledge to Action?* Oxford: Oxford University Press.

Erwin, J. and Douglas, P. (2000) Six sigma's focus on total customer satisfaction. *Journal for Quality and Participation*, 23(2): 45–9.

Feigenbaum, A. (1961) *Total Quality Control*. New York: McGraw-Hill.

Gershon, P. (2004) *Releasing Resources to the Front Line: Independent Review of Public Sector Efficiency*. London: The Stationery Office.

Goldratt Consulting Group (2005) Healthcare the TOC way. *http://www.healthcare-toc.com/TOCFORHEALTH.htm* (accessed 12 December 2005).

Goldratt, E. M. (1988) Computerised shop floor scheduling. *International Journal of Production Research*, 26(3): 453.

Golembiewski, R., Proehl, C. and Sink, D. (1982) Estimating success of OD applications. *Training and Development Journal*, 72: 86–95.

Greenwood, T., Bradford, M. and Greene, B. (2002) Becoming a lean enterprise: A tale of two firms: Both an aircraft manufacturer and an oral surgeon are reaping efficiencies from following the principles of lean transformation. *Strategic Finance*, 84(5): 32–40.

Grol, R., Baker, R. and Moss, F. (eds) (2004) *Quality Improvement Research: Understanding the Science of Change in Health Care*. London: British Medical Journal Books.

Groonroos, C. (1984) *Strategic Management and Marketing in the Service Sector*. London: Chartwell-Bratt.

Hackman, J. R. and Wageman, R. (1995) Total quality management: Empirical, conceptual and practical issues. *Administrative Science Quarterly*, 40(2): 309–42.

Hammer, M. and Champy, J. (1993) *Reengineering the Corporation: A Manifesto for Business Revolution*. New York: HarperCollins.

Haraden, C. and Resar, R. (2004) Patient flow in hospitals: Understanding and controlling it better. *Frontiers of Health Services Management*, 20(4): 3–15.

Hill, D. (2001) Physician strives to create lean, clean health care machine. *Physician Executive*, 27: 5.

Hines, P., Holweg, M. and Rich, N. (2004) Learning to evolve: A review of contemporary lean thinking. *International Journal of Operations and Production Management*, 24(10): 994–1011.

Horton, S. (2004) Increasing capacity while improving the bottom line. *Frontiers of Health Services Management*, 20(4): 17–23.

Iles, V. and Sutherland, K. (2001) *Organisational Change: A Review for Health Care Managers, Professionals and Researchers*. London: National Co-ordinating Centre for NHS Service Delivery and Organisation.

Institute for Healthcare Improvement (2003) *Optimizing Patient Flow: Moving Patients Smoothly through Acute Care Settings*. Boston: Institute for Healthcare Improvement.

Institute of Medicine and Committee on Quality Health Care in America (2001) *Crossing the Quality Chasm*. Washington, DC: Institute of Medicine.

Ishikawa, K. (1979) *Guide to Total Quality Control*. Tokyo: Asian Productivity Organisation.

Joint Commission on Accreditation of Healthcare Organisations (2005) Failure mode effect and criticality analysis. *http://www.jcaho.org/accredited*+organizations/patient+safety/fmeca/index.htm (accessed 11 March 2005).

Juran, J. (ed.) (1951) *The Quality Control Handbook*. New York; McGraw-Hill.

Kaplan, G. S. and Rona, J. M. (2004) Seeking zero defects: Applying the Toyota production system to health care. *16th National Forum on Quality Improvement in Healthcare*, Orlando, Florida.

Kenagy, J. W., Berwick, D. M. and Shore, M. F. (1999) Service quality in health care. *JAMA*, 281(7): 661–5.

Kerfoot, D. and Knights, D. (1995) Empowering the 'quality worker'? The seduction and contradiction of the total quality phenomenon. In A. Wilkinson and H. Willmott (eds) *Making Quality Critical*. London: Routledge.

Kerr, D., Bevan, H., Gowland, B., Penny, J. and Berwick, D. (2002) Redesigning cancer care. *British Medical Journal*, 324(7330): 164–7.

Kolb, D. A. (1984) *Experiential Learning: Experience as the Source of Learning and Development*. New York: Prentice-Hall.

Langley, G. J., Nolan, K. M., Nolan, T. W., Norman, C. L. and Provost, L. P. (1996) *The Improvement Guide*. San Francisco: Jossey-Bass.

Locock, L (2003) Healthcare redesign: meaning, origins and application. *Quality and Safety in Health Care*, 12(1): 53–8.

Lubitsh, G. (2004) The impact of theory of constraints (TOC) in an NHS trust. Submitted to *Journal of Management Development*.

Lugon, M. and Secker-Walker, J. (eds) (1999) *Clinical Governance: Making it Happen*. London: Royal Society of Medicine Press.

McLaughlin, C. P. and Simpson, K. N. (1999) Does TQM/CQI work in healthcare? In C. P. McLaughlin, and A. D. Kaluzny, *Continuous Quality Improvement in Health Care: Theory, Implementation and Applications*. Gaithersburg: Aspen.

McNulty, T. and Ferlie, E. (2002) *Reengineering Health Care: The Complexities of Organisational Transformation*. Oxford: Oxford University Press.

Mabin, V. J. and Balderstone, S. J. (2003) The performance of the theory of constraints methodology: Analysis and discussion of successful TOC applications. *International Journal of Operations and Production Management*, 23(6): 568–95.

Marshall, T., Mohammed, M. and Rouse, A. (2004a) A randomised controlled trial of league tables and control charts as aids to heath service decision-making. *International Journal for Quality in Health Care*, 16: 4.

Marshall, T., Mohammed, M. A. and Rouse, A. (2004b) A randomized controlled trial of league tables and control charts as aids to health service decision-making. *International Journal of Quality Health Care*, 16(4): 309–15.

Maxwell, R. J. (1984) Quality assessment in health. *British Medical Journal*, 288: 1470–2.

Middleton, S., Barnett, J. and Reeves, D. (2001) What is an integrated care pathway? *What is?* 3(3): 1–8.

Mohammed, M. A. (2004) Using statistical process control to improve the quality of health care. *Quality and Safety in Health Care*, 13(4): 243–5.

Mohammed, M. A., Cheng, K. K., Rouse, A. and Marshall, T. (2001) Bristol, Shipman, and clinical governance: Shewhart's forgotten lessons. *The Lancet*, 357(9254): 463–7.

Mohammed, M. A., Rathbone, A., Myers, P., Patel, D., Onions, H. and Stevens, A. (2004) An investigation into general practitioners associated with high patient mortality flagged up through the Shipman inquiry: Retrospective analysis of routine data. *British Medical Journal*, 328(7454): 1474–7.

NHS Modernisation Agency (2005a) 10 high impact changes for service improvement and delivery. *http://www.wise.nhs.uk/NR/rdonlyres/6E0D282A–4896–46DF-B8C7–068AA5EA1121/654/HIC_for_web.pdf* (accessed 12 December 2005).

NHS Modernisation Agency (2005b) NHS Institute for Innovation and Improvement supersedes the Modernisation Agency. *http://www.wise.nhs.uk/cmsWISE/aboutUs/AboutMA.htm* (accessed 12 December) 2005.

Nielsen, D. M., Merry, M. D., Schyve, P. M. and Bisognano, M. (2004) Can the gurus' concepts cure healthcare? *Quality Progress*, 37(9): 25–6.

Nolan, T. W. (1998) Understanding medical systems. *Annals of Internal Medicine*, 128(4): 293–8.

Øvretveit, J. (1997) A comparison of hospital quality programmes: Lessons for other services. *International Journal of Service Industry Management*, 8(3): 220–35.

Øvretveit, J., Bate, P. and Cleary, P. (2002) Quality collaboratives: Lessons from research. *Quality and Safety in Health Care*, 11: 345–51.

Parasuraman, A., Zeithaml, V. A. and Berry, L. L. (1988) SERVQUAL: A multiple item scale for measuring consumer perceptions of service quality. *Journal of Retailing*, 64(1): 14–40.

Plsek, P. (1999) Quality improvement methods in clinical medicine. *Pediatrics*, 103(1): 203–14.

Pollitt, C. (1993) The struggle for quality: the case of the NHS. *Policy and Politics*, 21(3): 161–70.

Reason, J. (1997) *Managing the Risk of Organisational Accidents*. Aldershot: Ashgate.

Reeves, C. A. and Bednar, D. A. (1994) Defining quality: Alternatives and implications. *Academy of Management Review*, 19(3): 419–56.

Revere, L., Black, K. and Huq, A. (2004) Integrating six sigma and CQI for improving patient care. *TQM Magazine*, 16(2): 105–13.

Robertson, P. J. and Seneviratne, S. J. (1995) Outcomes of planned organisational change in the public sector: A meta analytic comparison to the private sector. *Public Administration Review*, 55(6): 547–58.

Schon, D. A. (1988) *Educating the Reflective Practitioner. Toward a New Design for Teaching and Learning in the Professions*. San Francisco: Jossey-Bass.

Seddon, J. (2005) Watch out for the toolheads. *www.lean-service.com* (accessed 1 February 2005).

Sehwail, L. and DeYong, C. (2003) Six sigma in health care. *International Journal of Health Care Quality Assurance*, 16(6): 1.

Senge, K. A., Roberts C., Ross R. B. and Smith B. J. (1994) *The Fifth Discipline Fieldbook*. London: Nicholas Brearley.

Shewhart, W. A. (1931) *Economic Control of Quality of Manufactured Product*. New York: Van Nostrand.

Shingo, S. (1986) *Zero Quality Control: Source Inspection and the Poka-Yoke System*. Cambridge, MA: Productivity Press.

Shortell, S., Levin, D., O'Brien, J. and Hughes, E. (1995) Assessing the evidence on CQI: Is the glass half empty or half full? *Journal of the Foundation of the American College of Healthcare Executives*, 40: 4–24.

Slack, N., Chambers, S. and Johnston, R. (2004) *Operations Management*. Harlow: FT/Prentice Hall.

Snee, R. D. (1990) Statistical thinking and its contribution to total quality. *American Statistician*, 44(2): 116–21.

Stiles, R. A. and Mick, S. S. (1994) Classifying quality initiatives: A conceptual paradigm for literature review and policy analysis. *Hospital and Health Services Administration*, 39(3): 309.

Taguchi, G. (1986) *Introduction to Quality Engineering*. New York: Asian Productivity Organisation.

Vinzant, J. C. and Vinzant, D. H. (1999) Strategic management spin-offs of the Deming approach. *Journal of Management History*, 5(8): 516–31.

Walley, P. (2003) Designing the accident and emergency system: Lessons from manufacturing. *Emergency Medical Journal*, 20(2): 126–30.

Walley, P. and Gowland, B. (2004) Completing the circle: from PD to PDSA. *International Journal of Health Care Quality Assurance*, 17(6): 349–58.

Walshe, K. and Boaden, R. (eds) (2006) *Patient Safety: Research into Practice*. Maidenhead: Open University Press.

Webb, J. (1995) Quality management and the management of quality. In A. Wilkinson and H. Willmott (eds) *Making Quality Critical*. London: Routledge.

Wilkinson, A. (1992) The other side of quality: soft issues and the human resource dimension. *Total Quality Management*, 3(3): 323–9.

Wilkinson, A. and Willmott, H. (eds) (1995) *Making Quality Critical*. London: Routledge.

Womack, J. P. and Jones, D. T. (1996) *Lean Thinking*. London: Simon and Schuster.

Zbabada, C., Rivers, P. A. and Munchus, G. (1998) Obstacles to the application of TQM in healthcare organisations. *Total Quality Management* 9(1): 57–67.

Zimmerman, R. S. (2004) Hospital capacity, productivity and patient safety – it all flows together. *Frontiers of Health Services Management*, 20(4): 33–8.

Websites and resources

Agency for Healthcare Research and Quality. *http://www.ahrq.gov/*
Canadian Council on Healthcare Accreditation. *http://www.cchsa.ca*
European Society for Quality in Healthcare. *http://www.esqh.net*
Healthcare Commission. *http://www.healthcarecommission.org.uk*
Institute for Healthcare Improvement. *www.ihi.org*
International Society for Quality in Healthcare. *http://www.isqua.org.au/*
Joint Commission for the Accreditation of Healthcare Organisations. *http://www.jcaho.org/*
Quality Improvement Scotland. *http://www.nhshealthquality.org/*
National Institute for Clinical Excellence (NICE). *http://www.nice.org.uk/*

NHS Institute/Modernisation Agency. *http://www.institute.nhs.uk/ http://www.wise.nhs.uk/cmswise/default.htm*

NHS Productive Time Programme. *http://www.dh.gov.uk/PolicyAndGuidance/HumanResourcesAndTraining/ProductiveTime/fs/en*

27 Research, evaluation and evidence-based management

Kieran Walshe

Introduction

This chapter is about how healthcare managers and policymakers use evidence when they make decisions, and it argues that by making more effective use of evidence from research and evaluation, managers and policymakers could make better decisions. It is not difficult to find examples of bad decisions – which not only look like mistakes in retrospect, but which flew in the face of evidence available at the time. For example, mergers between healthcare organisations have often been justified on the grounds that the new, larger organisation would be more efficient, with lower administrative costs and savings from the rationalisation of clinical services, buildings and facilities. In the UK the late 1990s saw an epidemic of acute hospital mergers and reconfiguration based on little or no real evidence (Edwards and Harrison 1999), and more recently the Department of Health has mandated mergers among primary care organisations across England (DH 2005). In fact, the research evidence suggests that such mergers rarely achieve their explicit objectives, that there are often as many diseconomies as economies of scale and that after merger it takes years for the new organisation to become properly integrated and begin to realise any of the potential advantages of its scale (Fulop et al. 2002). There are even a number of well-documented examples of frankly disastrous mergers that have come close to destroying the unfortunate organisations which have been pressed into merging (Kitchener 2002). So why, faced with all this evidence, do managers and policymakers continue to have such faith that organisational mergers 'work'? The unpalatable truth may be that managers do not know about the evidence; do not understand, trust or believe it if they do know it exists; and allow other factors such as ideology, fashion and political convenience to predominate in the decision-making processes in their organisations (Abrahamson 1996; Marmor 2001; Smith et al. 2001).

This chapter first explores the growth of the evidence-based healthcare movement in the 1990s and the increasing role played by research evidence in clinical decision making. It then argues that while managerial and clinical decision making are very different processes, decision making by managers and policymakers can and should be more directly informed by research evidence. Next, the chapter explores how evidence is created in research, and then examines how healthcare managers and policymakers can find, appraise and apply relevant evidence. It concludes by suggesting that the technical challenges of providing the right evidence, at the right time, in the right format for managers to use are not negligible but are also not insuperable. However, making better use of evidence requires a real cultural shift among managers – towards a more scientifically informed, intellectually rigorous way of thinking and behaving.

The rise of evidence-based healthcare

In the 1990s, there was a widespread international change in the way that healthcare professionals, researchers, and health systems thought about and used research evidence about research in clinical decision making, which has been labelled as the rise of the 'evidence-based healthcare movement' (Davidoff et al. 1995; Sackett and Rosenberg 1995). It was driven in part by a growing realisation of what is sometimes termed the 'research–practice gap' – that healthcare interventions which we knew to be effective took a long time to enter common clinical practice, while other interventions which we knew did not work also took a long time to be discarded by clinicians (Antman et al. 1992). The Institute of Medicine (1999) described these as problems of underuse, overuse and misuse, and there was no shortage of practical and high-profile examples. Thrombolytic therapy for myocardial infarction – a drug treatment for people with heart attacks which, if given promptly reduces the likelihood of the person having another heart attack in the future and significantly reduces mortality – became the 'poster child' for the EBM movement because there was good evidence that it had taken a decade or more for physicians to adopt it after the research evidence for its effectiveness was incontrovertible (Birkhead 1999). But just as high-profile examples of overuse, underuse and misuse can be identified in the clinical domain, we can also find cases in the managerial arena as Table 27.1 shows.

In retrospect, we saw a real shift in the 1990s in the paradigm that dominated our thinking about how health services research was conducted; how research findings were disseminated or communicated to healthcare professionals and organisations; and how those findings were implemented and used to change clinical practice (Lemieux-Charles and Champagne 2004). This shift is mapped out in Table 27.2 and can be summarised as a move away from seeing all these matters as issues primarily for individuals – researchers and practitioners – to seeing them as issues which organisations and healthcare systems needed to grapple with; and a shift from allowing these issues to be treated passively and reactively, leaving them almost wholly unmanaged and uncontrolled, to

Table 27.1 The research–practice gap

	Clinical domain	Management and policy domain
Overuse	• Prophylactic extractions of asymptomatic impacted third molars (wisdom teeth) • The widespread/general use of screening for prostate cancer	• Organisational mergers as a response to problems of service quality, capacity or financial viability in healthcare organisations
Underuse	• Smoking cessation through nicotine replacement therapy • Compression therapy for venous leg ulcers	• The replacement of physicians with other health professionals in providing many routine health services especially in settings like primary care and accident and emergency departments
Misuse	• Pressure-relieving equipment in the prevention of pressure sores • Selection of hip prostheses in hip replacement surgery	• The adoption and implementation of total quality management or continuous quality improvement initiatives

Source: Adapted from Walshe and Rundall (2001).

being much more proactive and strategic in setting direction, managing implementation and monitoring progress.

The idea that evidence should play a bigger part in decision making has an intuitive appeal and it quickly began to appear in a much wider literature, in public policy fields such as housing, social care, criminal justice and education (Davies et al. 2000) and in other areas of management (Tranfield et al. 2003). After the UK General election in 1997, the New Labour government announced that 'what matters is what works', signalling a move away from ideologically driven policymaking to a more pragmatic and technocratic approach in which evidence of effect and impact would play a much later part (Cabinet Office 1999). The realities of this ambitious announcement have been more complex and contingent, but the Cabinet Office and National Audit Office have both produced reports and materials on using evidence in policymaking, and the Economic and Social Research Council (ESRC) has supported the creation of a Centre for Evidence Based Policy and Practice (see website resources section at end of chapter).

Health policy and management have been on the front line of this developing movement. Clinicians challenged to justify the adoption of a new surgical technique or new pharmaceutical have often responded by arguing that the same evidentiary standard should be applied to management decisions – like proposals to change or reconfigure services, to introduce new organisational structures, or to change payment or incentive systems (Hewison 1997; Kovner et al. 2000). It is a difficult argument to resist. While some commentators have asserted that policy and management decisions are different in some important and fundamental ways which mean they are not simply amenable to technocratic, rationalist analysis (Klein 2000), and while others have cautioned about the unthinking transfer of methods and techniques for research synthesis and

Table 27.2 The paradigm shift of evidence-based healthcare

	From	To
Research strategy	No national leadership of healthcare research, funding fragmented across many research funders with poor communication and coordination	Growing strategic lead at a national level, coordination of research activity and funders leading to a more coherent overall research agenda
Research direction	Researcher led, tied to academic agendas, little coordination	Needs led, tied to health service priorities, focused on major service areas/needs, well coordinated
Research quality	Much ad hoc, piecemeal, small-scale, poor quality research, sometimes repetitive, not well managed or reviewed	Coherent research programmes made up of well-planned, larger research projects of high quality.
Research methods	Inflexibility about methods, with frequent mismatches between research questions and methods used	More appropriate use of research methods, from experimental methods to qualitative approaches, depending on the research questions
Research outputs	Publications in peer-reviewed academic journals seen as researchers' primary goal	Changes in clinical practice seen as primary aim of research, with publication as one step towards that goal
Dissemination of research findings	Journals, textbooks, expert opinions, and narrative reviews	Online databases, summaries of evidence, clinical guidelines, secondary journals, systematic reviews
Mode of access to research findings	'Pull' access, reliant on clinicians seeking information by accessing libraries, journals, databases, etc.	'Push' access, with relevant research findings delivered to clinicians proactively, as close to the relevant point of care as possible
Practitioner understanding of research findings	Focused on reports of individual research studies	Focused on meta-analyses and systematic reviews of relevant, appraised research
Practitioner attitudes to research	Uninformed, suspicious of methods and motives, lacking skills in research appraisal and interpretation	Informed, accustomed to using and participating in research, skilled in appraising and applying research to own clinical practice
Major influences on clinical practice	Personal clinical experience, precedent, tradition, expert opinion.	Clinical epidemiology, empirical evidence, research
Responsibility for implementing research findings	Left to individual clinical professionals and clinical teams, with little corporate interest or involvement in decision making	Seen as a key organisational function, supported by investments in information resources, etc., with corporate involvement and oversight alongside clinical team in decision making

Source: Adapted from Walshe and Rundall (2001).

application from the biomedical to the managerial arena, few would argue that there is not scope to improve the quality of managerial decisions and policy choices by bringing robust evidence to bear (Lomas 2005).

Evidence-based management and policymaking

Table 27.3 summarises and compares the clinical and managerial domains in terms of their approaches to producing and using evidence in decision making. In broad terms, they have very different cultures and the clinical culture places much greater value on empiricism and science, while the managerial culture gives priority to personal experience and experiential learning. They draw on quite different literatures. The clinical literature is better organised and structured, easier to search and more positivist and oriented toward generalising research findings, while the management literature is less coherently defined and organised, less amenable to searching and synthesis and makes fewer claims to generalisability. The decision-making process is different too. Clinicians make many homogeneous decisions to which it is sensible and simple to apply algorithmic approaches (guidelines, protocols and procedures) to define and standardise the process and to embed the use of evidence. In contrast, managers' decision are more heterogeneous and less clearly bounded and are often made in combination with others (Walshe and Rundall 2001).

In short, while the principles of evidence-based decision making should clearly apply in the managerial and policymaking arenas, their practical application is likely to be rather different. The challenges are less concerned with the technical and logistic problems of delivering the right evidence in the right place at the right time to support the decision-making process, and more about changing attitudes and beliefs among both researchers and managers, promoting linkage and exchange between the two communities and creating a culture in which the value of good evidence is recognised and a capacity to make use of it in decision making (Lomas 2000).

The Canadian Health Services Research Foundation (CHSRF), created in 1997 with funding from a government endowment of CD\$126 million, has pioneered work in this area and unusually for a research institute defines its purpose as to 'support the evidence-based decision making in the organisation, management and delivery of health services through funding research, building capacity and transferring knowledge' and aims to 'establish and foster linkages between decision makers (managers and policymakers) and researchers' (CHSRF 2004). CHSRF has tackled this ambitious mission on several fronts. They fund programmes of research which have to have co-funding from healthcare organisations, a requirement which is designed to ensure that researchers have managerial commitment and support for their work and have to engage with the practice community. They also support training for managers in research

Table 27.3   The clinical and managerial domains compared

	Clinical practice	Health care management
Culture	• Highly professionalised, with a strong formal body of knowledge and control of entry to the profession resulting in coherence of knowledge, attitudes and beliefs • High value placed on scientific knowledge and research, with many researchers who are also practitioners (and vice versa)	• Much less professionalised, with much less formal body of knowledge, no control of entry, and great diversity among practitioners • Personal experience and self-generated knowledge highly valued, intensely pragmatic • Less understanding of research, some suspicion of value, and of motives of researchers • Divide between researchers and practitioners, with little interchange between the two worlds
Research and evidence	• Strong biomedical, empirical paradigm, with focus on experimental methods and quantitative data • Belief in generalisability and objectivity of research findings • Well organised and indexed literature, concentrated in certain journals with clear boundaries, amenable to systematic review and synthesis	• Weak social sciences paradigm, with more use of qualitative methods and less empiricism • Tendency to see research findings as more subjective, contingent, and less generalisable • Poorly organised and indexed research literature, spread across journals and other literature sources (including grey literature), with unclear boundaries, heterogeneous and not easy to review systematically or synthesise
Decision making	• Many clinical decisions taken every day, mostly by individual clinicians with few constraints on their decisions • Decisions often homogeneous, involving the application of general body of knowledge to specific circumstances • Long tradition of using decision support systems (handbooks, guidelines, etc) • Results of decision often relatively clear, and some immediate feedback	• Fewer, larger decisions taken, usually by or in groups, with many organisational constraints, often requiring negotiation or compromise • Decisions heterogeneous, and less based on applying a general body of knowledge to specific circumstances • No tradition of using any form of decision support • Results of decision and causal relationship between decision and subsequent events often very hard to determine

Source: Adapted from Walshe and Rundall (2001).

appraisal and research application and training for researchers aimed at developing research capacity and researcher skills in in knowledge translation and utilisation. They invest directly in the process of linkage and exchange through events, workshops and forums in which researchers, policymakers and practitioners are brought together to discuss issues of common concern, and through publications like their evidence briefings and 'mythbuster' series, designed to provide clear, credible and comprehensible summaries of the evidence on a topic for a practitioner audience (Box 27.1).

The work of CHSRF provides an eloquent proof of principle, showing that it is possible to bring evidence to bear on the worlds of managers and policymakers, and that research can make a real and important contribution to decision making. More importantly, its experience supports the contention that action at a health system level is needed to promote linkage and exchange between the research and practice communities, to change cultures and attitudes, and to build capacity on both sides in knowledge translation and utilisation. For other countries, the work of CHSRF has been held up as a model to follow or learn from (NAO 2003). In the UK, the NHS service delivery and organisation (SDO) research programme, established in 2000 by the Department of Health, has adopted some of the principles and ideas of CHSRF in setting its research agenda and communicating research funding to managers and others in the NHS.

Box 27.1   About the Canadian Health Services Research Foundation

- The Canadian Health Services Research Foundation (a) funds management and policy research in health services and nursing; (b) supports the synthesis and dissemination of research results; (c) supports the use of research results by managers and policymakers in the health system.
- It provides research funding opportunities for both researchers and decision makers to investigate specific health-system questions (including investigator-initiated and commissioned research, as well as policy syntheses).
- It provides training opportunities for senior decision makers in nursing, medicine, and health administration to learn to find and apply research in their daily work and to facilitate evidence-based decision making.
- It supports training and personnel development for new researchers as well as for established researchers in our own field and those in other fields who would like to apply skills from other domains to health-system challenges.
- It provides user-friendly research results and descriptions of ongoing projects.
- It offers services and resources to both decision makers and researchers, to support communication and networking, and disseminating and using research.
- It holds and co-sponsors skill-building events and activities where researchers and decision makers work together to find better ways to enhance research results and put them to work.
- It recognises excellence and achievement in doing, supporting, communicating and using research results, through its Health Services Research Advancement Award.

Creating evidence: the role of research

The traditional complaint of clinicians and managers alike is that they cannot pursue evidence-based practice because the right evidence to support their decision making is not available. While in some cases this may be an excuse for inaction, it is certainly true that the conventional processes of research outlined in Table 28.2 often delivered research which was interesting to researchers rather than research useful to practitioners, health organisations or health systems.

Now, research funders make increasing use of research 'horizon scanning' or 'listening' processes designed to help them identify or predict the issues on which research is needed, and then to set their priorities accordingly (Lomas et al. 2003). For example, the NHS SDO programme has conducted and subsequently updated a broad consultation which identified its main research themes through, among other things, a large-scale email survey of key stakeholders asking them to respond to five key questions (NCCSDO 2000, 2002):

1 What is the single most important change to the organisation of the NHS services that you would like to see?
2 What do you think will be the major issues facing the NHS in five years time?
3 Would you like to see any further R&D work on the current themes, over and above the work outlined below?
4 What new themes should the NHS SDO R&D Programme be addressing now to inform the next five years?
5 Have you used any research evidence on service delivery and organisation in healthcare to effect change in services? If yes, what were the key elements that encourages you to act on its finding?

The results of this exercise in horizon scanning are summarised in Box 27.2, which sets out the research themes which resulted.

Of course, this is just the start of the process. Research funders have to convert these broad themes into researchable, focused questions and decide on what methodologies or approaches are best suited to tackling them. Some questions may need new primary research, involving empirical fieldwork that gathers data to try to answer the questions, but others may be better answered by seeking and summarising the findings from existing research through a process of synthesis (Pawson 2002; Lavis et al. 2005). Research funders also have to think pragmatically about the timescale for the research, and the point at which it will deliver meaningful research findings to decision makers. Commissioning and undertaking research can be a laborious and time-consuming process, taking anything from six months to three years before the products are available. If policymakers and practitioners need the evidence more quickly than researchers can deliver it, some compromise needs to be made in research design and process to try to match timescales while maintaining the rigour and validity of the research.

Box 27.2 NHS service delivery and organisation research programme themes

Organising the NHS around the needs of the patient	Access, adapting to local needs, self-management, choice, empowerment and consumerism, role of carers
User involvement	Formal mechanisms, empowerment and evaluation
Continuity of care	Organisational boundaries, partnership working, professional boundaries
Co-ordination/integration across organisations	Structural and financial issues, financial changes, shifting the balance of power, integrated care organisations
Workforce issues and interprofessional working	Interprofessional working, changing roles, recruitment and retention, staff morale, education and training
Resources	Effects of increased investment, financial systems, evaluation of benefits of investment
Implications of the communications revolution	Development of electronic records, the need for patient held records, and the development of improved information systems
Relationship between organisational form, function and outcomes	Development of organisational roles and boundaries, and tensions between central and local control
Evaluation of major policy initiatives	Developing new models of service delivery, development of nationally comparable service models
Management of change	The changing role of the patient, scale and pace of change, management styles in change management, benefits of change

---

Finding the evidence: what do we know?

Most policymakers and managers are not in a position to commission research when they face a decision – and do not have the time to wait for research findings anyway. Therefore, what matters most is their ability to access, appraise and apply the findings from existing research to the situations or decisions they face. The first step is finding that research.

Unfortunately, while a huge investment has been made in organising the clinical evidence base, particularly through the worldwide Cochrane Collaboration and its associated library of systematic reviews, randomised controlled trials and other evidence, the literature on management and policy issues remains fragmented, heterogeneous, distributed and difficult to access. There is no single portal or gateway to use and so it is very important to work out a clear search strategy. Ideally, that search strategy would achieve three things: it would be sensitive (which means it finds all the relevant research and does not miss anything out); specific (which means it does not find any irrelevant or unrelated research); and realistic (which means it can be done in the time and with the resources available). In reality, there is an inevitable tradeoff to be made between sensitivity, specificity and realism, depending in part on the circumstances and context for the decision. If resources and time are short, then 'quick and dirty' searching is needed, while if there is more space for reflection and analysis, a more sophisticated and comprehensive search can be undertaken. Obviously, the more important and significant the decision, the more should be invested in the search for evidence.

Table 27.4 sets out four main sources of evidence to which managers might turn, broadly in the order in which they could or should be searched: evidence databases; bibliographic databases; key research agencies; key journals.

The place to start is the evidence databases, though as has already been observed, no one has yet tackled the immense task of providing a proper portal to the evidence on healthcare management and policymaking. Table 27.4 suggests three sources. First, the Cochrane Library, although mainly focused on clinical interventions, contains some reviews and other data relevant to organisational issues (Lavis et al. 2006). For example, it holds evidence on the impact of stroke units on the management of stroke, and reviews of interventions to change professional practice like the use of financial incentives and educational programmes. Second, the NHS National Electronic Library for Health (NeLH) provides a superb and searchable portal to a wide range of resources from NHS organisations and research programmes, including clinical guide-

Table 27.4   Research findings: some key sources

Evidence databases	Cochrane Library NHS National Electronic Library for Health NHS Centre for Reviews and Dissemination WHO Health Evidence Network
Bibliographic databases	Medline ABI-INFORM/Proquest Health Management Information Consortium (HMIC)
Key research agencies	Canadian Health Services Research Foundation NHS service delivery and organisation (SDO) research programme US Agency for Healthcare Research and Quality UK Department of Health Policy Research Programme
Key journals	*Health Affairs* *Health Services Research* *Health Services Management Research* *Journal of Health Services Research and Policy* *Milbank Quarterly* *Frontiers of Health Services Management*

lines, official reports, research reports and other materials. Third, and with a more international orientation, the World Health Organisation's Health Evidence Network provides an integrated, searchable interface to the evidence and information from a wide range of agencies in many countries, as well as undertaking its own syntheses on questions raised by members of the network.

The next step – and one that many practitioners will find more difficult – is to access the relevant bibliographic databases which index the contents of academic and practitioner journals, and also provide some coverage of books, official reports and other materials. Here, recommendations are much more difficult to make as there are dozens of such databases with overlapping and complementary coverage, but three particular examples are cited. The first port of call for many people will be Medline – the database of medical and health-related literature created and maintained by the US National Library of Medicine. While it is somewhat Americocentric, it has by far the best overall international coverage both of clinical and policy/management materials in the health sector and it is freely available through the NLM's PubMed service. However, much of the relevant literature on management issues is not health-sector specific and will have been published in more generic business and management journals. To access the literature on issues like leadership, organisational design and development, quality improvement and many other topics it is very important not to confine the search to the health-related literature covered by Medline. The most useful database in this area is ABI Inform (also known as Proquest) which gives comprehensive coverage of the business and management literature. However, neither ABI Inform nor Medline cover what some people call the 'grey literature' – publications from healthcare organisations, health ministries and agencies, think tanks, government departments, and others. In this area, for the UK, the Health Management Information Consortium database (HMIC) provides by far the best coverage. It combines the catalogues of collection at the UK Department of Health's library services and the King's Fund and is particularly useful because it indexes and abstracts UK practitioner journals like the *Health Service Journal* and official reports and publications, though its coverage is very UK focused.

For most purposes, the search strategy is likely to stop after accessing evidence and bibliographic databases, but some may find it useful to search the information resources provided by key research agencies like CHSRF, the NHS SDO research programme, the US Agency for Healthcare Research and Quality, and so on. Searching these sites for research on a specific issue is likely to be a frustrating and unproductive experience, but browsing them to get a better sense of the research resources, themes and issues they have covered is certainly worthwhile. Similarly, few managers will have the time to undertake hand searches of key journals like those listed in Table 27.4, but it can be very useful to scan the contents pages of past issues to understand their coverage, or to subscribe to the contents page services most journals now offer, so that summary details of each new journal issue are received by email as it is published.

Searching some or all of these sources is made much easier with some informed and trained support from a knowledge officer, information scientist or librarian who understands the search structures and terminology used. It is common for untrained searchers either to cast their search too broadly – using terms which return hundreds or even thousands of 'hits' – or too narrowly, so that they get little or nothing and miss relevant materials. But finding the evidence is only one step in the process – the next challenge is knowing whether to trust it and what it means.

Appraising the evidence: what does it mean?

Just because research is published in a prestigious journal or produced by a government agency does not mean it should be taken on trust. Many agencies have a political or organisational agenda, covert or overt, and the authors of the research may have been influenced by their own beliefs and values. However stringent the quality control and peer review process, badly designed, poorly conducted research studies still get published even in the best journals. Moreover, the findings from research are not always clear and unambiguous – they can be open to interpretation or difficult to understand. Even if the findings are clear, it is important to consider how generalisable or transferable they are – in other words, to what extent they can be applied to a particular organisation or context, and whether there are important differences between the setting for the research and the setting in which it is to be applied. The ability to appraise research evidence critically and carefully is essential (Coomarasamy and Khan 2004). There are three key questions to be asked in appraisal:

1 Can I trust this research? Has it been conducted properly, using the right research methods, to tackle a meaningful set of research questions?
2 What does this research mean? What are the findings, and how much confidence can I place in them?
3 How can this research be applied to our local situation? Is it appropriate to generalise or transfer from the setting in which the research was conducted, and what implications are there from any differences in setting?

Of course, the way these questions might be asked would be different for different sorts of research. Appraising a qualitative study involving interviews with health professionals may require different criteria from those used to appraise a quantitative experimental study such as a randomised controlled trial. But the three issues remain the same – trust, meaning and application. Table 27.5 sets out a critical appraisal framework which

Table 27.5   Appraising research evidence: key questions to ask

	Randomised controlled trial	Qualitative study
Can you trust this research?	Did the trial address a clearly focused issue? (Are the population, intervention and outcome studied clear?)	Was there a clear statement of the aims of the research? (what were they trying to find out, and was it relevant and important)
	Was the assignment of patients to treatments randomised?	Is a qualitative methodology appropriate? (Does research seek to understand/ illuminate experiences or views?)
	Were all patients entered into the trial properly accounted for at its conclusion? (Look at completion of follow–up and whether groups analysed by intention to treat).	Was the sampling strategy appropriate to address the aims of the research? (Consider where sample selected from, who and why, how and why, sample size, non participation.)
	Were patients, health workers and study staff blind to the treatment?	Was the data collection appropriate to address the aims of the research? (Consider where and how collected, how recorded, whether methods modified during study.)
	Were the groups similar at the start of the trial?	Was the data analysis appropriate to address the aims of the research? (Consider whether method is clearly explained, how it was done, how categories/themes were derived from data, if credibility of findings tested, whether all data taken into account.)
	Aside from the experimental intervention, were the groups treated equally?	How well were research partnership relations handled? (Did researchers critically examine their own role, bias and influence? how was research explained to participants? how and where was data collected?)
What does it mean?	How large was the treatment effect? How precise was the estimate of the treatment effect?	Is there a clear statement of the findings? (Are they explicit and easy to understand?)
	Were all the important outcomes of the intervention considered?	Is there justification for data interpretation? (sufficient data to support the findings, selection of data for paper explained).
How can it be applied locally?	Can the results of this study be applied to your local population? (Consider what differences might exist and how significant they might be.)	How transferable are the findings to a wider population? (Consider context of study, sufficient details to compare to other settings, whether all relevant outcomes considered.)
	Are the benefits of this intervention worth the costs and/or harms, for your local population?	How relevant and useful is the research? (Address the research aim, add new understanding, suggest further research, relevance to your setting.)

Source: Adapted from the CASP, JAMA and EBM tools, all available from the SCHaRR Netting the Evidence Website (see web resources)

could be used to analyse a randomised controlled trial (RCT) or a qualitative study. Similar sets of questions can be produced to appraise other kinds of study – case study designs or economic evaluations, for example – and to appraise secondary research such as systematic reviews.

Applying the evidence: informed decision making?

The final step – and perhaps the most difficult one – is to use the evidence in a local context as part of the decision-making process (Lavis et al. 2005). Experience and research both suggest that it is unrealistic to expect this to be a simple or linear process in which the evidence – packaged or presented as a product by researchers – directly shapes an individual decision. It is more likely that evidence plays a more indirect and longer term part, shaping the context in which decisions are made and contributing to an iterative local debate in which evidence, values, politics, resources and other priorities all play a part. It is unlikely that for most health management or policy issues the research evidence will offer unambiguous or universal prescriptions for action. Rather, it is more probable that any recommendations will be contingent and will offer a range of possible courses of action with different potential benefits and costs.

Researchers may find their engagement in the decision-making process exciting and rewarding, as they see their endeavours having a real-world impact on health services and organisations. However, they may equally find the process alien and uncomfortable, and be disappointed by the way their carefully created and presented research findings are dealt with rather sceptically or abruptly, and other considerations accorded greater value. Researchers also need to consider how they are viewed by other stakeholders in the decision-making process – as honest brokers, offering information as a currency in the debate to all parties, or as yet another vested interest, allied to one side or another and using evidence as ammunition. The challenge for researchers is to engage closely with policymakers and practitioners while at the same time maintaining some distance. The researcher should not lose the disinterested and objective perspective on issues which they bring to the debate and for which they will be valued.

Conclusion

The quality of management and leadership in healthcare organisations is a fundamental determinant of the quality of service they provide to patients. Well-managed and effectively led organisations provide an environment in which high quality clinical care is both clearly valued and more capable of being delivered consistently. The decisions made by managers in organisations and, at a health system level, by policymakers inevitably influence organisational capacity, capability and behaviour.

There is no doubt that the more effective use of research evidence in the decision-making process could make for better decisions, less prone to fashion, ideology or personal conviction and more likely to be considered, rational and, in the longer term, more beneficial. But we are a long way from that position now. We have at the moment separate and divided research and practice communities, with different and conflicting notions of what constitutes evidence, and how to use it in decision making. Managers and researchers need to learn to speak each other's languages, to understand and respect each other's expertise, and to trust and value the contribution each can make to improving healthcare organisations and health systems.

Summary box

- By making more effective use of evidence from research in decision making, managers and policymakers in healthcare organisations and health systems could improve the quality of decision making which would have direct benefits for the quality of health services.
- The rise of the evidence-based healthcare movement has led to a shift in the paradigm for knowledge creation, translation and utilisation in many sectors, to place greater emphasis on the use of evidence in decision making.
- There are important differences between the clinical and managerial or policymaking domains which mean that the way evidence is collated and used may be very different. There is a real need to change attitudes and beliefs among researchers and managers, and to promote linkage and exchange between the two communities.
- Some research funders, such as the Canadian Health Services Research Foundation and the NHS service delivery and organisation research programme are showing that research can make a more significant contribution to health management and policy development.
- Managers can make some immediate progress in their own organisations by searching for, appraising and applying evidence in their own decision making. There are a growing number of sources of evidence available intended to support a more evidence-informed approach to management.
- Managers and researchers need to learn to speak each other's languages, to understand and respect each other's expertise, and to trust and value the contribution each can make to improving healthcare organisations and health systems.

Self-test exercises

1 Undertake an audit of the evidence resources available in your organisation to support managers. Visit your postgraduate centre, library, information services department and other potential resources. Explore what training is available in searching, critical appraisal and

other areas. Find out whether information scientists/librarians are available to support you in accessing evidence. Consider whether there are important gaps in provision and, if appropriate, draw up a short report to discuss with colleagues.

2 Choose an issue or topic of current relevance to your organisation – something on which important decisions are being made in the near future. Search some of the sources of evidence described in the chapter and listed in the website and resources section. Appraise the evidence you find using the framework set out in Table 27.5. Consider how the information from this process could be used by decision makers in your organisation.

References and further reading

Abrahamson, E. (1996) Management fashion. *Academy of Management Review*, 21(1): 254–85.

Antman, E., Lau, J., Kupelnick, B., Mosteller, F. and Chalmers, I. (1992) A comparison of the result of meta-analysis of randomised controlled trials and recommendations of clinical experts. *Journal of the American Medical Association*, 268: 240–8.

Birkhead, J.S. (1999). Trends in the provision of thrombolytic treatment 1993–1997. *Heart*, 82: 438–42.

Cabinet Office (1999) *Modernising Government*. London: The Stationery Office.

Canadian Health Services Research Foundation (CHSRF, 2004). *Annual Report*. Ottowa: CHSRF.

Coomarasamy, A. and Khan, K.S. (2004) What is the evidence that postgraduate teaching in evidence based medicine changes anything? A systematic review. *British Medical Journal*, 329: 1017–22.

Davidoff, F., Haynes, B., Sackett, D. and Smith, R. (1995) Evidence-based medicine. *British Medical Journal* 310(6987): 1085–6.

Davies, H. T. O., Nutley, S. M. and Smith, P. C. (eds) (2000) *What Works? Evidence-based Policy and Practice in Public Services*. Bristol: The Policy Press.

Department of Health (DH, 2005) *Commissioning a Patient Led NHS*. London: DH.

Edwards, N. and Harrison, A. (1999) The hospital of the future: Planning hospitals with limited evidence: A research and policy problem. *British Medical Journal*, 319: 1361–3.

Fulop, N., Protopsaltis, G., Hutchings, A., King, A., Allen, P., Normand, C. and Walters, R. (2002) Process and impact of mergers of NHS trusts: Multicentre case study and management cost analysis. *British Medical Journal*, 325: 246–52.

Hewison, A. (1997) Evidence-based medicine: What about evidence-based management? *Journal of Nursing Management*, 5: 195–8.

Institute of Medicine (1999) *The National Round-Table on Health Care Quality: Measuring the Quality of Care*. Washington, DC: Institute of Medicine.

Kitchener, M. (2002) Mobilizing the logic of managerialism in professional fields: The case of academic health center mergers. *Organization Studies*, 23(3): 391–420.

Klein, R. (2000) From evidence-based medicine to evidence-based policy? *Journal of Health Services Research and Policy*, 5(2): 65–6.

Kovner, A.R., Elton, J.J. and Billings, J. (2000) Evidence-based management. *Frontiers of Health Services Management*, 16(4): 3–46.

Lavis, J., Davies, H.T.O., Oxman, A., Denis, J.L., Golden-Biddle, K. and Ferlie, F. (2005) Towards systematic reviews that inform health care management and policy-making. *Journal of Health Services Research and Policy*, 10(3): S35–48.

Lavis, J., Gruen, R., Davies, H. and Walshe, K. (2006) Working within and beyond the Cochrane Collaboration to make systematic reviews more useful to healthcare managers and policymakers. *Healthcare Policy*, 1(2): 21–33.

Lemieux-Charles, L. and Champagne, F. (2004) Using knowledge and evidence in healthcare: Multidisciplinary perspectives. Toronto: University of Toronto Press.

Lomas, J. (2000) Using linkage and exchange to move research into policy at a Canadian foundation. *Health Affairs*, 19(3): 236–40.

Lomas, J., Fulop, N., Gagnon, D. and Allen, P. (2003) On being a good listener: Setting priorities for applied health services research. *Milbank Quarterly*, 81(3): 363–88.

Lomas, J., Culyer, T., McCutcheon, C. et al. (2005) Conceptualising and combining evidence for health system guidance. Ottowa: CHSRF.

Marmor, T. (2001) Fads in medical care policy and politics: The rhetoric and reality of managerialism. London: Nuffield Trust.

National Audit Office (NAO, 2003) *Getting the Evidence: Using Research in Policy Making.* London: NAO.

NCCSDO (2000) *National Listening Exercise: Report of the Findings.* London: NCCSDO.

NCCSDO (2002) *Refreshing the National Listening Exercise: Report of the Findings.* London: NCCSDO.

Pawson, R. (2002). Evidence based policy: The promise of realist synthesis. *Evaluation*, 8(3): 340–58.

Sackett, D.L. and Rosenberg, W.M. (1995) The need for evidence-based medicine. *Journal of the Royal Society of Medicine*, 88(11): 620–4.

Smith, J., Walshe, K. and Hunter, D.J. (2001) The redisorganisation of the NHS. *British Medical Journal*, 323: 1262–3.

Tranfield, D., Denyer, D. and Smart, P. (2003) Towards a methodology for developing evidence informed management knowledge by means of systematic review. *British Journal of Management*, 14: 207–22.

Walshe, K. and Rundall, T. (2001) Evidence based management: From theory to practice in healthcare. *Milbank Quarterly*, 79(3): 429–57.

Websites and resources

Cabinet Office. Policy hub website providing resources on evidence-based policymaking: *http://www.policyhub.gov.uk/*

Canadian Health Services Research Foundation. *http://www.chsrf.ca/*

Critical Appraisal Skills Programme. *http://www.phru.nhs.uk/casp/casp.htm*

ESRC Centre for Evidence-Based Policy and Practice. *http://www.evidencenetwork.org/*

National Electronic Library for Health. Pages on evidence-based decision making: *http://www.nelh.nhs.uk/ebdm/*

NHS Centre for Reviews and Dissemination. *http://www.york.ac.uk/inst/crd/*

SCHaRR Netting the Evidence. *http://www.shef.ac.uk/scharr/ir/netting/*
US Agency for Healthcare Research and Quality. *http://www.ahrq.gov/*
World Health Organization's Health Evidence Network. *http://www.euro.who.int/HEN*

28 Conclusions: complexity, change and creativity in healthcare management

Judith Smith and Kieran Walshe

Introduction

This book has demonstrated in a most vivid manner the complexity of the task facing healthcare managers in the twenty-first century, especially in relation to the rapidly changing nature of the context in which healthcare is delivered and managed. Healthcare is, as Chapter 2 demonstrated, an intrinsically political domain in which every citizen has some sort of interest and where managers are just one group of stakeholders within a complex web of actors who influence the development and implementation of health policy. The fundamental complexity of healthcare as a sector is increasing on account of four main factors as set out at the start of this book in Chapter 1:

- the demographic shift (ageing population accompanied by rising incidence of chronic disease)
- the pace of technological innovation
- changing user and consumer expectations
- rising costs.

These factors are woven throughout the chapters of the book, emerging at different points when authors assess the current state of play for their particular area of healthcare management. In this final chapter, we examine the specific nature of the challenge facing healthcare managers as they seek to deal with the inherent complexity and change within health systems, and we describe the creativity that is thus called for in order for healthcare management to be truly effective. As academics who both started their professional life as healthcare managers and who spend a lot of time involved in the development of the current and future generation of managers, we felt we had to conclude the book by setting out what this analysis of healthcare management actually means for the task of being a healthcare manager today. Hence we make no apology for the conclusions resting on a form of 'job specification' for a healthcare manager – a manager who needs to be highly creative when managing change within a highly complex environment.

Managing in the face of complexity

The implications of this increasing complexity for the role and activities of healthcare management are evident in the challenges associated with making decisions about funding healthcare (see Chapter 3). These challenges operate at both a macro (national or system-wide) and local level, with managers being at the forefront of developing proposals on resource allocation and advising their political masters as to how funding should be used and with what anticipated results. As such, managers are clearly often in a difficult and unpopular place – at the heart of difficult decisions about how a country, region, district, hospital or primary care service is going to divide up and allocate resources when faced with many competing demands. The manager's role as a potentially unpopular decision maker is not confined to financial resources. As Chapter 4 illustrated, managers face new challenges in relation to how the different sectors of healthcare are configured – what might have been traditionally understood as community- or hospital-based care is now contested as technology increasingly enables the shift of care away from hospital settings. Similarly, societal moves towards increased expectations of public services mean that healthcare managers find themselves under constant pressure to try and support the design of services that are much more clearly patient focused and not so much influenced by the convenience and priorities of professional staff (Chapter 4).

In making decisions about resource allocation and service configuration, managers constantly face the challenge of how to respond to new and emerging technological advances, about whose efficacy and efficiency data may be initially in short supply. Chapter 5 set out the intricacy of processes for assessing new technologies and setting funding priorities, along with the rise of health economics as a discipline that can assist managers in making investment (or disinvestment) decisions. These processes, and an understanding of health economics and priority setting, are areas where healthcare managers now need to have some understanding and expertise in a way that would have been much less pressing even a decade ago. Technological advances increasingly drive approaches to the design and delivery of healthcare, and being able to identify and interpret the implications of emerging technologies is now a vital skill for the healthcare manager.

A further dimension to the complexity of the task facing healthcare managers, and perhaps the most difficult one in relation to its enormity, is that of the changing epidemiology of almost all countries' health. As pointed out in Chapter 6, the rising incidence of chronic disease throughout developed countries of the world, and the increasing availability of treatments to treat such conditions, means that 'people living with long-term conditions' now represent the greatest single public health management challenge for countries in the OECD. For countries in the developing world, the impact of diseases such as HIV/AIDS are the foremost epidemiological challenge, posing challenges for health managers in relation to the design and delivery of services across the spectrum from health promotion to palliative care.

If the rising incidence of chronic and infectious diseases is the greatest public health challenge to healthcare managers, finding ways of tackling deep-seated and often increasing inequalities in the health status of populations must be the next most knotty public health management challenge. As Chapters 5 and 16 explained, the only route to addressing the causes of ill health and inequality lies in managers finding much more effective ways of working in partnership with other agencies such as housing, social care, education and regeneration. In order to do this, managers will need to adopt a more holistic approach to their understanding of 'health' along with new strategies for addressing multi-sectoral and highly complex social problems that in turn impact on people's (poor) health.

Given that the context of healthcare management in the twenty-first century is characterised by a high level of complexity, the major challenges facing healthcare managers when seeking to manage that complexity can be summarised as shown in Box 28.1.

Box 28.1   Major challenges for healthcare managers

- Developing the political acumen and astuteness to understand, influence and manage within the health policy process.
- Having robust and transparent approaches to making healthcare funding decisions.
- Having sophisticated and sensitive approaches to making decisions about the redesign of services across healthcare systems.
- Understanding and using new approaches to the assessment and prioritization of new health technologies.
- Developing new approaches to the management of chronic disease and long-term conditions.
- Having coherent and sophisticated plans for tackling infectious diseases.
- Being able to adopt a range of strategies that enable healthcare funders and providers to work in close partnership with other agencies whose activities impact on health status.

Managing in the face of change

If the context of healthcare management is defined by its complexity, the nature of the healthcare management task would seem to be characterised by the need to deal with and accommodate change. In the chapters that focus on specific sectors of healthcare management (Chapters 7, 8 and 9), it was made clear that primary care is becoming more 'managed' and organised as its importance to overall health gain is realised, acute care is being redefined by technological and staff training advances together with a stronger focus on clinical governance and patient safety, and mental health services are being constantly challenged in relation to having a stronger user focus and less of a medical or institutional bias. It is striking that in each of these sectors the most evident management challenge is in relation to trying to change the centre of gravity of the particular service, bringing about a reorientation towards a stronger client or patient focus (mental health and acute services) and in primary care towards a broader public health and less medical model of provision.

There are a number of areas of healthcare management that tend to receive relatively little policy and management development attention, often remaining 'in the wings' whilst other functions that are more closely related to the direct delivery of patient care take centre-stage. These neglected and perhaps for some people, less exciting, areas of management include: service and capital development (Chapter 10); health planning and strategy (Chapter 11); healthcare commissioning and contracting (Chapter 12); and healthcare information technology and systems (Chapter 13). However, it is clear from a careful reading of these chapters that these management functions are at the epicentre of much of the current change within healthcare systems, change which is in itself a reflection of the complexity of the wider context of healthcare. As the nature and focus of health services change, so the requirement for buildings and equipment evolves, and increasingly globalised economies mean that capital and service planning can rarely be contained at a national level in the twenty-first century (Chapter 10). Complexity calls for sophisticated strategy and planning within healthcare organisations and for wider populations, and the intricacies of political and policy influences set out in Chapter 2 make the process of strategy development ever more challenging (Chapter 11). The complexity of decision making about resource allocation and service design that is explored earlier in the book (Chapters 3 and 4) becomes a very real and pressing management activity in the chapter on healthcare commissioning and contracting (Chapter 12).

Healthcare commissioning and contracting are probably only partially understood by a majority of people working with health systems. Yet Chapter 12 makes it clear that the responsibilities facing commissioners are crucial to determining the nature, level and quality of health services people receive, and the environment within which health professionals can practise. Once again, this area of management is defined by change – for health systems look to their funders or commissioners to develop the levers and incentives to bring about desired changes to patterns of service delivery and hence commissioning is where new forms of primary, acute and mental healthcare will ultimately be enabled and incentivised.

Healthcare information technology (IT) and systems are the area of management where complexity and change perhaps converge in the most dramatic manner (Chapter 13). Technological change is for most people particularly evident in the IT sector (and indeed in all our daily working lives) and its increasingly complex nature has far-reaching implications for how health services are organised and delivered and for the management of many of the most basic (and yet crucial) systems within healthcare organisations; for example, medical records, transmission of test results, prescribing of drugs and communication between departments and organisations. For managers, changes and developments in IT pose a range of challenges, not least in relation to how such developments will impact on how healthcare staff work, services will be delivered and patients will access the health system. As with most management activity, the people element of this challenge is likely to be the most exacting for managers – how to maximise the benefits of new information technology and systems. This leads us to consider the other main area of change that challenges healthcare managers – how to change the ways in which people work at an individual, group and organisational level.

The challenge of healthcare management in the face of changes to the ways in which people are organised and developed was explored in Chapters 14, 15, 16 and 17. The overall scale of the healthcare workforce was examined along with an exploration of how human resource management can be used as a way of bringing about new ways of working – new ways that are needed in response to the changing and complex context within which healthcare is delivered (Chapter 14). Specific areas in which healthcare managers have to use their skills in bringing about change were also examined, including the ways in which managers and clinicians work together (Chapter 15) and governance arrangements are established and managed for healthcare organisations (Chapter 16). In these two latter cases, it was made clear that managers will need to be able to persuade and influence colleagues whilst setting overall parameters and standards of conduct for teams and organisations – more directive approaches being unlikely to work in such complex and political settings. Similarly, when seeking to develop and manage the relationship between healthcare organisations and partner agencies (an activity that we have already noted is vital to health improvement and public health work), the healthcare manager will need sophisticated interpersonal skills that enable the building of trust alongside robust processes of accountability for delivering on agreed objectives across organisations.

In a climate of continuous change, there is a clear need to measure organisational performance and put in place 'dials' from which managers, staff, users and others can read the important indicators of the organisation's activity. There has been a proliferation of approaches to performance measurement in healthcare in recent years, but Chapter 18 organised these into an analytical framework that offers managers a way of ordering their approach to performance measurement and thus bringing some way of taking stock amidst rapid change within complex services. When managing in the face of change, healthcare managers face the challenges shown in Box 28.2.

> **Box 28.2   Managing in the face of change**
>
> - Having the necessary skills to be able to bring about changes in the overall model and orientation of care towards one that is more person focused.
> - Being able to develop robust plans for capital and service development in an increasingly globalised world.
> - Finding new ways of developing strategy within a political context that continues to become more complex.
> - Developing appropriate levers and incentives to use within funding and commissioning, and thus bring about desired changes to healthcare provision.
> - Creating the wider culture and environment where IT developments can be maximised.
> - Enabling human resource management that is focused on developing the new ways of working that are needed in a changing world.
> - Having the necessary powers of influence and persuasion to work with clinicians and board members in an effective manner.
> - Using these skills of influence and persuasion to develop strong partnership working with other agencies in a manner that also assures the delivery of joint objectives.
> - Developing a clear set of measures by which stakeholders can assess the performance of healthcare organisations and thus look for further improvements.

Managing with creativity in order to improve care

In a context of heightened complexity and constant change – a context that seems set to define healthcare management for the foreseeable future – healthcare managers need to be highly skilled and have well-developed emotional intelligence if they are to bring about the improvements in health and care that represent the ultimate aim of their profession. In concluding her book on NHS leaders in 1989, Rosemary Stewart, probably the foremost UK researcher of healthcare management in the 1970s and 1980s, exhorted healthcare managers as follows:

> The NHS needs leaders who can enthuse others with high goals for what they can achieve. Do not have too grand an idea of leadership. You do not have to be charismatic but you must care – and care deeply – about what you want to achieve. You must show that you care in what you do because you are a model for other people's actions. . . . Above all, you must inspire trust: that is a key aspect of successful leadership in the NHS because there are so many individuals and groups who may be suspicious of you and your intentions. (Stewart 1989: 185)

This relationship between having an advanced set of skills and yet a commitment to the ultimate aim of improving health and care seems to us to continue to be an apt summary of the task facing modern healthcare managers. Stewart, however, rightly points to the fact that healthcare management is a profession that tends to attract mistrust, criticism and even derision – in comparison with jobs such as medicine and the law which typically command a much greater degree of public respect and even deference. The healthcare manager is never going to become a popular figure within communities and society, for he or she is, as we have seen in this book, charged with making some of the most difficult and sometimes unpalatable decisions about health funding and provision. However, what the healthcare manager must be is someone who, as in Stewart's words, inspires trust and credibility.

The final nine chapters of the book set out the 'toolkit' for managers to use in developing this trust and credibility – credibility that is concerned not only with acquiring practical skills such as managing projects, process improvement and resources, but also with the personal integrity that comes from having a well-developed sense of personal awareness and effectiveness, and a commitment to respecting the integrity of colleagues in teams and organisations. In acquiring an appropriate combination of skills and personal qualities to enable effective practice, healthcare managers need, above all else, the ability to be creative in their approach to how they foster personal, team and organisational development. Rosemary Stewart asserted that 'A good leader should also be an effective manager. You will not be effective unless you are able to understand and manage yourself and your job' (Stewart 1989: 185). This message underpins Chapter 21 with its many pointers about how to understand and manage one's own practice as a manager.

The importance of developing emotional intelligence and understanding one's own and other people's leadership styles and behaviour was made clear in Chapter 19. The challenge for the healthcare manager in relation to matching behaviour and management style to specific situations and needs underlined the importance of managers being about to be creative and adaptive in their practice. Chapter 20 took this analysis of individual style and behaviour further and explored the implications for organisational design and development, again underlining the need for managers to be able to interpret and make sense of organisations for those with whom they work, acting as an interpreter and 'sensemaker' of organisational pressures and life. Perhaps one of the most immediately practical and challenging chapters of the whole book is the one that focuses on personal effectiveness and development (Chapter 21), asking managers to examine their style of working and to find ways of developing the creativity and reflective practice that is crucial for effective leadership and development as set out in Chapters 19 and 20.

For managers currently working within health services, Chapters 22 to 26 set out a wealth of evidence-based practical guidance for how actually to do the business of management in a complex and rapidly changing context. Whether seeking advice on how to manage projects, develop a business plan, or improve team working, it is clear that managers need to have the skills to set up robust processes which are at once transparent and accountable in an increasingly contested environment, but also flexible and dynamic and able to respond to change in a creative manner. Similarly, when challenged to improve the involvement of service users with the management of services (Chapter 25) or to find new ways of improving the quality and processes of care (Chapter 26), this combination of stronger and yet adaptable processes again emerges as a key message for healthcare managers.

Developing management practice that is properly evidence based and open to learning from research is something that all too often remains as aspiration rather than reality (Chapter 27). This book is itself intended as a contribution to the ongoing international effort to develop evidence-based management in healthcare, bringing together as it does the practical challenge of managing health and health services with the wealth of research evidence about what is needed to manage effectively in this complex and changing world. In order to manage in a creative manner that in turn enables care to be improved, managers need to develop a number of ways of practising (Box 28.3).

Box 28.3   Managing in a creative manner

- Inspire credibility and trust.
- Develop emotional intelligence and use this to understand others' style and behaviour.
- Interpret and make sense of organisations for those with whom they work.
- Develop as reflective and self-aware practitioners.
- Develop and keep updated fundamental management skills such as project and resource management.
- Be able to design and implement robust yet flexible processes for improving services and assuring proper user involvement.
- Focus their organisation on issues of diversity and inclusiveness.
- Practise in an evidence-based manner that remains open to change and challenge.

Overall conclusions

Concluding this book appeared at first to be a daunting task, with 26 substantive chapters covering so many aspects of healthcare management. Yet as it turns out, the task has not been as difficult as we imagined, for a reading of the totality of the book's contents has revealed a strong and consistent message in relation to the complexity of the context, the changing nature of the task, and the degree to which creative and thoughtful responses are required, rooted in a commitment continually acquire to and update practical management skills. We have devoted our careers to first of all managing and then latterly researching and seeking to develop the management of healthcare, and we have a strong belief in the need for ever more effective and skilled management of health services. The challenge set by Rosemary Stewart in 1989 remains pertinent today, and all good leaders of healthcare need to be first and foremost good managers. This book seeks to add in some small way to the process of developing healthcare management as an international community of professionals dedicated to improving the health and care of people who are often vulnerable and unable to act for themselves within the wider health system and society. If the book helps you to understand better and hence practise the craft of healthcare management in a creative way that ultimately improves care, we will have achieved what we intended.

Reference

Stewart, R. (1989) *Leading in the NHS: A Practical Guide.* Basingstoke: Macmillan.

Index

Related books from Open University Press

Purchase from www.openup.co.uk or order through your local bookseller

PATIENT SAFETY
RESEARCH INTO PRACTICE

Kieran Walshe and Ruth Boaden (eds)

In many countries, during the last decade there has been a growing public realization that healthcare organisations are often dangerous places to be. Reports published in Australia, Canada, New Zealand, United Kingdom and the USA have served to focus public and policy attention on the safety of patients and to highlight the alarmingly high incidence of errors and adverse events that lead to some kind of harm or injury.

This book presents a research-based perspective on patient safety, drawing together the most recent ideas and thinking from researchers on how to research and understand patient safety issues, and how research findings are used to shape policy and practice. The book examines key issues, including:

- Analysis and measurement of patient safety
- Approaches to improving patient safety
- Future policy and practice regarding patient safety
- The legal dimensions of patient safety

Patient Safety is essential reading for researchers, policy makers and practitioners involved in, or interested in, patient safety. The book is also of interest to the growing number of postgraduate students on health policy and health management programmes that focus upon healthcare quality, risk management and patient safety.

Contributors
Sally Adams, Tony Avery, Maureen Baker, Paul Beatty, Ruth Boaden, Tanya Claridge, Gary Cook, Caroline Davy, Susan Dovey, Aneez Esmail, Rachel Finn, Martin Fletcher, Sally Giles, John Hickner, Rachel Howard, Amanda Howe, Michael A. Jones, Sue Kirk, Rebecca Lawton, Martin Marshall, Caroline Morris, Dianne Parker, Shirley Pearce, Bob Phillips, Steve Rogers, Richard Thomson, Charles Vincent, Kieran Walshe, Justin Waring, Alison Watkin, Fiona Watts, Liz West, Maria Woloshynowych.

Contents
List of contributors – Preface – Introduction – Part 1: Perspectives on patient safety – Clinical perspectives on patient safety – Sociological contributions to patient safety – Psychological approaches to patient safety – The quality management contribution to patient safety – Technology, informatics and patient safety – Patient safety and the law – Part 2: Approaches to evaluating patient safety – Developing and using taxonomies of errors – Incident reporting and analysis – Using chart review and clinical databases to study medical error – Techniques used in the investigation and analysis of critical incidents in healthcare – Learning from litigation: The role of claims analysis in patient safety – Ethnographic methods in patient safety – Evaluating safety culture – Part 3: Patient safety in practice – Patient safety: education, training and professional development – Pathways to patient safety: The use of rules and guidelines in healthcare – Team performance, communication and patient safety – Conclusions – and the way forward – References – Index.

2005   256pp   0 335 21853 9 (Paperback)   0 335 21854 7 (Hardback)